Third Edition

Hormonal Balance

How to Lose Weight by Understanding Your Hormones and Metabolism

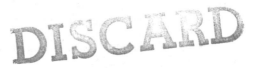

Scott Isaacs, M.D.

Foreword by Neil Shulman, M.D.

Bull Publishing Company
Boulder, Colorado

Published by Bull Publishing Company

P.O. Box 1377

Boulder, CO, USA 80306

www.bullpub.com

Library of Congress Cataloging-in-Publication Data

Isaacs, Scott, 1967-
Hormonal balance : how to lose weight by understanding your hormones and metabolism /
    Scott Isaacs ; foreword by Neil Shulman. -- 3rd ed.
       p. cm.
    Includes bibliographical references and index.
    ISBN 978-1-936693-22-1
    1. Hormones--Popular works. 2. Weight loss--Endocrine aspects--Popular works. 3.
    Endocrine glands--Diseases--Popular works. 4. Metabolism--Popular works. I. Title.
    QP571.I833 2012
    612.4'05--dc23

31088100759123

                                                        2012012063

NOTE TO READERS: The information in this book is for informational and educational purposes only. It is not intended to serve as medical advice or to be any form of medical treatment. You should always consult with your physician before starting any diet or exercise program. Any use of the information is at the reader's good judgment and sole responsibility. This book is not intended to diagnose or treat any medical condition and is not a substitute for a physician.

First Edition
17 16 15 14 13 12   10 9 8 7 6 5 4 3 2 1

Interior design and project management: Dovetail Publishing Services
Cover design: Shannon Bodie, Lightbourne, Inc.

This book is dedicated to my lovely wife, Fiona, who has helped me with every aspect of this book, especially giving me the love and support I needed to make it a reality.

Contents

Acknowledgments

I thank all my patients, past and present, for the knowledge they have given me about successful weight loss and the privilege of being involved in their care.

Thank you to Hossein Gharib, M.D., Lewis Blevins, M.D., Adriana Ioachimescu, M.D., PhD, Nelson Oyesiku, M.D., PhD, Vin Tangpricha, M.D., PhD, Victoria Musey, M.D., James Early, M.D., and Guillermo Umpierrez, M.D., for their continued expertise with countless "curbside consultations." Thank you to Neil Shulman, M.D., Randy Kessler, and Robyn Spizman for their help with this book. A hearty thanks to Bobbie Christmas for her help writing and editing this book. I thank Jim Bull and Claire Cameron from Bull Publishing, who first published this book a decade ago and continue to support the project with this updated third edition. Thank you to Karin Slaughter for being an inspiration and teaching me how to concentrate on writing. I also thank my office staff: Janet Baldwin, R.N., Misty Roland, L.P.N., Fran Ritter, R.N., Deborah English, Annie Goode, Bethany Burton, and Shundalyn Vanderhorst. I give a special thanks to my officer manager Bethany Knott, who has helped keep my office running smoothly while I took time off to write this book. I thank Jillian Michaels, Isadore Rosenfeld, Lance Armstrong, and Robin Meade for their support in promoting our message of better health through hormonal balance.

I thank my mother and father Sheryle and Howard Isaacs. A special thanks to Sheryle Isaacs for many of the recipes used in this book. I give an extra special thanks to the two loves of my life: my wife Fiona Isaacs and my daughter Arabella Isaacs. Thank you for everything!

Foreword

By Neil Shulman, M.D.

Hormonal Balance is a very important resource in today's world, where the number one preventable cause of early death and suffering in the United States and many countries throughout the world is *obesity*.

The everyday person needs to understand the interface between obesity and hormones. This updated book provides a unique opportunity to understand and improve the overall health crisis due to the obesity epidemic. The book should be required reading for a wide spectrum of folks: from primary and secondary school teachers to family doctors and other health professionals. It is an essential guide for everyone, because a truly global understanding of the obesity epidemic and how to help ourselves, our families, and our friends avoid obesity is not simply a matter of going on a diet or exercising. It involves having a true understanding of all potential contributors to the problem. Whether psychological, disease induced, diet induced, or the result of lack of exercise—every case of obesity is unique and dependent on individual factors. In order to reduce the obesity epidemic, we all need to understand the big picture of what is causing the obesity we experience personally or see in our friends, relatives, and clients. Hormones play a key role.

Scott Isaacs, M.D., has written a very important book that can make a major impact on the health of many of us. He wants to empower all of us to help rein in the disastrous consequences of the obesity epidemic. He wants to empower all of us. He has written and updated, with inclusion of new groundbreaking discoveries, a very reader-friendly, comprehensive book. He is a caring, compassionate doc. He has acquired his broad base of knowledge by training in endocrinology, diabetes, and metabolism as well as by treating patients, training health professionals, and conducting research.

I have had the opportunity to work with many wonderful humanitarians, helping to organize a Global Humanitarian Summit, associate producing the movie *Doc Hollywood* based on my novel and starring Michael J. Fox, working with more than 120 doctors and nurses on our book *Your Body's Red Light Warn-ing Signals,* and helping to demystify medicine for kids by performing as a goofy doctor on public television's, *What's in a Doctor's Bag?,* inspired by one of my children's books. With this background, I can say that Scott Isaacs is one of the brightest, most caring, and dedicated humanitarians whom I have met.

Introduction

Since the first edition of *Hormonal Balance* was published in 2002, research on the subject of hormones and obesity has exploded. Literally thousands of scientific articles have been published on every conceivable aspect of this topic. New discoveries are being made every day.

Despite these scientific breakthroughs, we are still fat.

Government studies estimate that nearly 75 percent of Americans are either overweight or obese. If you aren't overweight, you're in the minority. And obesity-related illness, like heart attacks, strokes, high blood pressure, diabetes, and even certain cancers, has become the number one preventable cause of early death in the United States.

We continue to see the rise and fall of fad diets. No-fat, no-carb, low-carb, Jenny Craig, Nutrisystem, Sugar Busters, Atkins, South Beach . . . the more we diet, the fatter we get.

Studies have shown that about 98 percent of people who lose weight on a diet will regain the weight or even more within five years.

Why?

Hormonal imbalance.

If you want to be part of the 2 percent of dieters who experience permanent weight loss, your hormones have to be balanced. Through hormonal balance, you will be able to lose weight and keep it off forever.

What is hormonal balance? It depends on whom you ask. A gynecologist will tell you it's about the female hormones—estrogen, progesterone, and prolactin. A urologist will tell you it's all about testosterone. A diabetologist will tell you it's about balancing your insulin, glucagon, and blood sugar. An endocrinologist will tell you that it is having all your hormones balanced. This is because all your hormones affect one another. It's one big circle. When one hormone is out of balance, it has profound effects on all your hormones. They are all connected. Hormonal balance means having the right amount of every hormone. It means having a body that's healthy and resilient.

Hormonal balance improves just about every aspect of your life. With balanced hormones, your body will be lean and efficient. You won't have excessive hunger or cravings, and your metabolism will work to keep your body at a healthy weight. You will feel more energetic but without stress or anxiety. Your mood will be elevated. You will have deep, restful, rejuvenating sleep every night. You will have a sharp mind. Hormonal balance means feeling better and living longer.

As you read this book you'll learn how all your hormones work together to control your appetite, body weight, and metabolism. You'll learn about the subtle or not so subtle signs and symptoms of hormonal imbalance and what you can do to get your body's system of communication back on track.

Virtually all of the information that was in the first edition of *Hormonal Balance* still holds true today. You won't see any new philosophies or dieting principles in this edition. The purpose of the third edition of *Hormonal Balance* is to incorporate new research on hormones that affect your body weight, appetite, body composition, and metabolism. I've included all the best new medications and supplements available to treat the various hormonal conditions as well as bringing to light some ineffective and even dangerous products that falsely claim to help you lose weight through hormones.

The new edition reveals important new information about traditional hormones and newly discovered hunger hormones that influence the body and the brain to explain why we feel hungry and why we crave food.

Hormones are the misunderstood part of our whole weight-obsessed culture. Yes, you can lose weight on a diet—but you might not be healthy, and you'll probably put it all back. Underneath all the meal suggestions, exercise programs, and everything else in the dietary lexicon are little messengers within your body: your hormones. Your hormones—and there are hundreds of them—carry messages from your brain to your body and from your body to your brain. When you eat certain foods, some hormones kick in, telling you whether you want more food, where that food is going to go, what effect it will have on the body and on the brain. When you exercise, hormones go to work, directing the body to move energy stores here, consume energy stores there, boost this part of the body, shut down that part.

It's a very delicate dance.

And it's very easy to throw off. If one of your glands—those are the places in your body that produce hormones—shuts down, becomes overactive, or develops a tumor; if your consumption of a particular food throws off your body chemistry; if depression, pregnancy, any kind of emotional, psychological, or physical turmoil occurs, the body goes a little haywire.

Sometimes, it's self-correcting. It might be off for a few minutes or a few days, but pretty soon things return to normal. But sometimes it's a "new normal." The body has gotten used to its condition, and you eat more, or metabolize less, or alternate between those two extremes. That's when you start to gain weight.

And, lest we think that "new normal" can only be caused by an "extreme" situation—like tumors or gland failure—consider the aging process. If you could consume pizza and beer every night during your college years without gaining an ounce, you've probably found you can't do that any more.

What's the reason? Hormones. Many hormones decline with age, slowing metabolism. It's a fact of nature. But that doesn't mean we have to be captive to weight gain.

The hormonal changes that cause weight gain and occur because of weight gain are complex. The myriad of diet books and hormone books that are currently available are incomplete. Most of these books focus on the hormone insulin as the major hormone that makes you fat. Books on other hormones, such as estrogen, thyroid, and growth hormone, are also available, but none of these really gets to the heart of the matter. All your hormones work in concert to control your metabolism, body composition, and body weight. I wrote this book because I became frustrated with the incomplete messages these other books provided.

The information contained in this book is the most up-to-date scientific information about your body's hormones. Most of the topics in this book have been the major focus of national and international medical meetings. There are hundreds of scientific studies to back up this information; many of these are listed in the bibliography of this book. Some of the information I present in this book is pretty technical, but I have made every effort to walk you through the concepts step by step so you understand all the variables involved.

In 1994 the hormone leptin was discovered. This opened the door to a new science of hungry hormones that has become one of the most important areas of medical research today. We now know about dozens of hungry hormones that influence appetite, cravings, metabolism, and body weight.

The third edition combines these recent scientific discoveries with my experience over the past fifteen years as an endocrinologist and weight loss specialist. My intention with *Hormonal Balance* is to bring hope and some new solutions to overweight people who suffer needlessly because of hormonal imbalance.

This edition contains a lot of new information about environmental endocrine disruptors, which are chemicals in our environment that mimic hormones, causing hormone imbalance, increased appetite, and weight gain. Endocrine disruptors can affect many different hormones that can lead to increased appetite and weight gain.

Since the publication of the first edition of *Hormonal Balance,* thousands of people have seen permanent weight loss success following the Hormonal Health Diet. This diet is a balanced and nutritious way of eating that will allow you to lose weight without feeling hungry or deprived. This section at the end of the book—"Practical Strategies for Intelligent Weight Loss"—contains all the information you need to lose weight effectively and permanently. There is a new 7-day meal plan, with delicious recipes. I've also included a symptom guide to help you track and understand symptoms that may be keys to a hormone disruption.

You can control your hormones. You can control your metabolism. Follow the lessons in this book, and you will be on your way to a lifetime of health and hormonal balance.

PART

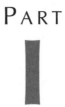

Losing Weight Now

CHAPTER

1

Balance Your Hormones to Lose Weight

You are probably reading this book because you are frustrated about your weight. You have read every book, tried every diet, and you are aware of the health benefits of weight loss. You have probably lost weight on a diet but gained it back, or you struggle to keep it off. You are discouraged and don't know what to do next.

It is not your fault.

Weight problems do not develop because of lack of motivation, overeating, or not enough exercise. Weight problems occur because your hormones have evolved over thousands of years to force your body to gain weight. Your hormones keep you fat so you can survive when food is scarce. In the developed world, food is not scarce. Your hormones don't know that. This book will help you understand, eat, and live in harmony with your hormones so you can lose weight and keep it off permanently.

Obesity is one of the greatest health challenges our species has ever faced. According to the World Health Organization, there are more than one billion overweight and 300 million obese adults in the world. There are more than 120 million overweight adults in the United States. Seventy percent of Americans have an unhealthy body weight. This number has almost doubled in the past fifty years and is expected to increase further. Obesity costs an estimated $300

In This Chapter

▶ Why Losing Weight Is So Hard

▶ How Hormones Control Your Weight

▶ Diagnosing Hormonal Disorders

▶ Are Genetics Linked to Obesity?

7

billion in medical bills and lost productivity each year. One in five children and one in three young adults under the age of twenty-four are obese. Worldwide, 92 million children are at risk from becoming overweight in the next decade. Obese children are seven times more likely to be severely obese by their early thirties. Children and teens typically have accelerated weight gain as they enter adulthood and are especially susceptible to the profound health risks of excess weight.

The obesity epidemic is out of control.

Our comfortable couches, our reliance on fast food, our speedy cars and road systems and spread-out cities that mean we never have to touch a foot to the ground—they help make us fat. We spend billions of dollars on diet books; we throw $100 bills at bottles of diet pills; we scarf up diet supplements, diet magazines, and turbo-quick diet weight loss plans; we sign up for subscriptions at health clubs that we never use, book appointments with doctors whom we ignore, and make half-hearted attempts at starting exercise programs that we don't continue.

And still we are fat and getting fatter every day.

Why is this? Why can we not lose the weight? Why can we not be the thin, svelte, sexy, beautiful human beings we picture ourselves to be? The human body is a terrifically complex machine. Each piece of the machine has an impact on every other piece of the machine, and the machine is continually analyzing input from inside and outside and adjusting itself accordingly. If one part of the machine goes "off," other parts can follow.

Becoming overweight can be a result of the human machine getting off track. And one purpose of this book is to help you understand why it gets off track and how it gets off track—reasons that are greatly influenced by our hormones. And, finally, it tells you how to maintain your body so that it doesn't get off track at all and your weight is under safe and healthy control.

Hormonal Balance reveals important information about hormones that influence the body and the brain, explaining why we feel hungry and why we crave food.

Make This Diet Your Last Diet

In a study of more than 180,000 dieters, it was concluded that 83 percent of people who start a diet pick one that is virtually guaranteed to fail. Ninety-eight percent of people who lose weight on a diet gain it all back within five years. Some gain more than that.

You can be among the other 2 percent.

Obesity is not a problem of willpower. It's a lot more complicated than that. Fortunately, the past few years have brought a change in the way doctors and scientists view obesity. Previously, most thought of obesity, except in the rarest of patients, as a question of willpower. Obese people ate too much. They didn't exercise. They didn't have a balanced diet or a regular workout program. They could lose the weight if only they'd have some guts and determination. Today, nine out of ten doctors now believe that losing weight is as emotionally and physically difficult as quitting smoking.

In a study of nearly 1.5 million people published in the *New England Journal of Medicine* in 2011, it was concluded that being overweight or obese dramatically increases the risk of dying early. Obesity has passed cigarette smoking as the number one preventable killer because it's connected with a host of medical problems ranging from heart disease and high blood pressure to diabetes, arthritis, gall bladder problems, Alzheimer's disease, and even cancer. Due to our

Conditions Made Worse by Being Overweight

Absenteeism from work	Gallstones	Plantar fasciitis
Academic discrimination	Gastroesophageal reflux disease (GERD) and heartburn	Polycystic ovary syndrome (PCOS)
Acanthosis nigricans (see chapter 6 on insulin resistance)	Gestational diabetes	Prediabetes
Arthritis	Gout	Pulmonary hypertension
Breast cancer	Heart attacks	Sciatica
Colorectal cancer	Hernias	Skin infections
Congestive heart failure	High blood pressure	Skin tags
Death	High cholesterol	Sleep apnea
Decreased work productivity	Impaired quality of life	Social discrimination
Diabetes	Increased surgical risk	Stroke
Employment discrimination	Kidney failure	Urinary incontinence
Fatty liver disease and cirrhosis	Low back pain	Uterine cancer
	Low testosterone (in men)	Varicose veins

growing waistlines, experts predict that by 2050, one in three Americans will have diabetes. Despite this, 74 percent of doctors believe that overweight people are in denial about their weight.

Americans are experiencing more weight-related ailments than ever before. The *New England Journal of Medicine* reported in 2010 that even a small amount of weight gain increases the risk for dying. Every pound you gain increases your risk of dying. Overweight people have a 13 percent increased risk of dying early, and the risk increases to 44 percent once a person becomes obese. The study reported that those with higher body weight are at even higher risk for dying.

Body Mass Index (BMI)*	Increased Risk for Death
25–29.9 kg/m^2	13%
30–34.9 kg/m^2	44%
35–39.9 kg/m^2	88%
40–49.9 kg/m^2	251%

Pharmaceutical companies get rich making the vast array of medications needed to treat the medical problems caused from being overweight. I'm not putting down medical science; these medications have extended our lives and prevented certain death for many people. But it's a sign of the times that instead of treating the root causes of our problems, we treat many individual diseases with drugs. In fact, these diseases—which are known as "diseases of civilization"—were almost unheard of generations ago among our lesser-weight ancestors. And doctors have discovered that even a miniscule amount of weight loss—say, 5 or 10 pounds—can reduce our risk for many of these diseases.

The key to permanent weight loss? Hormonal balance. Hormonal balance can help you lose the weight you need to prevent, alleviate, or even cure many of the ailments caused from being overweight.

Your Hormones Control Your Weight

Your hormones regulate your appetite, cravings, metabolism, and body weight. Many overweight people have an intuitive sense that something's wrong in their bodies. My patients often have symptoms that can be attributed to a number of

---

*For more on the body mass index see "Practical Strategies for Intelligent Weight Loss" beginning on page 327.

hormone problems. In fact, it is not unusual for me to diagnose multiple hormonal abnormalities in the same person. That's because hormones don't go out of whack in a vacuum. When one hormone is out of balance, it can lead to other hormone problems like a chain reaction.

Hormones not only regulate weight, but also mood and emotion and the desire for food (or lack of desire for food). The ability to process food is intimately related to hormone levels in the body. This complex interplay of hormones ultimately determines your appetite and body weight. This has nothing to do with willpower.

Listen to Dr. Bjorntorp of the University of Goteburg, Sweden:

With visceral fat accumulation multiple endocrine perturbations are found, including elevated cortisol and androgens in women, as well as low growth hormone and, in men, testosterone secretion. These hormonal changes exert profound effects on . . . metabolism and [fat] distribution. Cortisol and insulin promote [fat] accumulation . . . while testosterone and growth hormone and . . . estrogens exert opposite effects.

What does this mean? Hormones have powerful interactions with your fat cells and have a major influence on your weight. And insulin, cortisol, growth hormone, and testosterone are only a few of many hormones involved.

Hormones are as fundamental as life itself. All living creatures have hormones. They are powerful molecules that control your metabolism. Hormones regulate how much fat you have and where you have it; they control your appetite; they affect your energy level; they influence your mood, your emotions, even your desire to exercise. Hormones determine the size and strength of your muscles. And hormones help determine your body weight.

Hormonal Disorders Can Be Hard to Diagnose

Doctors learn about hormonal disorders in medical school. But the medical school curriculum teaches that hormonal disorders are usually rare. Not only is this not true, but it does a disservice to endocrinologists, who study hormones and hormonal disorders, and patients, who are told that the problem lies elsewhere. Medical schools do teach about hormonal disorders in their extreme cases but may not teach about less severe cases of the same disorders. The flaws of medical education don't stop there. In med school, the blood test is emphasized as the be-all and end-all. Symptoms may be brushed aside if blood tests are "normal." But blood tests can be wrong. Many people with hormonal problems can have normal blood test results.

In real life, hormonal disorders can occur in many ranges and are due to many things. Some hormonal disorders are caused by tumors (sometimes cancer, sometimes not) of glands—the glands pump out tons and tons of a particular hormone. Other hormonal disorders are caused by complete failure of a gland. Other problems can occur when hormones aren't made properly or don't function the right way.

Medical schools don't teach much about the hormonal disorders caused by a mild overproduction or a mild deficiency of a hormone. They also don't teach much about receptor problems or other ways that a hormone could go haywire. The result: over the years, many doctors forget to look for any type of hormonal disorder. Why should they? They've practically been trained to ignore them. But that can have costly effects for patients in more ways than one. Many overweight patients seek advice from their physicians. They are usually told their hormones are normal. "It's not your hormones," doctors say. "Just eat less and exercise more." Meanwhile, the doctor may think to herself, "This poor obese patient. I know that the odds are less than 2 percent that they will ever lose weight, so why even bother to try?" This attitude has become so prevalent that doctors now openly debate the utility of trying to have their patients lose weight at all.

Sometimes doctors miss severe hormone problems because physicians are not in the frame of mind of looking for them. I have seen many of these missed cases. For example, the average patient with Cushing's syndrome (a disorder resulting in excess cortisol production and weight gain) sees multiple doctors and waits about ten years before getting an accurate diagnosis. Doctors may ignore subtle complaints and attribute your problems being overweight, getting older, or feeling depressed. They forget to consider that perhaps your symptoms may be clues to the *cause* of your weight gain, not the result of it.

Many hormonal disorders will make you gain weight, and all the dieting in the world will not help until the hormonal disorder is corrected. Maybe a simple blood test won't find it, but other testing methods can—and hormonal testing techniques continue to improve. We can detect hormones in blood, urine, and even saliva. But even there, a well-trained doctor will know what else to ask for, because tests can only go so far: they should be given at certain points of the day, test certain parts of the body, and have other requirements that many doctors aren't aware of.

This book explains symptoms of various hormonal disorders. Your symptoms will help you determine whether you may have a hormonal disorder. This book demystifies hormone tests and helps you to interpret the results of tests. It is not meant to be a substitute for your physician. It is to be used as a guide to help answer questions and is intended to bring about your awareness of symptoms so that you can make your physician aware of them.

The Genetics of Weight Gain

There have been great strides made in determining the genetics of obesity. To date, many genes have been attributed to the control of body weight. More than 500 genes have been associated with obesity, with 30–40 genetic sites identified as having a very strong link. These genes influence the complex biology of body weight by controlling appetite, metabolism, and body fat distribution. Genetic researchers emphasize that weight gain generally occurs when people burn fewer calories than they consume. Genes, personal choices, and a society that encourages high-calorie foods and discourages exercise all play a role in body weight. But, genetic differences may explain why some people gain weight despite healthy lifestyles while others stay lean without exercising much or paying much attention to what they eat. Researchers believe that we can learn a lot from people who are genetically resistant to gaining weight.

Because of our genes, our hormonal systems are almost identical to those of our ancient ancestors. Very little has changed over the generations. Unfortunately for us, our environment has changed even though our hormones have not. No longer do we need to forage for nuts and berries; no longer do we need to kill our dinner or go without. We have food that's quick, easy, and high in calories, and cars to get us to the restaurant or grocery store.

"Becoming obese," says obesity expert Dr. James Hill of the University of Colorado, "is a normal response to the American environment." It's an environment created by the industrial revolution. Before the industrial revolution and all its advances in agriculture, transportation, and processing, granulated sugar was an extravagance. Ice cream was a delicacy. Anything requiring refrigeration existed only for the wealthy (or those in very cold climates). It all changed almost overnight, given the context of human history: suddenly, high-calorie, high-fat, high-refined sugar foods were inexpensive and readily available.

And we *like* those foods. We want more; we want more for our money. Think of "supersizing." A double cheeseburger for 99 cents! A 48-ounce Coke for only a dime more than a 32-ounce Coke!

Seems like a bargain, right? But does "more" mean "better"? We are paying a price for all that cheap food. Sugars and fats bombard our delicate hormone systems. Our genes can't keep up with the changes.

Many nutrition experts today recommend that we eat the way our ancestors did thousands of years ago. Dean Ornish, creator of the diet that bears his name, has said that thousands of years ago "it was survival of the fattest."

But things have changed. Back then the problem was finding enough food to avoid starvation. And different cultures had different diets. The Inuits of northern Canada had (and have) a high-protein, high-fat diet, the better to insulate their bodies during the long, hard winter (the body burns more calories to generate body heat). The ancient tribes of Africa, Mexico, and India adhered to a whole-grain, high-carbohydrate diet. The bottom line is the same: the healthiest diets of the world promote hormonal balance and lean bodies.

Cold Virus Linked to Obesity

Adenovirus, a virus that causes the common cold, may contribute to obesity, according to researchers at the University of California, San Diego. Although research is still preliminary, it is thought that this virus and perhaps others may be a contributing factor to weight gain. The virus appears to infect fat cells, making them grow bigger.

But today, we look for a "one-size-fits-all" solution. That's why so many diet books contradict each other. Different authors select the diet of a particular ancient culture to match the diet they're writing about. This anthropological basis for dieting falls short in that it does not take hormones into consideration at all. Obesity today is caused because the food of our civilization disrupts the delicate hormonal balance we are genetically programmed to have.

"Genetics loads the gun. Environment pulls the trigger," says obesity guru George Bray. Well, we can't change our genetics (not yet, anyway). But we can change our hormones. And you can change your hormones without eating like a caveman. This book shows you how.

Chapter Review

Losing weight is not always a matter of willpower or how much you eat or exercise. This chapter explored how hormonal balance influences the body and the brain and why hormonal imbalance helps explain feelings of hunger and craving for food.

In addition, the chapter pointed out that despite great public awareness of obesity and its consequences, millions still deny the ultimate impact of excessive weight on their health and well-being.

The chapter also explained why it is difficult for physicians without the necessary background and training to diagnose hormonal imbalance as the root cause of weight gain. Finally, the chapter noted the link between inherited genetics (including evolutionary genetic history) and the current obesity crisis.

In the next chapter you'll learn how metabolism affects your weight. I give you some basic information about the brain's role in regulating hormonal levels, and I discuss how stress is linked to weight gain and diet failure. You'll also get some practical tips on how to treat and control hormonal imbalance.

Chapter 2

How Metabolism Affects Your Weight

Metabolism is a critical determinant of your weight. How can two people eat the same amount of food and one gains weight while the other does not? It's metabolism. A fast metabolism burns off the weight, while a slow metabolism applies the food directly to your hips. Hormones and metabolic rate help explain the paradox that exists between those who pig out and never gain weight and the calorie counters who gain weight even when they only smell doughnuts. Think of your body as an engine. Metabolism is the rate at which the engine runs. Hormones are the push on the accelerator. Step on the gas and raise your metabolism.

Hormones Regulate Your Metabolism

Most of us have very efficient metabolisms. This means that the food—the fuel—you eat is efficiently burned, conserving as much as possible. But unlike cars, where the more efficient the better, an efficient metabolism means you need less food to maintain your metabolism. So the more efficient your metabolism, the less food you need to consume. And what happens to that extra food? It's stored as fat.

Why do most of us have such efficient metabolisms? The answer is genetics.

In This Chapter

▶ Boosting Metabolism to Burn More Calories

▶ How the Brain Regulates Hormonal Levels

▶ The Links among Stress, Weight Gain, and Failed Diets

▶ How to Treat and Control Hormonal Imbalance

We have been genetically selected for our efficient metabolisms. Keep in mind that, until very recently, food was scarce. Many people died of starvation. There was no such thing as a fat caveman. The key to survival was a slow metabolism: save every excess calorie as fat, because you'll need it during the famine. The world revolved around agriculture, and agriculture was far less refined in those days. Any natural event—and, of course, there were no weather forecasts—could wipe out a year's crop and influence the crops for years to come. So only those individuals with efficient, slow metabolisms survived. Those people who would be considered naturally thin in today's environment would have died in the famines of centuries past.

There are some individuals who have inefficient metabolisms who have survived the centuries. You know these people. These are the ones who eat and eat and never get fat. Their internal processes are so inefficient that they need to take in as much fuel-food as possible just to keep their bodies going. There is never enough left over to be stored as fat. At one time this was a survival disadvantage, but times have changed. The metabolically inefficient are able to eat large quantities of food and never get fat.

But what about the rest of us? Are we doomed to keep piling fat on until the next famine? Of course not. There is a lot you can do to change your metabolism, and changing your metabolism will improve your health. If your metabolism is efficient and slow, you are sluggish and tired all the time. When you boost your metabolism, you burn calories more quickly. Your energy levels are raised, and you feel great.

Unfortunately, there are no medications that can safely boost metabolism. These medications have been researched, but they tend to have an annoying side effect: they can be fatal.

Maybe you're thinking you can do the job with exercise alone; after all, if you burn the calories, you'll lose weight, right? Well, you will. But there are limits. Most people exercise one, or a maximum of two, hours each day. But a revved-up metabolism works 24/7. Take jogging: you'll need to jog about 35 miles to lose just one pound. But boost your metabolism via your hormones and your weight will come off consistently and stay off the right way. As you read this book, you'll learn about your hormones. You'll learn how hormones work together, how one hormone can influence another (or several), and how the most efficient system for losing weight is the one in balance.

Here are a few ways you can boost your metabolism:

■ **Turn down the heat.** Researchers from University College of London have discovered that higher temperatures indoors may be lowering metabolism and contributing to weight gain. When the body is kept warm, it doesn't need to burn as many calories. Conversely, when we are exposed to the cold, metabolism increases to generate more body heat. Turning down the thermostat just a couple of degrees can raise metabolism, helping you burn an extra 100 calories a day.

■ **Spice up your meals.** Warming spices like chili peppers, cinnamon, ginger, cloves, mustard, vinegar, and garlic can give a little boost to your metabolism.

■ **Exercise every day.** Exercise not only raises metabolic rate while it is happening, but for up to 24 hours after you finish. By exercising every day, you keep your metabolism higher all the time.

■ **Build muscle.** Increasing the amount of muscle in your body is one of the best ways to boost metabolism.

You Need More Brown Fat

There are different types of fat. Fat is actually a series of different types of tissues with different functions. In chapter 6, I discuss how the location of fat matters and that fat in the belly is the unhealthiest type of fat, which leads to many of the problems we associate with obesity, including insulin and leptin resistance. But location is not the only factor that distinguishes different types of fat.

There are two colors of fat: brown fat and white fat. The fat we are most familiar with is white fat, which comprises most of the fat in the body. White fat is a storage depot for excess calories and provides insulation. White fat produces inflammation, an unhealthy situation for the body. Brown fat is a healthy type of metabolically active fat. Brown fat is named as such because it contains a lot of energy-generating mitochondria, which gives rise to the color. Brown fat is considered "good" fat because it burns calories and generates body heat.

Through complex brain–hormone interactions, the body controls its own temperature. A higher body temperature is the result of increased metabolism. It's like running an engine; the harder it runs, the hotter it gets. The hormones that raise metabolism, in fact, do so mainly by increasing thermogenesis. Low body temperature means lowered metabolism; we've seen this is an indicator of low thyroid function. People with more brown fat have higher body temperatures and higher metabolisms because they burn more calories to produce body heat.

Brown fat produces a specialized blood protein known as *thermogenin* that allows for the production of body heat. Brown fat is controlled by nerves and stress hormones. The stress hormones epinephrine and norepinepherine, released from nerve cells and the adrenal gland, activate brown fat, increasing thermogenesis. A special receptor for these hormones is found only in brown fat. It is called a *β-3 receptor.* (Other tissues in the body have β-1 and/or β-2 receptors). Stimulation of the β-3 receptor increases metabolism. It does this by increasing heat production and fat breakdown. And the hormones epinephrine and norepinephrine work by stimulating β-receptors.

Newborn babies have the highest concentrations of brown fat, but until recently it was thought that adults didn't have any brown fat. In 2009, scientists discovered the presence of brown fat in adults. This was considered a major medical breakthrough when the research was published in the *New England Journal of Medicine.* Less than one percent of the body's fat is brown fat. Most brown fat is located in the front of the neck, shoulders, and around the collar bones. Brown fat also hides in deeper layers of fat, and the number of brown fat areas varies among individuals. Thinner people and younger people tend to have the most brown fat. Although you lose brown fat as you get older and as you gain weight, it doesn't go away completely. In the past, it was thought that once you lost your brown fat, it was gone forever. However, this is clearly not the case. Everyone has the potential of making more brown fat.

Now researchers are working feverishly to find ways to help people make more of this calorie-burning fat. Researchers are investigating different types of medications and even stem cell transplants as ways to induce brown fat production. Animal studies show that lowering room temperature just a few of degrees will make them lose weight by boosting their metabolism. Cold also makes white fat act more like brown fat, which burns more calories.

You can make more brown fat by cooling your body down. Even a small decrease in the temperature your body is exposed to will induce your body make more brown fat cells. From a survival perspective, when the body is cooled, it has to make more brown fat to generate enough body heat to keep from freezing to death. Researchers have speculated that warm temperatures may

Ways to Increase Brown Fat

Turn your thermostat down.

Exercise in cold weather.

Exercise in water (swimming, water aerobics, walking in the water).

Sip on cold water all day long.

be contributing to our obesity epidemic. Turning down the thermostat just a couple of degrees could help boost your metabolism because you need to burn more calories to stay warm.

Exercise done in the water is particularly good at drawing out body heat, forcing your body to burn more calories. You don't need to make yourself so cold that you feel uncomfortable or shiver. Swimming is one of the best fat-burning exercises. Swimming is extremely relaxing and a great form of aerobic exercise. But any water exercise is a great way to cool your body and burn extra calories. Submersing yourself in water that's cooler than body temperature will cool you down, causing you to make more brown fat to keep you warm. Try walking in a pool, using a kick board, or taking a water aerobics class. You don't have to be a great swimmer to use water to help you burn extra calories.

Just as healthy brown fat can be part of the cycle to help lose weight, dysfunctional brown fat can get in the way. And, ironically—or perhaps not so ironically, considering the continual feedback loops of the body—obesity can cause brown fat dysfunction. If you are very overweight, your brown fat tissue cannot produce heat properly, so your metabolism is lowered, and it becomes even harder to lose weight, ad infinitum.

Since the only place β-3 receptors are located is in brown fat, this makes it the ideal target for a metabolic enhancement drug. Theoretically, there should be very few side effects, because only the β-3 receptor is being affected. This would likely be the magic drug we've all waited for. And, indeed, several major pharmaceutical companies are investigating β-3 receptor stimulator medications as a way of enhancing metabolism and helping with weight loss. Unfortunately, they are not as great as they might seem. It turns out that the original β-3 research was done on mice. And, as we continue to have to remind ourselves, mice are different than humans. Humans do have β-3 receptors, but we lose most of them within the first six months of our lives. After that, there just aren't many β-3 receptors at all. Studies of β-3 medications on humans have been, as expected, disappointing. Newer compounds still under investigation hold promise, but no one knows whether these medications will really work.

Another area hotly investigated by drug companies, thermogenins made by brown fat tissue are responsible for body heat production. Thermogenins are regulated by blood proteins known as *uncoupling proteins*. The more uncoupling proteins in your system, the higher your metabolism. There are three types of uncoupling proteins: the prosaically named UCP-1, UCP-2, and UCP-3. UCP-2 and UCP-3 are most promising for weight loss, but so far research has been limited to mice. Scientists have been working on ways to increase uncoupling proteins as a form of increasing metabolism and causing weight loss. There are also medications under development that mimic UCPs; these could be injected and would speed metabolism.

More Than Just Insulin

You may be familiar with the hormone insulin and its links to body weight. You also may have heard that too much insulin makes you fat and leads to diabetes. That's what the experts say, anyway. Dozens of books have been published on the subject of lowering insulin levels. These books offer solutions on how to improve the way insulin works in the body and ultimately lose weight.

Insulin is only a small part of the complete hormonal picture. Dozens if not hundreds of hormones are involved in the regulation of your body weight. Glands like the adrenal gland, the thyroid gland, the pituitary gland, the ovary, the testicle, even fat cells all make hormones that influence your body weight and body composition. There are many hormonal disorders that can cause you to be overweight. This book explains conditions like hypothyroidism, Cushing's syndrome, polycystic ovary syndrome, male hypogonadism, menopause, growth hormone deficiency, insulin resistance, and even stress and depression. All of these conditions can slow your metabolism, increase appetite, and make you gain weight. Once you identify specific hormonal deficiencies or excesses, you can alter your diet, add certain vitamins or herbal products, or even go on medications to help balance your hormones.

Hormones contribute to obesity, and obesity creates a hormonal imbalance that slows metabolism and perpetuates the obese state. Now, insulin does have an effect. Improper insulin action leads to high insulin levels, resulting in hunger and weight gain. But there's also the thyroid. Low thyroid hormone or inefficient processing of thyroid hormone slows metabolism and causes weight gain. Also, problems with testosterone and growth hormone cause weight gain, loss of muscle mass, and increased fat mass. In women, low estrogen levels increase fat in the belly, but high estrogen levels increase fat in the hips and buttocks. High cortisol levels increase fat in the belly and cause tremendous weight gain. Various genetically controlled hunger hormones, like leptin, ghrelin, cholecystokinin, resistin, adiponectin, and others, affect your appetite, metabolism, and body weight. Hungry hormones have powerful actions on the hunger centers in the brain. Finally, food affects your hormones. Food is a powerful drug that triggers a vast array of hormonal, chemical, and brain effects.

But you're not hostage to your hormones. You can achieve hormonal balance. With hormonal balance you will experience weight loss and increased energy, but the benefits do not stop there. Hormonal balance can dramatically reduce your susceptibility to medical problems and can improve a wide variety of complaints. With hormonal balance, you will optimize your metabolism and you will lose weight. And by learning the principles of your body's hormones, you can tailor the optimal nutrition plan for yourself and your family members. Put simply, hormonal balance can save your life.

Your Hormonal Identity

You are an individual. Your fingerprints are not like anyone else's fingerprints; your sense of humor is not like anyone else's sense of humor; your taste in music, in clothing, in colors or animals or people is not like anyone else's tastes in those things, or most any other thing.

Your hormones are not the same as anyone else's hormones.

But keep in mind that hormones control all facets of life. In addition to body weight and metabolism, hormones control mood, energy level, sex drive, the menstrual cycle, and your biological clock. Hormonal balance will help you achieve health, wellness, physical and mental well-being, and optimal metabolism. And *your* hormones, in particular, reflect your internal chemistry. Hormones are the reason why some people remain youthful and vital later in life and others quickly deteriorate both mentally and physically.

The answer to achieving a healthy body weight is in your hormones.

You may not know what your hormonal identity is, but this book will help you find it. Subtle clues—from physical symptoms to physical traits—all give us clues to our hormonal identity. In addition, hormonal testing, *when done properly,* may also help us to discover our hormonal identity. Each chapter in this book offers methods of determining your hormone status for a particular hormone. Your levels may be too high, too low, or right where you want them. I show you how to have them right where you want them all of the time.

Hormones Change with Age

Want to know why you get fatter when you age? Want to know why your muscles start to droop, your sex drive diminishes, your sleep gets a little harder to come by?

The answer: your hormones.

Many of our vital hormones are at a fraction of what they were when we were young. These low levels, once considered a normal part of aging, are now considered by many physicians to be abnormal. We don't accept anymore that aging means falling apart and crawling into that long goodnight. Doctors are now treating hormonal deficiencies, and a new branch of medicine, called anti-aging medicine, has evolved. Anti-aging physicians routinely prescribe hormones as a way of reversing some of the effects of aging. It's a whole new paradigm for medicine. Aging is discussed throughout this book because hormones, aging, and metabolism are so closely related. We become older; our metabolism slows; we gain weight. But that need not be the end of the story. I show you how you can reverse some of the hormonal changes that occur with aging.

The Endocrine System: Your Body's Hormones

The endocrine system is the body's way of communicating and controlling bodily functions. Virtually every part of the body is regulated by hormones. The word *hormone* has an interesting etymological root: The word comes from the Greek, meaning "to stir up" or "to urge on." Classically, a hormone is a substance produced by a gland and secreted into the bloodstream that has its action at a distant location in the body.

We now know that almost every organ, not just traditional glands, make hormones. Nerve cells, fat cells, intestinal cells, liver cells, even heart cells and kidney cells all make hormones. Many of the "classic" hormones are controlled by the pituitary gland—referred to as the *master gland*—in the brain (see Figure 2.1). These include thyroid hormone, androgens, estrogens, cortisol, and growth hormone. The pituitary gland makes its own set of hormones that control these glands. The pituitary gland is controlled by a portion of the brain known as the *hypothalamus*. Higher centers in the brain, influenced by your thoughts, mood, emotions, and other hormones, control the hypothalamus.

Ultimately, then, your brain controls your hormones. But: your hormones also control your brain.

Your hormones are continually in a state of flux. They are never steady, always going up or down. Your brain "listens" to your hormones to figure out what

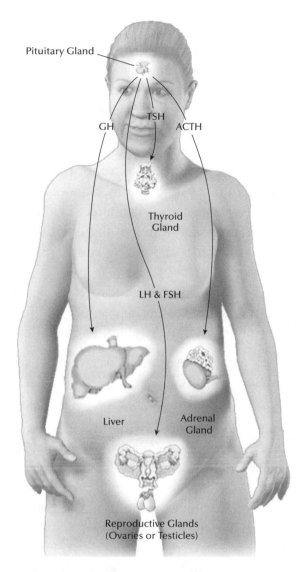

Figure 2.1   **The Endocrine System I: Control by the "Master Gland"**

The pituitary gland, also known as the *master gland,* produces hormones that regulate other glands in the body. Thyroid stimulating hormone (TSH) regulates hormone production from the thyroid gland. Adrenocortitrophic hormone (ACTH) regulates adrenal gland hormone production, including cortisol and dehydroepi-androsterone (DHEA). Lutenizing hormone (LH) and follicle stimulating hormone (FSH) regulate gonadal (ovaries and testicles) hormone production, including estrogen, progesterone, testosterone, and androstenedione. Growth hormone (GH) regulates the production of insulin-like growth factor-1 (IGF-1) in the liver. Hormones made by the target glands send signals back to the pituitary gland.

to do. High hormone levels give signals to the brain telling it to shut down production of a particular hormone. Low hormone levels do the opposite, telling the brain to make hormone levels surge. The rhythms are not always predictable, either. Some hormones follow a regular 24-hour cycle known as a *circadian rhythm*. But those rhythms aren't in sync. Cortisol, for example, peaks at 7:00 to 8:00 A.M. Growth hormone, on the other hand, peaks at about 3:00 A.M. If you are not sleeping well, it will have a detrimental effect on your hormonal rhythms.

Many hormones are not under the control of the pituitary gland. Insulin is not controlled by the pituitary gland, but imbalances of thyroid, growth hormone, cortisol, estrogen, or testosterone can affect insulin. Various other hormones, such as fat hormones, pancreatic hormones, gut hormones, and other hormones that don't come from traditional "glands," are not regulated by the pituitary gland. (See Figure 2.2.)

Many things can go wrong with hormones. There can be too much or not enough; the receptors might not work, there might be proteins in the blood binding up specific hormones . . . the possibilities are endless.

How Do Hormones Work?

Hormones, in the great scheme of things, are tiny. A single drop of blood contains literally thousands of hormones. The hormones travel through the blood and other bodily fluids, serving as chemical messengers. The message directs the body at the receiving end—known, logically enough, as a "receptor"—to do something. (See Figure 2.3.) Receptors are special proteins that can recognize and bind a particular hormone, and when hormone and receptor merge in a cell, a chain of events begins. Think of a lock and a key. The key (hormone) unlocks the lock (receptor), "directing" it to open or close, as the case may be. It changes the lock's status from locked to unlocked, or vice versa.

The keys—the hormones—are made by glands. The pituitary gland makes special hormones that control many of the glands (think of the pituitary gland as the chief executive officer of the key company). And, the brain makes other hormones that control the pituitary gland (like the chairman of the board). So, ultimately, everything is controlled by the brain. But in nature's delicate balance, a system known as *feedback* exists. Hormones made by the glands have reciprocal influences on the brain and pituitary gland. In other words, your brain controls your hormones, and hormones control your brain. The situation works both

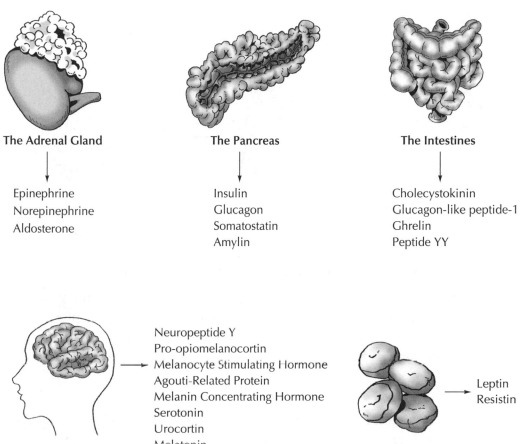

The Adrenal Gland

Epinephrine
Norepinephrine
Aldosterone

The Pancreas

Insulin
Glucagon
Somatostatin
Amylin

The Intestines

Cholecystokinin
Glucagon-like peptide-1
Ghrelin
Peptide YY

Neuropeptide Y
Pro-opiomelanocortin
Melanocyte Stimulating Hormone
Agouti-Related Protein
Melanin Concentrating Hormone
Serotonin
Urocortin
Melatonin

The Human Brain

Leptin
Resistin

Fat Cells

**Figure 2.2   The Endocrine System II: Hormones Functioning
Independently of the Pituitary Gland**

Many hormones are not under control of the pituitary gland. The adrenal
gland produces the stress hormones epinephrine and norepinephrine as well
as aldosterone (a steroid hormone that regulates blood pressure). The pancreas
makes several important hormones including insulin, glucagon, somatostatin, and
amylin. The stomach and intestines make ghrelin, cholecystokinin (CCK), peptide
YY, enterostatin, and glucagon like peptide-1 (GLP-1). Fat cells make leptin,
TNF, IL-6, resistin, and adiponectin. The brain makes many hormones including
orexins, endocannabinoids, neuropeptide Y (NPY), proopiomelanocortin (POMC),
melanocyte stimulating hormone (MSH), Agouti-related protein (AgRP), galanin,
endorphins, GABA, melanin concentrating hormone (MCH), serotonin, urocortin,
and melatonin.

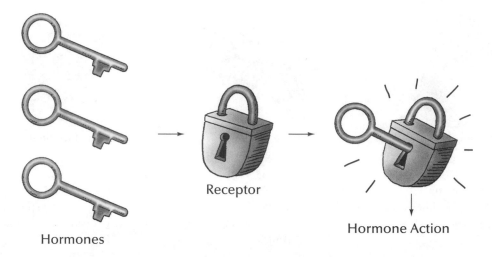

Receptor

Hormone Action

Hormones

Figure 2.3 Hormones and Receptors: How Hormones Work

The specific hormone molecules are like specific "keys." Only the appropriate hormone corresponds to a receptor (lock). When a hormone and receptor interact, it sets forth a chain of events that ultimately leads to the actions associated with each specific hormone.

ways because, as messengers, hormones can tell parts of the body what to do— and then they have to obey a part of the body telling *them* what to do.

After all, every living cell has hormone receptors, and hormones control every living cell. They do so by working through the most fundamental component of living beings: DNA. Glands "secrete" hormones into the bloodstream. There they travel to every nook and cranny of your body until they locate their specific receptor. Virtually every cell in the body has receptors for a wide variety of hormones.

Stress Disrupts Hormonal Balance

We are living in stressful times. The great recession has lead to an increased level of stress among our society as a whole. In general, stress means pressure or strain on the body because of physical, psychological, or emotional reasons. Certainly many generations have uttered those words, but think of what our generation faces: instantaneous communication. Constant availability. "Just-in-time" production methods. Even our children, once largely free of the stresses of adult life, now make "play dates." Our lives have been sped up in ways previous generations never could have imagined.

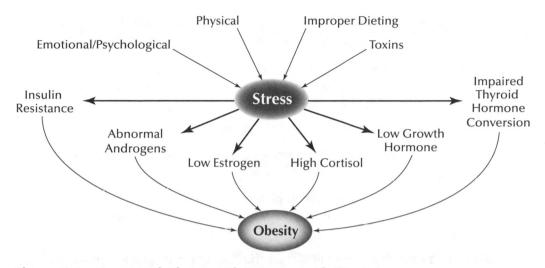

Figure 2.4   Hormonal Changes That Occur with Stress

Stress disrupts the body's hormonal system by creating insulin resistance, lowering sex hormones (estrogen and testosterone), lowering growth hormone, and increasing cortisol levels. Stress also reduces the body's ability to convert thyroid hormone to an active form. Each one of these hormonal changes slows metabolism and causes weight gain.

We cope, or try to. *Allostasis* is the term scientists use to describe how the body copes with stress. We take vacations and get away from it all. But most of the year, there it is: all the stress we live with. And then there are other stresses: the death of loved ones, the heartbreak of ending or losing a relationship, even the "good-for-you" hunger of a crash diet (which, of course, isn't really good for you at all).

Usually, two things happen. The first is that our body goes into conservation mode. Metabolism slows, and even the normal diet we were adhering to makes us put on weight. The second is we look to one of the most familiar items in our lives for consolation: food. And often not just food, but chocolate bars, sugary sodas, and supersized containers of french fries. "Comfort food," it's sometimes called. Why do we do this? Because of our hormones. Any kind of stress—whether mental, physical, or emotional—can disrupt hormonal balance in our bodies in ways that make us gain weight. (See Figure 2.4.)

Stress causes the brain, pituitary gland, and adrenal glands to pump out stress hormones. These hormones cause the biological reactions we associate with stress, from rapid heartbeat to a rise in blood sugar to slowed digestion.

How Chronic Stress Affects Your Health

Digestive system: Stress causes abnormal stomach acid production and stomach pain. It causes irritable bowel syndrome with symptoms like nausea, diarrhea, or constipation.

Obesity: Stress increases appetite and alters hormonal balance.

Immune system: Weakening of the immune system makes you more likely to get infections.

Nervous system: Stress causes anxiety, depression, insomnia, and an inability to enjoy life. Stress can also impair memory and the ability to make decisions.

Cardiovascular system: Stress increases the risk for heart attacks and strokes

---

They prepare us for the "fight-or-flight" response. Now, all of us experience stress. Our bodies have adapted to handle the normal hormonal surges that occur with stress. This acute, short-term stress does not cause you to gain weight. Chronic, long-term stress, however, is something else entirely. Too much stress causes longer-term elevations of stress hormones that cause weight gain.

Many diets make you lose weight in such a way that it creates a tremendous stress on your body. This is one of the main reasons why so many people who lose weight on a diet ultimately gain it all back. Chronic stress also causes the body to shift its focus away from its normal activity. Stress causes the immune system to wane, muscles to shrink, and, in general, a lousy feeling throughout your body.

Why Do Most Diets Fail?

When you go on a diet, your metabolism is dramatically altered. When your body is losing weight, it is "stressed"—causing hormonal disruptions that slow metabolism and boost appetite.

This is why 98 percent of diets ultimately fail.

How does this happen? Think of a famine. When you go on a diet, your body doesn't realize that you are doing this for its own good. Your body thinks it is starving. Your body cannot tell the difference between a diet and a famine. It is all about survival. Your body slows its metabolism, making it even more efficient. Eventually your body succumbs to this hormonal pressure, and your diet ultimately fails.

I show you how to prevent this from happening. You can teach your body that weight loss does not mean you are starving to death. By eating to outsmart your hungry hormones, you can lose weight consistently, and you will *keep the weight off.* In fact, it is possible to lose weight and maintain—or even increase—your metabolism. It all relies on outsmarting your hormones.

Hormone Problems Can Be Treated

Hormone treatments cover a wide range. For some people, dietary changes are enough. For others, specific vitamins and/or minerals may also be helpful. For yet others, medications may be required. Fortunately, hormones and hormone treatments come in many forms: pills, patches, shots, gels, and creams. And they work in many ways. Some boost the body's natural supply of certain hormones, while others work by stimulating a particular gland to make more of its own hormone.

Treatment with hormones goes back to the nineteenth century, when French physician Charles Edouard Brown-Sequard injected himself with an extract of crushed dog and guinea pig testicles in order to test the effects of testosterone. At the time, the good doctor was seventy-two years old, and like many seventy-two-year-olds, aging had taken a toll on his appetite and sex drive. However, after the injection—and to the amazement of his colleagues—the extract had the same effect as modern-day testosterone.

While testosterone medications are derived from different sources nowadays, not all hormone medications have strayed from an animal form processed for human consumption. For example, a popular thyroid hormone medication, Armour Thyroid, consists of ground pig thyroid glands. And a popular estrogen medication is made from the urine of pregnant mares. But hormones come from a variety of sources, and natural does not always mean better than synthetic. Moreover, some hormones work better when taken by mouth; others get digested in the stomach; and others work only if taken by injection, patch, cream, gel, or other creative delivery device.

In today's health care environment, the average doctor only has about 10 minutes to spend with each patient. He simply doesn't have enough time to go into as much detail as this book. So this book is written as a guide for you and your doctor. This book is also recommended for doctors and other health care providers as a guide to up-to-date treatments for hormonal problems. My goal is to demystify hormone treatments for both patients and professionals. Whether you're already taking hormones—or merely considering it—I believe this book will be very helpful to you.

Hormone Weight Loss Products and Hormone Preparations

Health food store shelves are filled with herbal products that make claims to affect your hormones and/or your weight. In a clever bit of marketing, herbal products are now referred to as *nutraceuticals*—"functional foods," including vitamins and minerals, that are available from health food stores and drug stores without a prescription. Nutraceuticals are not under as strict regulation as prescription medications. The quality control is highly variable. Many of them have not been properly tested. Prescription medications are held to a much higher standard. This is not to put down nutraceuticals completely; many of them show great promise.

But know what you're getting. Many nutraceuticals are derived from plants, but some are hormone preparations made from ground animal glands or brains. The labels can be disguised (*bovine* means cow, *porcine* means pig), and consumers may end up buying something that, at worst, can hurt, not heal.

Think of this: Many nutraceutical products make weight loss claims. And many of these products claim to affect your metabolism and/or your hormones. The important point is that these products, although considered "natural," can be just as potent as prescription medications and should be treated as such.

In this book, I talk about many nutraceutical products. I help you put things into perspective. I tell you what products are worthwhile, what products are garbage . . . and what products are dangerous. This book points out specific instances when a common vitamin or mineral affects your hormones. Many of us eat too much processed food that is lacking in vitamins and minerals vital for proper hormonal balance. In addition, many crops are grown in nutrient-poor soil, so that even fresh fruits and vegetables may be lacking in specific vital nutrients. Hormones require specific vitamins and minerals in order to be made or processed efficiently.

Hormonal Balance: Your Guide to a Healthy Life

It all comes down to hormonal balance. Whether you want to lose a significant amount of weight, get in shape, or even want to reverse the effects of aging, hormonal balance is critical. We've come to assume that once out of control, hormones are always out of control—that we are powerless against these messengers circulating throughout our bodies. That isn't true, even if you've already suffered from a hormonal ailment. You can control your hormones. You can control your metabolism. Follow the lessons in this book, and you will be on your way to a healthier, thinner, well-tuned version of you.

Chapter Review

While no current medications offer a proven, foolproof way to boost your metabolism, this chapter offered some practical tips and techniques to help you take charge of your body's metabolism.

Simple steps such as lowering the heat levels in your house or even eating more spicy foods—in addition to getting more exercise—were offered as viable options to boost your calorie burning metabolism.

The chapter also discussed an individual's unique individual "hormonal identity" and how this is linked to difficulties controlling weight. The dramatic changes that age brings to hormonal levels were also highlighted.

The brain's role in regulating hormonal levels was discussed in detail. In particular, the importance of the pituitary gland (also known as the *master gland*) was highlighted. Stress was also cited as a factor in weight gain, because continuous high levels of stress tend to disrupt normal hormonal levels.

Finally, the chapter pointed out why simple actions such as changes in diet are sometimes not enough to rebalance your hormonal levels. It concluded by offering a number of the best available treatments, including pills, patches, shots, gels, and creams.

The next chapter discusses the links between the foods you eat and hormonal imbalance. It offers some practical diet and weight control strategies and suggestions you can put in place now that will help you begin to take charge of your weight.

CHAPTER

3

Understand How Food Affects Your Hormones

Every bite of food that you put in your mouth affects your hormones. Whether you eat junk food, healthy food, large quantities or small quantities, even if you starve yourself, your hormones are affected. Hormones can even be affected by the *sight or smell* of food. Every time you eat, a chemical reaction takes place between your hormones and the food. Hormones control your digestive system, and, in turn, your digestive system produces its own set of hormones. Hormones control your appetite, and hormones control your cravings. The hormone traditionally linked to food is insulin. But insulin isn't the only hormone affected by food, nor is it necessarily the most important. In this chapter, I explain how the components of food—carbohydrates, proteins, and fats—affect your hormones.

Sometimes hormones in food can affect us without our even knowing about it. Hormone use in the livestock industry is commonplace, and those hormones are ingested by us when we eat the cows, pigs, sheep, and chickens that have eaten them. The toxins and chemicals that get into our foods frequently contain substances that mimic hormones.

In This Chapter

▸ Why Eating Slowly Creates a "Full" Feeling

▸ Surprising Facts about Healthy Carbohydrates

▸ Fruits and Vegetables: Five of Each Is the Key

▸ Why Smaller Meals Are Better Than "Three Squares"

35

Slow Down to Control Appetite

Taking a long time to eat or eating foods that are digested slowly allows time for the "I am full" signal to reach your brain. Most of us eat faster than our hormones are able to react. The result is eating more than your body needs. Eating slowly can be difficult. Have you ever noticed how a dog eats his food? Dogs eat as fast as they can. Humans have these same basic instincts: we have to fight against these instincts when we eat slowly. It is hard to do.

Slowly digested foods help you slow things down because you can eat them at a normal pace and still have time for your brain to get the right signals. Foods that are chewy or crunchy make your body work harder from the very start. To increase chewiness, your best bet is to eat whole foods instead of chopped or processed foods, like a whole apple instead of apple sauce or a salmon steak instead of canned salmon.

> **Eat Foods That Are Digested Slowly or Take a Long Time to Eat**
>
> Beans
>
> Chewy foods
>
> Complex carbohydrates (vegetables, fruits, whole grains)
>
> Crunchy foods
>
> Lean proteins (chicken, beef, seafood)
>
> Low-fat dairy products
>
> Smoothies
>
> Thick, water-based soups

Foods that are low in calories but hearty, heavy, and thick are great for appetite control. These foods tend to contain a lot of fiber and water, increasing the bulk of the food without increasing calories. They take up more room in your belly, wake up appetite-controlling gut hormones (see chapter 5), and help you feel full and satisfied. There have been several studies showing that the weight of the food, not the calories, is the main determinant of how full you feel. This means that if you eat the same amount of a high-calorie food or a low-calorie food, you will feel just as full.

Liquid calories have an appetite-stimulating effect. But foods with high water content have the opposite effect. I recommend avoiding all liquid calories—juice, soda, and even skim milk. Drinks are just empty calories and won't help you lose weight. Smoothies, thick soups, and other foods with high water content, however, are slowly digested and are more filling.

Crunchy Foods

Apples	Edamame	Radishes
Bell peppers	Frozen grapes	Roasted chickpeas
Carrots	High-fiber breakfast cereal	Turnips
Celery		Whole-grain crackers
Cucumbers	Jicama	Zucchini (raw)
	Lettuce	

Eating a balanced diet that is high in fruits and vegetables has an added benefit because the vitamins and minerals nourish and satisfy the body. If the body doesn't get enough of a particular vitamin or mineral, the result can be excessive hunger or cravings. Taking a vitamin doesn't help reduce appetite and cravings the way that eating vegetables and fruits does.

"Eat foods that will repair, nourish and support every cell in your body so your body will work for you and not against you."

—Jillian Michaels

Chewy Foods

Baked apples	Corn on the cob	Mushrooms
Barley	Frozen bananas	Quinoa
Cantaloupe	Frozen peas	Shrimp
Cooked oatmeal (not instant)	Frozen strawberries	Wild rice
	Honeydew	
	Lean meat and poultry	

Fiber Slows Digestion

If you want to slow your digestion, fiber is the way to go. Like starch, fiber is an undigestible carbohydrate. That's bad, right? Nope. It's a good thing. Fiber helps you feel full and satisfied. Fiber slows down the breakdown of carbohydrates. This, in turn, lowers blood sugar. Fiber also plays a major role in maintaining good health in a variety of other ways:

- Fiber makes you feel full. Soluble fibers swell in the stomach and bowels, enhancing the release of anti-hunger hormones and reducing the release of hunger hormones. And since the body cannot digest fiber, the fiber harmlessly makes its way through the digestive system, eventually passed out into the stool.

- Fiber nourishes your colonic mucosa, the innermost layer of the large intestine, and has a role in the prevention of colon cancer, constipation, and other colonic diseases.

- A high-fiber diet reduces bad cholesterol and raises good cholesterol.

- Fiber lowers the glycemic index of foods.

- High-fiber diets have been shown to help people lose weight.

Not all fiber is created equal. Soluble fibers are foods like beans and steel-cut oats, as well as pectin, found in apples. Insoluble fibers are foods like whole wheat or bran, foods often found in certain cereal grains. You need to eat 25–35 grams a day of fiber each day, minimum, in your diet. The best way to get fiber in your diet is to eat lots of fresh vegetables and fruits.

Carbohydrates Are an Important Part of a Healthy Diet

Scientifically, carbohydrates or "carbs" are simply any compound that contain hydrogen and oxygen—the elements of water—combined with carbon. They are the most common organic compounds found in nature and are the substances produced by green plants during photosynthesis.

Carbohydrates in one way or another are the focus of many diets. In most of these plans, breads, pasta, sugary foods, and grains are off-limits. You can lose weight on a "low-carb" or "no-carb" diet, but you are likely to gain all the

Carbohydrate Chemistry

The terms *sugar* and *starch* are very non-specific. I'd like to provide a more detailed, scientific description of carbohydrates, to help you understand exactly what a carbohydrate is and how sugars and starches are made up of the same building blocks.

Monosaccharides are the building blocks of all carbohydrates. All carbohydrates are made up of these three simple sugars:

1. *Glucose.* The most abundant monosaccharide. It has the strongest effect in stimulating production of insulin. The terms blood sugar and blood glucose are interchangeable.

2. *Fructose.* Half of what makes up table sugar, fructose is best known as the primary sugar found in fruit.

3. *Galactose.* No, not the kind of sugar they use on Star Trek, but a form of sugar only found in milk and milk products.

Disaccharides occur when two monosaccharides come together to form a simple sugar. During digestion, the disaccharides are broken down into monosaccharides by special enzymes in the intestine. The two primary disaccharides are

1. *Sucrose.* Made of equal parts glucose and fructose, sucrose is found in fruits and table sugar.

2. *Lactose.* Made of equal parts galactose and glucose, lactose is only found in milk and milk products. Lactose is digested by the enzyme lactase. People with lactase deficiency have problems digesting milk.

Polysaccharides are created by many monosaccharides linked together in very complex arrays. However, they're still nothing more than a string of monosaccharides. Polysaccharides are also known as starch or complex carbohydrates.

weight back. The truth is that carbohydrates are an important component of any healthy diet.

Carbohydrates are often referred to as two kinds: simple and complex. Simple carbohydrates are known as sugars; complex carbohydrates are known as starches. Regardless of what kind they are, carbohydrates—in the form of sugar, wheat, rice, grains, fruits, and vegetables—are the principal components of nearly every human's diet and the primary source of energy in our diet.

Though many fad diets emphasize low- or no-carbohydrate intake, carbohydrates are an important part of your diet and are necessary for hormonal balance. When you are losing weight, it is essential that your body get ample supplies of carbohydrate in order to prevent muscle breakdown. Processed carbohydrates and sugar, however, can make blood sugar and insulin spike, which often has a rebound effect, resulting in low blood sugar and carbohydrate cravings.

A Carbohydrate's Journey

What happens when you eat carbohydrates? It's a seemingly complex process, but it only takes a matter of hours—sometimes less—to occur. Let's run through it step by step. Carbohydrates are broken down into simple sugars in the intestines—glucose, fructose, and galactose. The sugars are transported through the intestinal lining into the blood stream. This carbohydrate-rich blood flows to the liver. This is very important, because the liver does not treat all carbohydrates the same. Glucose zips straight through the liver, raising blood sugar very quickly. Fructose and galactose, however, are slowly converted into glucose by the liver before reaching the bloodstream. Fruits, vegetables, whole grains, and dairy products that have fructose and galactose are ultimately converted into glucose by the liver, but this takes time. The result is that these foods cause less spiking of blood sugar and insulin.

Once glucose gets into the bloodstream, it is detected by the pancreas, which responds by pumping out insulin. Foods high in sugar and processed carbohydrates make it to the bloodstream quickly, resulting in a spike of insulin followed by a blood sugar crash. Complex carbohydrates, protein, and fat take time to be broken down, delivering glucose to the bloodstream in a slow, controlled manner, resulting in a more natural and healthy insulin response. Insulin moves glucose from the blood into cells. Without insulin, your cells would starve. When you have insulin resistance, a condition discussed in chapter 6, insulin doesn't work properly, and more insulin needs to be produced to get the glucose into the cells. Eating too much sugar magnifies insulin's response to food. This has been shown to increase the production of new fat cells and raise cholesterol and triglyceride levels.

Your Diet Should Contain about 40 Percent Healthy Carbohydrates

For the past several decades, there has been great public interest in the composition of the American diet. The high calorie and fat content of the typical diet has been linked to a wide variety of diseases, including heart attacks, strokes, diabetes, liver disease, kidney failure, and cancer. In the fervor to cut back on calories from fat, many people end up increasing their consumption of carbohydrates.

Diet experts continue to debate the perfect balance of carbohydrates, protein, and fat. My belief—and the belief of many other physicians and nutrition experts—is that a diet should contain a healthy balance of 40 percent carbohydrates, 30 percent protein, and 30 percent fat. Exact percentages aren't critical, however.

Best Carbohydrates for Hormonal Balance

Dairy products	Beans
Fruits	Vegetables
Nuts and seeds (in limited amounts)	Whole grains

Eat Less Sugar

If you want to balance your hormones, you need to eat more complex carbohydrates and less sugar. The average American now consumes more than 20 teaspoons of sugar every day. Compared to 1977, consumption of sugar has increased as much as 92 percent in adolescents. Sweeteners like high-fructose corn syrup and other types of sugar make up as much as one-third of the carbohydrate content of the typical American diet. Think about that: 33 percent of everything the average American consumes is simply sugar. Thirty-three percent! That's the brown sugar in your "fat-free" "whole-grain" muffin, the sugar added to the "mango salsa" on your "heart-healthy" grilled grouper, the sugar in that "energy" bar. That's the sugar in soft drinks, coffee drinks, ketchup, snack cakes, and even salad dressings. And if you don't think you're eating so much sugar, check the labels of some of your favorite products. Sugar includes honey, molasses, dextrose, sucrose, maltose, and the worst offender, high-fructose corn syrup (now sometimes labeled as "corn sugar"). White foods, like mashed potatoes, pasta, rice, and bread, are processed carbohydrates that are basically sugar and should also be limited in your diet.

Many low-fat or no-fat products have hit the shelves in recent years: fat-free chips, fat-free ice cream, and even fat-free chocolate cookies. But these foods aren't calorie-free because they are so much higher in sugar. In fact, many fat-free or low-fat foods have more calories than the regular versions.

Eat Slowly Digested Carbohydrates

In their most basic form, complex carbohydrates, or starches, are strings of simple sugars that come in many different arrangements. Ounce for ounce, all carbohydrates have the same number of calories (4 calories per gram). They differ, however, in the speed at which they are digested. This has profound effects on blood sugar and insulin production. All carbohydrates are eventually converted by the body into glucose. Healthy carbohydrates are digested and broken down slowly, providing a more gradual source of sugar to the body. Unhealthy carbohydrates, though, are rapidly digested and cause huge sugar and insulin spikes.

> **Beans Are a Slow Carbohydrate**
>
> The complex carbohydrates found in beans are very good because they are encased in protein. In order to digest this super-healthy starch, your body must first digest the protein. Beans provide a stable, constant source of energy that can last many hours.

Ways to Slow Down Carbohydrates

Cook vegetables a little less. The more a carbohydrate is cooked, the quicker it is digested. This is because heating breaks down the chemical bonds of the food, making it easier for your body to absorb the carbohydrates. Raw foods are digested more slowly. You don't have to eat only raw foods, but try cooking your vegetables a little less, so they retain a little crunch.

Eat fewer processed foods. Processing a food includes milling grain into flour, mashing potatoes, juicing or drying fruit. Processing concentrates sugars and makes food easier to digest. Eating less processed food will help you feel fuller with fewer calories.

Eat slowly. If you eat sugar or processed carbohydrates, make sure to eat them slowly. This slows the rate at which carbohydrates hit the bloodstream and allows your body's hormones to react in a controlled manner. Insulin, for example, won't surge as much if you take a long time to eat a sugary food. Eating slowly also gives your body time to receive the stop-eating signals from anti-hunger hormones.

How to Make a Potato Healthier

There is a chemical process called *retrogradation* that makes a potato harder to digest. When food is heated and then cooled, then heated again, the process can modify starches and make them harder to digest. So after you bake a potato, place it in the refrigerator overnight, then reheat it the next day. It will be digested more slowly than it was after first baking. Leftovers, in other words, are a *good* thing.

Don't overchew your food. Eating slowly doesn't mean chewing slowly. Back in the 1800s, many families followed the teachings of clergyman Sylvester Graham. Today, Graham would be considered prescient in many ways: a vegetarian, he encouraged his followers to eat fruits and vegetables, avoid fried foods, and invented an unsifted wheat flour that has taken his name (as has a cracker made from that flour). But one of his pronouncements was dead wrong. He believed, rightly so, that Americans ate too fast. His answer, however, was that one should chew food at least thirty-two times (one chew for each tooth) before swallowing, and many more times if possible. This process, and some of the philosophy behind it, became known as "fletcherism," after one of Graham's followers.

Unlike eating slowly, which is a healthy way to help you feel full, excessive chewing liquefies and almost completely digests the food in your mouth. The saliva contains an enzyme that breaks down carbohydrates, so we start to digest sugars and starches before we swallow. By the time the overchewed food hits the stomach and intestines, it's ready to be instantly absorbed into the bloodstream—creating a huge insulin surge. (And, as nineteenth-century Americans found out, excessive chewing also leads to colossally boring meals. When do you get a chance to talk?)

Combine protein with carbohydrates. Starches are digested more slowly if you combine them with protein. Protein will even slow down the digestion of sugar and white flour. Make an effort to eat protein at every meal.

Don't take enzyme supplements. Enzyme supplements speed up digestion. This is exactly what you don't want.

Whole Wheat Bread

Although wheat bread is healthier than white bread, it still contains flour, which is a processed carbohydrate. You don't need to avoid bread altogether, but when you do eat bread, make sure it is made with whole wheat flour and has at least 4 grams of fiber per slice. Don't eat soft whole wheat bread with enriched flour because it is basically white bread colored brown.

Limit Foods Made with Flour

Starch or carbohydrates are frequently considered the culprit in failed weight loss attempts. It is not that starch is bad for you, but of all the macronutrients—starch, protein, and fat—it is the most overeaten. Additionally, starchy foods in meals and snacks too often are accompanied by fat or sugary condiments, such as butter and jellies.

You don't need to eat any flour on the Hormonal Health Diet because you can get all your carbohydrates from vegetables and fruits, but if you do eat foods made from flour, make sure to choose foods made from whole-grain flour. Grinding of grains makes them easier to digest, so finely milled flour is digested more quickly than whole wheat flour or simple cracked wheat. In general, the more something is processed, the less healthy it is. You should make an effort to eat more whole grains and avoid processed grains, especially food made with flour. Even whole wheat flour is a processed carbohydrate and is not as healthy as whole grain. Even when you eat whole wheat flour for weight loss, you should eat no more than two servings daily.

Whole Grains You Can Eat Instead of Foods Made with Flour

Barley	Bulgur	Millet	Wheatberries
Brown rice	Corn	Oats	Wild rice
Buckwheat	Couscous	Quinoa	
	Flaxseed	Spelt	

Maximum Daily Limit of Foods Made from Flour (for Weight Loss*)

Bagel	1 small	High-fiber cereal	1 cup
Biscuit or roll (low-fat)	2 small	Macaroni noodles (cooked)	1 cup
Bread	2 slices	Matzo	2 × 5-inch squares
Breadcrumbs	½ cup	Melba toast	8
Cooked cereal	1 cup	Pasta	1 cup
English muffin	1	Pita bread	2 small
Flat bagel	1	Tortilla	2 small

*You can increase by 20–50 percent for weight maintenance (see Practical Strategies for Intelligent Weight Loss on page 327).

A Rating System for Carbohydrates

The *glycemic index* is a rating system for carbohydrates that dates back to 1981, when Dr. David Jenkins and Dr. Thomas M. S. Wolever published a paper detailing the concept that not all carbohydrates are created equal. The glycemic index can be misleading. When used in the proper context, however, the glycemic index can be a useful way to rate different carbohydrates beyond just "simple" or "complex."

The glycemic index is a number that is determined by measuring blood sugar levels in healthy volunteer subjects who have been fasting and then eat a portion of food that contains 50 grams of carbohydrate. The amount of food can vary, as long as it contains this constant amount of carbohydrate. The average blood sugar levels from a group of volunteers are compared to those from a standard high-carbohydrate food (typically a pure glucose beverage or white bread that is assigned a score of 100). Carbohydrates that are digested quickly cause a rapid rise in blood glucose level and have a high glycemic index. Carbohydrates that are digested slowly release glucose into the bloodstream slowly and thus have a low glycemic index. Foods with a glycemic index score of 70 or above are considered to be high, scores between 56 and 69 are moderate, and scores of 55 or less are considered low. The glycemic index can be affected by a number of variables. Acidity lowers the glycemic index; so does a high amount of fiber. The way in which food is cooked also affects the glycemic index. The glycemic index is based

Calories Count

Although the glycemic index is important, calories still count. Even if you eat low-glycemic index foods, if you eat too many calories, you will gain weight.

Calories are measured in a laboratory, not in real people. A food is placed in a device known as a bomb calorimeter and is literally burned to a crisp. The amount of heat produced by the food is measured as calories. A true calorie is the amount of heat required to raise the temperature of 1 cubic centimeter of water by 1 degree Celsius; the calories we're familiar with, the ones noted on the nutrition information boxes listed on every supermarket food product, are actually kilocalories—1,000 calories. Either way, what's being determined is simply a measure of energy—not the effect a food has on the body.

See "Practical Strategies for Intelligent Weight Loss" beginning on page 327 to find out how many calories you should eat.

on eating one food at a time, and foods eaten in conjunction with each other—as we would in real life—affect the overall glycemic index.

There are criticisms of the glycemic index, including variability in the testing as well as the fact that the testing is based on eating only one food at a time, which is rarely done. The real impact of a mixed meal is completely different than the glycemic index score. The glycemic index is not based on a typical serving, but on the amount of a single food required to get exactly 50 grams of carbohydrate. For some foods, the portion is so huge that it is not a realistic serving size. On the other hand, the portions of other foods may be unrealistically small. Carrots, for example, have a high glycemic index despite being a very healthy food. This is because it takes a large volume of carrots (more than 4 cups of chopped carrots) to get to the 50 gram amount.

The *glycemic load* was developed to correct for the serving size problem of the glycemic index. The glycemic load measurements give a rating of the blood glucose response to the amount of carbohydrate in a "typical" serving of food. A glycemic load of 20 or more is considered high, between

	Glycemic Index	Glycemic Load
High	Above 70	Above 20
Moderate	56–69	11–19
Low	Below 55	Below 10

More Than Weight Loss
Many studies have been published proving the effect of consuming vegetables and fruits on the reduction of cancer, heart disease, and strokes, among other ailments.

11 and 19 is moderate, and 10 or below is considered low.

The experts do agree on some things. Slowly digested carbohydrates are more beneficial than quickly digested carbohydrates: beans and lentils are better than mashed potatoes and white rice, for example. Fruits are also an excellent carbohydrate because they're high in fiber, vitamins and minerals, and a healthy source of sugar. Studies have shown low-glycemic foods improve blood sugar levels and reduce the risk of getting diabetes, improve cholesterol, and increase "fecal bulk"—the size of the stool, a factor known to reduce the risk of colon cancer. See Table 3.1 for the glycemic index and glycemic load of certain foods.

Vegetables and Fruits: Have Five of Each Every Day

Many of my patients ask me if they should stop eating carbs. My answer is no. Most people need to eat more carbs, just the right kind—most important, vegetables and fruits. Vegetables and fruits are by far the best carbohydrates that you can eat. If there is such a thing as a "miracle food" for weight loss, vegetables and fruits are just that. I encourage you to eat lots of most fruits and vegetables—at least five servings of fruit and five servings of vegetables every day. Why? Pound for pound, vegetables and fruits are extremely low in calories. Vegetables and fruits are high in fiber and health-promoting phytonutrients and antioxidants.

It's worth repeating: you need to eat at least five servings of vegetables and five servings of fruits every day. I consider these numbers minimums. As far as vegetables and fruits go, more is better! If you eat a lot of vegetables and fruits all the time, you'll notice that you feel less hungry. It is better to eat fresh vegetables and fruits (although frozen or canned in unsweetened juice is also acceptable). Dried fruits, sweetened canned fruits, and fruit juices are high in calories and don't really count as a fruit.

Many people who are not used to eating vegetables and fruits have trouble eating five servings of each on a daily basis. I encourage you to

One Serving of Vegetables or Fruit	
Fruit	1 cup
Salad greens	2 cups
Vegetables (raw)	1 cup
Vegetables (cooked)	1/2 to 1 cup

Table 3.1   Glycemic Index and Glycemic Load of Selected Foods

	Glycemic Index	Glycemic Load
Breads		
Barley kernel bread, 50% barley flour	46	9
Barley flour bread, 100% barley flour	67	9
Bagel, white, frozen	72	25
Baguette, white, frozen	95	15
Bread stuffing	74	16
Coarse whole wheat bread	52	10
Gluten-free white bread (gluten-free wheat starch)	76	11
Hamburger bun	61	9
Melba toast	70	16
Oat bran bread	47	9
Pita bread	57	10
Rye kernel (pumpernickel) bread	50	6
Whole meal rye bread	58	8
White wheat flour bread	70	10
Crackers		
Breton wheat crackers	64	10
Puffed rice cakes	78	17
Rye crackers	64	11
Soda crackers	74	12
Stoned wheat crackers	67	12
Breakfast Cereals		
All-Bran	42	9
Bran Buds	58	7
Bran Flakes	74	13
Cheerios	74	15
Corn Flakes	81	21
Cream of Wheat	66	17
Golden Grahams	71	18

Table 3.1 Glycemic Index and Glycemic Load of Selected Foods

	Glycemic Index	Glycemic Load
Breakfast Cereals (*continued*)		
Grape-Nuts	71	15
Mini-Wheats, whole wheat	58	12
Müesli	49	10
Nutrigrain	66	10
Oat Bran	67	9
Quick Oats	66	17
Puffed Wheat	67	13
Raisin Bran	61	12
Rice Krispies	82	21
Shredded Wheat	75	15
Total	76	13
Wheat biscuits (plain flaked wheat)	70	13
Cereal Grains		
Buckwheat	54	16
Cornmeal	69	9
Sweet corn	53	17
Couscous	65	23
Millet	71	25
Pearl barley	25	7
Puffed Rice, Instant	69	29
Rice, brown	55	18
Rice, white	64	23
Pastas		
Fettucine	40	18
Linguine	46	22
Macaroni	47	23
Mung bean noodles	33	15
Spaghetti, white, boiled	42	20
Vermicelli, white boiled	35	16

Table 3.1   Glycemic Index and Glycemic Load of Selected Foods

	Glycemic Index	Glycemic Load
Fruits		
Apples, raw	38	6
Apple juice	41	11
Apricots, raw	57	5
Apricots, canned in light syrup	64	12
Apricots, dried	30	16
Banana, raw	51	13
Cantaloupe	65	4
Cherries, raw	22	3
Cranberry juice	68	16
Dates, dried	103	42
Figs, dried	61	16
Grapefruit juice, unsweetened	48	9
Grapes, raw	59	11
Kiwi fruit, raw	53	6
Lychee, canned in syrup and drained	79	16
Mango, raw	51	8
Oranges, raw	42	5
Orange juice	52	12
Papaya, raw	59	7
Peaches	42	5
Pears	38	4
Pineapple	59	7
Pineapple juice, unsweetened	46	15
Plums	39	5
Prunes, pitted	29	10
Raisins	64	28
Strawberries	40	1
Tomato juice	38	4
Watermelon, raw	72	4

Table 3.1 Glycemic Index and Glycemic Load of Selected Foods

	Glycemic Index	Glycemic Load
Vegetables		
Boiled potato	50	14
Carrots	47	3
French fries	75	22
Green peas	54	4
Mashed potato	91	18
Pumpkin	75	3
Sweet corn	62	11
Sweet potato	61	17
Tapioca	70	12
Taro	55	4
Yam	37	13
Legumes		
Baked beans	48	7
Beans, dried, boiled	29	9
Black-eyed peas	42	13
Butter beans	31	6
Chickpeas (garbanzo beans), boiled	28	8
Kidney beans	28	7
Lentils	29	5
Lima beans	32	10
Mung beans	31	5
Navy beans	38	12
Peas, dried, boiled	22	2
Pinto beans	39	10
Soybeans	18	1
Split peas	32	6

Table 3.1   Glycemic Index and Glycemic Load of Selected Foods

	Glycemic Index	Glycemic Load
Beverages		
Apple juice	40	12
Carrot juice	43	11
Coca-Cola	58	15
Cranberry juice cocktail	56	16
Gatorade	78	12
Grapefruit juice, unsweetened	48	11
Hot chocolate mix	51	11
Orange juice	50	13
Pineapple juice, unsweetened	46	16
Tomato juice	38	4
Dairy Products		
Custard	38	6
Ice cream, regular	61	8
Ice cream, reduced or low-fat	39	5
Ice cream, premium	38	3
Milk, full-fat	27	3
Milk, skim	32	4
Milk, chocolate	34	9
Pudding	44	7
Yogurt	36	3
Yogurt, low-fat with aspartame	14	2
Nuts		
Cashews	22	3
Peanuts	14	1

Source: *International Table of Glycemic Index* and *Overcoming Metabolic Syndrome.*

start slowly, adding one extra serving at a time. Keep adding servings until you get to ten or more a day. Eventually you will begin to feel bad if you do not get your ten servings of vegetables and fruits each day. When you fill your belly with these healthy foods, you will feel less hungry for the bad foods.

Take my advice and eat extra vegetables and fruits. Consider this: several studies have found that the more vegetables and fruit consumed in a day, the more weight lost. Increase your meal size with extra vegetables and fruits. If necessary, incorporate extra vegetables in to the foods you already eat. In one study, researchers found that adding extra vegetables to recipes helps people eat more of them, increasing weight loss. For some great ideas, I recommend Jessica Seinfeld's book *Deceptively Delicious.*

Starchy Vegetables

There is nothing wrong with eating starchy vegetables as part of a healthy balanced diet. But you should limit them to two or three servings daily.

Corn	Peas
Lima beans	Potato

Nonstarchy Vegetables Are Best

You should eat mostly nonstarchy vegetables that are lower in carbohydrates and better at satisfying appetite. As an added benefit, they are high in fiber and have a lot of antioxidant vitamins and minerals.

Nonstarchy Vegetables

Artichokes	Carrots	Mushrooms	Summer squash
Asparagus	Cauliflower	Mustard greens	Sweet potato
Baby corn	Celery	Okra	Swiss chard
Bamboo shoots	Collard greens	Onions	Tomatoes
Bean sprouts	Cucumbers	Pea pods	Turnip greens
Bell peppers	Eggplant	Pumpkin	Turnips
Bok choy	Green beans	Radishes	Zucchini
Broccoli	Hearts of palm	Salad greens	
Brussels sprouts	Kale	Sprouts	
Cabbage	Leeks	Sugar snap peas	

Vegetables High in Protein	
Asparagus	5 grams of protein per serving
Broccoli	5 grams of protein per serving
Brussels sprouts	4 grams of protein per serving
Shitake mushrooms	5 grams of protein per serving

Fruit Is Good for You

Despite the higher carbohydrate content compared to vegetables, fruits are unlimited on the Hormonal Health diet. Fruit contains healthy carbohydrates and is full of nutrients. Because of the high water and fiber content, fruit helps you feel full and gives you the healthiest form of sugar. However, fruit juices, dried fruit, and processed fruits are discouraged. Keep plenty of fresh fruit around. Most fruits will last in the fruit drawer of your refrigerator for a week or so. Mangos, melons, and pears may be left on the kitchen counter until they ripen (become softer and develop a sweet smell) and then moved to the refrigerator. You should eat mostly slow-carbohydrate fruit. It is okay to eat three or four servings of fast-carbohydrate fruit on a daily basis.

Eat Frequently to Balance Blood Sugar and Boost Metabolism

Our ancient hunter-gatherer ancestors lived from moment to moment, often off whatever nuts and berries they came across in their daily search for food. A big meal was a treat! It's only been in modern times, when even our agriculture

Slow-Carbohydrate Fruit (Eat Unlimited Amounts)			
Apples	Grapefruit	Oranges	Plums
Apricots	Guavas	Papaya	Raspberries
Blackberries	Honeydew	Peaches	Rhubarb
Blueberries	Kiwi fruit	Pears	Strawberries
Cantaloupe	Nectarines	Pineapple	Watermelon

Fast-Carbohydrate Fruit (Limit to Three or Four Servings Daily)	
Bananas	Grapes
Cherries	Mangoes
Figs	Tangerines

workers are governed by the time clock, that we've focused on eating three big meals a day, giving us the morning and afternoon to work.

Snacking on healthy foods is important to balance your blood sugar. Eating a huge portion of a so-called healthy food, such as beans or lentils, can prompt an insulin surge as easily as a Twinkie. So, if you eat frequently throughout the day, you will provide a continual source of calories and energy to your body. Once your body becomes accustomed to receiving a continual supply of food, your metabolism will increase. If you eat less often, the body freaks out. It thinks it's starving and slows metabolism, putting the body into survival mode. What happens then? You feel sleepy after a meal, and the food is turned into fat instead of burned as energy. The body is conserving energy, because even though it just got a huge meal; it is still in starvation mode and doesn't know when the next meal is coming. When you provide a continual source of calories to the body in the form of small frequent meals, the body relaxes: it goes out of starvation mode and starts using the calories instead of storing them. The result is less hunger, more energy and weight loss.

"Consume your snack before you feel ravenously hungry."

—Louis J. Aronne, M.D.

Snacking is a proven treatment for low blood sugar or hypoglycemia. Patients with hypoglycemia are instructed to avoid sugar and processed carbohydrates and to eat small meals throughout the day. Doing so prevents the insulin

Eat a Balanced Blend of Fruits and Vegetables

I recommend eating as many fruits and vegetables as you can, but balance is best. You should try to eat equal amounts of vegetables and fruits in addition to eating a variety of vegetables and fruits in a single day. Avoid eating too many servings of just one type of vegetable or fruit.

Hormone Disruption: Reactive Hypoglycemia

Have you ever experienced low blood sugar? Some people are afflicted with a condition called *hypoglycemia*. This happens when the sugar level in the blood drops below the point where it can fuel the body's activity. It usually occurs after eating large meals or high-glycemic index foods: blood sugar rises, insulin surges, and then—very rapidly—blood sugar levels decline. The hypoglycemia is caused by an "undershoot" when blood sugar levels fall below the level that existed *before* you ate. This reaction, known as *reactive hypoglycemia,* invariably occurs in response to eating the wrong kinds of foods.

A healthy diet keeps blood sugar levels more or less constant, increasing them at times when you need more energy, and letting them wane when you need less—but usually not to the point where they cause a negative reaction. Of course, almost none of us do that. Think about it: Have you ever eaten a huge meal? Have you ever ordered and consumed a rich dessert, often in an oversized serving, in a fine restaurant? Have you ever gotten home late at night, tired but not sleepy, and had a comforting bowl of ice cream? Have you ever quenched your afternoon carb craving with a bag of potato chips or a candy bar? All of these actions spiked your blood sugar.

When blood sugar drops rapidly, symptoms come on strong. You feel hungry (already!), sleepy, tired, and fatigued; your heart rate picks up and sweating increases. All you want to do is take a nap, which is the worst thing you can do—your metabolism slows to a crawl. But you probably can't sleep anyway; with your heart pounding and the extra sweating, you feel irritated, jazzed, and annoyed. Eating carbohydrates makes brain serotonin levels surge. Serotonin calms you and makes you sleepy, slowing your metabolism. This, of course, leads to weight gain and creates a vicious circle.

We all have these symptoms from time to time. We all like to eat, and we don't always eat what's good for us. What we can do is fight the appetite and the urge to sleep: we can take a walk, engage in some physical activity. We can do something to maintain or raise our metabolism and level out our blood sugar. Endocrinologists treat people with reactive hypoglycemia by having them eat low-glycemic index carbohydrates spread out in multiple small meals throughout the day. This type of eating reduces blood glucose surges and the insulin spikes that follow.

Hormone Disruption: Dangerous Hypoglycemia

Sometimes hypoglycemia can be a life-threatening condition. Problems with the islet cells in the pancreas can, on rare occasions, produce excessive amounts of insulin, resulting in life-threatening low blood sugar levels. A small tumor in the pancreas, known as an *insulinoma,* can cause severe low blood sugar levels. Unlike reactive hypoglycemia, the hypoglycemia caused by an insulinoma almost never occurs after a meal. Instead, this type of hypoglycemia occurs when you have not been eating. Without a continual source of food, blood sugar levels can drop dangerously. Low blood sugar can affect the brain, causing symptoms such as personality changes, confusion, and seizures or passing out. Once food is consumed, blood sugar rises and the symptoms disappear. The symptoms of an insulinoma can be subtle.

Many patients are not diagnosed for ten years or more, and they keep getting fat because of high insulin levels and because they keep eating, trying to fight low blood sugar. They learn that if they do not eat large amounts of food all of the time, they pass out. If you have symptoms of this disorder, you should see an endocrinologist to make sure you're not suffering from this potentially fatal, if rare, problem.

Recently, another type of hypoglycemia has been seen as a complication of gastric bypass surgery. The condition causes abnormal growth of insulin-producing cells of the pancreas known as *nesidioblastosis.* Patients who have had gastric bypass surgery who experience symptoms of hypoglycemia should discuss the condition with their physicians.

---

surge that comes with larger meals or high-glycemic foods, which in turn stops blood sugar from dropping in response to an insulin surge. Snacking supplies the body with nutrients in a gradual fashion, in the way it handles them best.

Since the publication of the first edition of *Hormonal Balance,* some people have criticized the concept of snacking. Critics argue that snacking makes you gain weight. Of course, eating unhealthy "snack foods" like chips and candy will make you gain weight, but snacking on healthy foods is one of the best things you can do to control your hunger hormones and your weight. In chapter 5, I explain how eating more than three meals a day helps control appetite by reducing ghrelin surges. Snacking doesn't mean you need to eat all the time. Not everyone

---

Hormone Disruption: Carbohydrate Cravings

Typical symptoms of carbohydrate cravings include:

▶ Feeling hungry all the time, especially two to three hours after a meal

▶ Feeling sleepy and sluggish in the afternoons

▶ Anxiety

▶ A feeling of calmness and satiation when eating sugars, candy, chips, pretzels, and other heavy-carbohydrate foods

This condition is caused by insulin and serotonin. As insulin rises and falls, a brain chemical called serotonin is released. You may have heard of serotonin; it's the neurotransmitter whose quantities are increased after taking antidepressant drugs, such as Prozac, Celexa, Lexipro, Zoloft, or Paxil. It makes you feel better and also provides a key signal to the brain: I am satisfied. I don't need to eat any more right now.

If insulin spikes too high, serotonin released is disrupted. When this happens, people become anxious, easily irritated, and generally out of sorts. Moreover, the brain hasn't received that key message to stop eating. So people continue stuffing their faces, often with carbohydrate-laden comfort foods, in an effort to finally feel that calm, satisfied feeling. See chapter 5 for more information on serotonin.

How do you avoid carbohydrate cravings? Don't give into the cravings. Eat healthy carbohydrates combined with protein whenever cravings set in.

---

needs to eat a mid-morning snack, for example. But, if you go more than three or four hours without eating, you'll experience rebound hunger that slows or stops weight loss. The bottom line is that snacking on healthy foods is an important behavior that you'll need to practice to achieve permanent weight loss.

Eat Lean Protein

Protein is an essential part of a balanced diet. Proteins, you may recall from high school biology, are made up of molecules called *amino acids*. Amino acids can be easily converted by the body into sugar and fat. Yes, you heard that right: protein can be turned into sugar and fat. So just like anything else, too much protein can make you gain weight. But, getting the right amount of protein at the right

Eat Protein at Breakfast

Protein at breakfast will help control hunger and cravings for the entire day. Studies have shown that eating protein at breakfast helps you eat less at lunch and dinner. Eat protein with breakfast to supply your body with a source of long-lasting glucose that will give you energy and prevent fatigue.

time of the day is an important element for hormonal balance.

I recommend that you eat about 0.4 grams of protein each day for every pound you weigh. So, a 150-pound person should consume about 55–60 grams of protein each day. However, this formula isn't perfect, because it doesn't take into account body composition. You should eat protein throughout the day, and eating protein in the morning is especially important. Many people are accustomed to all (or mostly) carbohydrate breakfasts such as juice and toast, cereal and skim milk (has minimal protein), pancakes or waffles and syrup. High-carbohydrate breakfasts cause sugar and insulin spiking and result in hunger, sleepiness, and carbohydrate cravings (usually in that order) later in the day.

Getting enough protein is a key element of the Hormonal Health Diet. Nowadays you will hear all the diet gurus pushing protein. That is because protein is filling and satisfying.

Grill, bake or broil meats to remove all possible fat. Egg whites are one of the best sources of protein. They are pure protein, without any fat or carbohydrates. On this diet plan you may have as many egg whites as you want. During any weight loss program, adequate protein eliminates hunger and prevents muscle loss. I recommend an egg white omelet as a delicious way to get in your protein. And egg whites can be used in recipes in many creative ways.

Egg whites are also one of the best proteins for making you feel full, building muscle, and giving you energy. Each egg white has 6 grams of protein. Each

Healthy Proteins

Beans	Clams	Fish	Pork, lean cuts	Tempeh
Beef, lean cuts	Crab	Lamb, lean cuts	Scallops	Tofu
Bison	Dairy products, low-fat	Lentils	Shellfish	Turkey breast
Chicken breast		Lima beans	Shrimp	Venison
Chickpeas	Egg whites	Lobster	Split peas	

Healthy Meat

Lean beef, pork, lamb (choose round or loin cuts)	Trim all visible fat	Consider alternative red meat like bison, ostrich, venison, elk
Chicken or turkey, breast with no skin	Have meat custom ground	
	Choose grass-fed over corn-fed	

egg yolk has 2 grams of fat that is all saturated fat. You can eat some egg yolks, but I recommend discarding nine or ten yolks for each dozen eggs.

Fat Is Okay in Limited Amounts

The Hormonal Health Diet contains 30 percent healthy fat. Healthy or unhealthy, it is important to understand that even a "good" fat is still fat, providing the same calories as a "bad" or saturated fat. So even though you need some healthy fat, eating too much fat—even if it is healthy fat—will make you fat.

Fat has become the most maligned of the nutrients and is blamed for causing obesity, cardiovascular disease, and other health problems. Ounce for ounce,

Low-Fat Dairy Products

You should eat at least two or three servings of low-fat dairy products daily. These products contain protein, healthy carbohydrates, calcium, and vitamin D and have been shown to help aid in weight loss. To help with weight loss, do not drink milk—any type of milk, including skim milk, soy milk, almond milk, or rice milk. Although milk has a healthy amount of nutrients, it contains empty calories. You gut doesn't react to the liquid calories in milk like it does when you eat low-fat dairy products. It is okay to use a small amount of milk in cof-

fee, tea, or cereal, or in recipes. Make sure you get enough calcium by eating enough low-fat dairy products, or take a calcium supplement (see chapter 9).

Fat-free cottage cheese

Fat-free cream cheese

Fat-free sour cream

Greek yogurt

Kefir

Low-fat frozen yogurt

Nonfat yogurt

Smoothies

Nutrients by Weight

All fats, whether saturated, trans, unsaturated, or a combination of all three, have the same caloric content.

Carbohydrates	4 calories per gram
Protein	4 calories per gram
Fat	9 calories per gram

fat is more than twice as high in calories as protein or carbohydrates. But fat is an essential part of our diet, and the right kinds of fats are necessary for hormonal balance. A balanced diet means a healthy blend of carbohydrates, protein, *and* fat. A diet that is very low in fat is not considered a healthy diet.

Fat has a number of benefits. Fat makes food more flavorful. It also makes the texture creamier. We like the taste of food when fat is in it. But, fat can help by slowing down the rate at which the entire meal hits the bloodstream, thus slowing digestion. And, fat causes the body to produce anti-hunger hormones—like cholecystokinin, leptin, glucagon-like peptide 1, and others—that tell your brain that it's time to stop eating. Fat helps you feel full.

Healthy fats are the poly- and monounsaturated fats. Polyunsaturated fats are omega-3 and omega-6 fatty acids and come mostly from fish and vegetables. Monounsaturated fats are omega-9 fatty acids found in nuts, chicken,

Essential Fatty Acids

Certain fats are, indeed, vital to our well-being. These are known as essential fatty acids (EFAs). Two EFAs, linoleic acid and lenolenic acid, are chief among the body's requirements. Linoleic acid is an omega-3 fatty acid, lenolenic acid an omega-6 fatty acid. Without EFAs, we fall victim to a variety of symptoms of essential fatty acid deficiency, including dry, flaking skin, hair loss, arthritis, weakness, incoordination of muscles, and numbness and tingling of the hands and feet.

vegetables, and fish. Chicken breast meat has primarily unsaturated fat, but chicken skin and thigh meat is higher in saturated fat. Grass-fed beef and meat from other grazing animals (like bison, elk, and deer) have a higher amount of unsaturated fat than grain-fed beef, which is very high in saturated fat. Nuts contain a lot of healthy monounsaturated fats, making them very high in calories. Eating too much healthy fat is not healthy and will make you gain weight. You need to eat healthy fats, but not too much. The fact that it has healthy fat doesn't mean you should eat a lot of it.

Foods with Healthy Monounsaturated and Polyunsaturated Fats (to Eat)

Avocados	Olives	Turkey breast
Chicken	Shellfish	Vegetable oils (canola, safflower, corn)
Fish	Soy products (soy oil, tofu, tempeh)	
Nut oils (peanut, sesame)		Vegetables
Nuts	Sunflower, pumpkin, and sesame seeds	
Olive oil		

Whenever you eat nuts, eat a small portion. I recommend eating nuts as part of a meal, combined with other foods, such as green beans with toasted almond slivers or a salad with chopped nuts. Many people who snack on a handful of nuts end up eating more than they planned. They start with a small portion, but then feel even hungrier. Nuts have so many calories packed in a small space that they don't fill you up right away. Nuts can even trigger binge eating.

Fish, especially fish that live in cold water (sardines, mackerel, herring, lake trout, and salmon), are very high in omega-3 fatty acids. Flax, soybeans, sunflower seeds, sesame seeds, peanuts, and walnuts are also good sources of this beneficial fat. Omega-3 fatty acids play a role in reducing insulin resistance (see chapter 6). By lowering blood triglycerides, these beneficial fats have also been found to reduce the risk of heart disease. The heart healthy benefits of omega-3 fatty acids have prompted the American Heart Association to recommend that everyone eat two 3-ounce servings of fish each week. But the fish oils sold in capsules deserve caution. Many over-the-counter products have inconsistent amounts of omega-3 fatty acids. Some products have been found to be contaminated with mercury. Overdoses have been linked to impaired immune function, elevations of vitamins A and D to toxic levels, and a worsening of diabetes.

Unhealthy fats are *trans fats* and *saturated fats*. These fats contribute to cholesterol problems and are linked to cardiovascular disease and other health problems. Unhealthy fats almost always come from one of three sources: animal products, tropical oils (like palm oil or coconut oil), or processed oils (like margarine or partially hydrogenated vegetable oil). Unsaturated fats can are converted to saturated fats by a process called *hydrogenation*—literally bubbling hydrogen gas through the oil. As hydrogen is added to the fat, it "saturates" the oil with hydrogen, changing

Foods That Contain Unhealthy Saturated and Trans Fats (to Avoid)

Candy bars

Chicken skin and dark meat

Commercially baked cake, cookies, muffins, and pastries

Fatty cuts of beef, ground beef, pork, and lamb

Fried foods (french fries, chicken nuggets, fried chicken, fried fish, doughnuts)

Margarine

Snack foods (microwave popcorn, chips, crackers)

Vegetable shortening

Whole-fat dairy products (butter, milk, cheese, and ice cream)

its chemical makeup. This process also creates a particularly dangerous form of unsaturated fat known as "trans fat." So even though trans fat is technically an unsaturated fat, it is even more toxic than saturated fat.

Fat Substitutes

Fat substitutes are fats the body cannot absorb, so they pass through the digestive system without entering the body. In large amounts, fat substitutes cause diarrhea and gastrointestinal pain. As I discuss in chapter 5, fat substitutes can confuse the brain, causing increased hunger and weight gain.

Fat Blockers

Orlistat, marketed under the brand name Xenical or Alli, works by blocking the digestion and absorption of some of the fat you eat. This medication does work; however, orlistat coupled with too much fat consumption can overload your intestinal tract with fat and cause gastrointestinal problems, including diarrhea and leakage of oily stool. It has been said that if you take orlistat and "cheat" on your diet that you are "punished" by these side effects, so it helps keep you eating healthy. There is a concern about deficiency of vitamins A, D, E, and K with the use of orlistat, and it is recommended that if you use this product you also take a multivitamin.

Natural foods partisans also have an obesity product, chitosan. Chitosan is made from crustacean shells and is supposed to block fat absorption. However, chitosan does not really work and blocks *zero* of the fat in your diet. The next time you see one of those infomercials for chitosan, don't be tempted. It's just a come-on and a rip-off. Another product, Nopal cactus, is claimed to have the same effect as chitosan but this has not been proven.

Chapter Review

A healthy diet—contrary to the dictates of many popular diets—should contain a balance of 40 percent carbohydrates, 30 percent protein, and 30 percent fat. This chapter explained the impact of these dietary components on the hormones that control appetite and food cravings.

A key concept in the chapter was the slow consumption of foods. Eating slowly allows time for the "I am full" signal to reach your brain. Specific examples were given of foods that bolster appetite control and encourage a full feeling, including foods with high fiber such as beans, steel-cut oats, whole wheat or bran. However, the best way to get fiber in your diet is to eat lots of fresh vegetables and fruits.

The chapter included extensive information on why carbohydrates are essential for hormonal balance and noted that healthy carbohydrates from vegetables, fruits, beans, whole grains, dairy products, and limited amounts of nuts and seeds should make up about 40 percent of your diet.

In addition, the chapter covered the essential recommendation of eating at least five types of fruits and five types of vegetables each day; these foods digest slowly and stave off feeling of hunger. Nonstarchy vegetables such as asparagus, bell peppers, cabbage, carrots, onions, and salad greens are best. Suggested fruits include apples, oranges, grapefruit, pineapple, and strawberries. However, consumption of fruits such as bananas, cherries, grapes, and mangos should be limited to three to four servings a day.

Finally, the chapter recommended eating smaller meals with snacks and suggested that eating the right foods frequently throughout the day increases metabolism and encourages your body to start using calories instead of storing them.

CHAPTER

4

The Hormonal Health Diet

Since the first edition of *Hormonal Balance* was published in 2002, many fad diets have come and gone. Meanwhile, the Hormonal Health Diet has stood strong as the best way to lose weight permanently by outsmarting the hormones that make you feel hungry. We have seen the fat-free craze, low-carb, no carb, blood type, caveman, cabbage soup, Mediterranean, and diets named for just about every other region of the world. The truth is that you can lose weight on almost any diet. The real challenge is taking the weight off and keeping it off for the long haul. I don't consider a diet successful if you take off weight and then gain it back. My goal is for you to be like my patients and the many others who have learned to eat to balance their hormones. You can be part of the elite 2 percent who lose weight and keep it off forever.

As an endocrinologist who specializes in the treatment of obesity, I have observed that some of my patients who successfully lose weight may struggle in the beginning. Eating and living a new way can feel uncomfortable and different. Even my most successful patients tell me that the new lifestyle felt stressful. Living and eating in a new way can feel stressful but shouldn't feel overwhelming. As I explain in chapter 11, too much stress can cause your adrenal glands to produce excess cortisol, which

In This Chapter

- ▶ Getting Used to a New "Normal" Diet
- ▶ Let Hormones Help You Feel "Full"
- ▶ How to Plan and Schedule Healthy Meals and Snacks

blocks weight loss. Understand that feeling uncomfortable is normal whenever there is change. The key is not to make too many changes all at once so that you revolt, quit the diet, and overeat. The diet in this chapter is the ideal diet for you to follow, but you don't have to be perfect to be successful. Even eating a few of the foods I recommend can be helpful. If you feel overwhelmed, start off with eating one healthy meal and build from there.

A New Normal

Eventually, eating this way will become an automatic part of your life, and you'll get used to a new normal. Over time, my patients say they feel completely normal at their healthy weight and they can't imagine going back to their old eating habits. In essence, they have reset their set points, their body's feeling of a "normal" at a specific body weight. In chapter 5, I explain how the hormone leptin controls your body's set point and how fixing leptin problems will help you reset your set point back to normal.

In order to lose weight permanently, all your hormones have to be balanced. Part II of this book will help you understand how all your body's hungry hormones control your appetite and weight. This second part of the book will help you determine whether you may have a hormonal disorder that is preventing you from losing weight and will give you important information you'll need to be able to work with your physician to get your hormones back on track. Treatments for hormonal disorders can range from simple lifestyle changes to medications or even surgical removal of a gland. It is important to understand how specific symptoms may be related to your hormones and may be a clue to a hormonal disorder affecting your weight.

Many of my patients have told me that they know what they should eat, but hunger or cravings get in the way of sticking with a diet for the long run. They get frustrated, go off the diet, and gain

Managing Hunger

To lose weight, most people think they need to eat less food. But in reality, the opposite is true. Instead of decreasing the amount of food you eat, which will lead to hunger and misery, it is better is to manage hunger by eating more healthy food. This helps you feel satisfied and is the best way to turn a *diet* into a *lifestyle*.

weight. This is known as yo-yo dieting. Even if you don't have a hormonal disorder, the Hormonal Health Diet will help you to outsmart your hormones so you can lose weight without feeling hungry or having cravings that block weight loss. The Hormonal Health Diet is not a fad diet. It is an approach that willpermanently change your way of eating and help you stay lean and healthy for the rest of your life.

Let Your Hormones Help You Feel Full

Until recently, no one realized that your stomach and intestines made hormones that regulate appetite. But now we know that the hormones produced by the gut are the way the body signals the brain that you should feel full. Your gut hormones, which I discuss in chapter 5, control this fullness feeling, also known as *satiety*. When you eat the right foods at the right time, gut hormones like ghrelin and peptide YY (PYY) send a message to your brain that you are full and satisfied. The key to success on the Hormonal Health Diet is letting ghrelin and PYY work in your favor by eating a lot of tasty, healthy foods that are filling and satisfying.

Throughout this book, you will read about many of the hormones and how they make you hungry and help you feel full. The Hormonal Health Diet is designed to let all your hunger hormones work in your favor instead of working against you. I show you how eating the right foods at the right times will help you suppress hunger hormones, preventing the out-of-control appetite that derails most people.

Highlights of the Hormonal Health Diet

Have a big breakfast with protein.

Have a healthy lunch.

Eat a protein snack in the afternoon.

Eat a healthy dinner with lean protein and lots of vegetables.

Eat a sweet low-calorie dessert.

Eat at least ten servings of vegetables and fruits every day.

Eat slow carbohydrates.

Eat lean proteins.

Eat healthy fats.

Drink 2 quarts of water daily.

Plan and Schedule Meals and Snacks

The third edition of *Hormonal Balance* reflects a small tweak in the Hormonal Health Diet. The morning snack is now considered optional. That's because I recommend eating a big protein breakfast to keep your hungry hormones under control until lunch. You've heard it before: breakfast is the most important meal of the day. This is true. Having breakfast is necessary to control your appetite all day long. You should eat a healthy balanced lunch, a protein snack in the afternoon, and a big dinner with lean protein and a lot of vegetables. Finish the day with a sweet, slow-carbohydrate dessert. The allowance of vegetables, fruits, and egg whites is unlimited. Remember, don't let yourself get hungry; eat until you feel full.

> ### Balance Carbohydrates, Protein, and Fat
>
> Carbohydrates, protein, and fat make up the key nutritional components of all food. The Hormonal Health Diet contains 40 percent carbohydrates, 30 percent protein, and 30 percent fat. Low-fat dairy products

Schedule the time you will eat all meals and snacks. Planning out your meals and snacks helps you eat at the right times to prevent you from getting too hungry. It may seem like a lot of work, but I assure you that a little planning is time well spent. I have seen many patients with the best intentions get derailed on a diet because they didn't take the time to plan out their meals and snacks. Eating on a schedule helps you prevent swings in ghrelin, which I discuss in chapter 5, and keeps you from overeating later in the day.

> ### Don't Forget to Eat!
>
> When you follow this diet you won't feel hungry, so at first, it may not feel natural to eat. For best results, do not miss any meals or snacks by eating on a schedule. Even if you don't feel hungry, you should eat all your meals and snacks on time. The idea is to prevent hunger, not to react to hunger.

Drink Enough Water

You should drink 2 quarts of water daily. Dehydration results in leptin resistance (see chapter 5) and can stop your body from losing weight. Keeping your body hydrated helps you burn fat by helping your metabolic hormones work properly.

Avoid All Liquid Calories

Do not drink any beverages that have calories, such as sodas, juice, sweet tea, alcoholic beverages, or milk. Liquid calories are empty calories because they don't satisfy your appetite. Liquids sneak through the digestive tract while your gut hormones remain oblivious to the extra calories.

Limit Use of Artificial Sweeteners

Do not drink diet soda or zero-calorie beverages with a sweet flavor. Experts believe that the artificial sweetness of diet beverages increases cravings for sugar. One study found that artificial sweeteners boost levels of the most potent brain hunger hormone, neuropeptide Y. All artificial sweeteners trick the brain with a sweet taste that doesn't have any sugar or calories. The brain expects sugar that never arrives in the gut. As a result, strong carbohydrate or sugar cravings can last for days. It is okay to use a small amount of artificial sweetener as a substitute for sugar in cooking, as long as the food item contains some calories. For example, you can add artificial sweetener to oatmeal or in a smoothie instead of using sugar. This lowers your sugar intake but won't give a sweet zero-calorie confusing message to the brain.

What You Should Drink

Coffee* (iced or hot); limit artificial sweeteners, sugar, or cream, but a small amount of fat-free milk is okay

Green tea

Herbal tea

Sparkling water or club soda

Tea* (iced or hot)

Water (add lemon)

*Caffeinated or decaffeinated. Limit to 4 cups of caffeinated coffee or tea (daily).

Minimize or Avoid Alcoholic Beverages

It is okay to drink an occasional alcoholic beverage as long as you aren't trying to lose weight. There have been many studies showing the health benefits of moderate drinking. But, despite these benefits, alcoholic beverages stimulate your appetite and add empty calories that slow weight loss.

Don't Use Fat Substitutes

Synthetic fat substitutes like olestra are promoted to help with weight loss, but they may have the opposite effect.

What You Should Not Drink

Alcoholic beverages	Milk
Diet soda	Soda
Fruit juice	Sweet tea
High-sugar sports drinks	

Fake fat confuses the brain, which thinks real fat is coming. The brain miscalculates the calories in the gut, resulting in an overproduction of hunger hormones. Appetite is increased, and the body is driven seek out the missing calories.

Start Every Day with a Big Protein Breakfast

Since the first edition of *Hormonal Balance* I have emphasized the importance of having a big breakfast with protein. Today, almost every nutrition expert gives the same advice. The time you invest planning for a healthy breakfast is an investment in your health that gives a big payoff. Skipping breakfast may save a few calories but will end up making you feel hungry, and you'll probably overeat later in the day. A big breakfast with plenty of protein will keep your metabolism higher because your body won't feel like it is starving. Your goal is to eat at least 30 percent of your calories for the day at breakfast. Your breakfast needs to have at least 30 to 40 percent low-fat protein, which is 30 grams of protein for a 150-pound person (for more information, see chapter 3).

Protein is a vital component of a healthy breakfast. When you eat a big breakfast with protein, it helps keep your appetite down at lunch and dinner. Even though you will eat more calories in the morning, you'll end up eating fewer calories by the end of the day. When you eat breakfast, your metabolism is revved up because your body doesn't think it is starving. Eating breakfast increases your productivity; your brain works better and you have more energy.

Eggs for Breakfast

Scramble up a lot of egg whites with one or two yolks, or boil the eggs and throw away most of the yolks. Try different breakfast egg recipes:

Make a vegetable into an omelet or frittata.

Try chopped asparagus, carrots, or broccoli.

Try an egg-white quiche.

Scramble egg whites with chunks of ham or turkey.

Add bits of smoked salmon to scrambled egg whites.

Add chopped sautéed mushrooms, peppers, and onions.

Stir in chopped herbs, like cilantro, parsley, basil, and oregano before cooking.

Use a tiny amount of oil to cook over low to medium heat.

You should not eat a breakfast that is high in processed carbohydrates, like toast and jam, cereal, or a bagel. Juice and milk are also problematic because they are liquid sugar that makes insulin spike. Research has found that high-carbohydrate breakfasts increase appetite. When you eat a breakfast with carbohydrates that aren't balanced by protein, blood sugar and insulin spike. This

Breakfast Foods You Should Not Eat

High-sugar breakfast cereals

Instant oatmeal

Jam, jelly, preserves (even sugar-free)

Pancakes

Toast made with low-fiber bread

Waffles (except whole grain)

results in carbohydrate cravings and makes you feel very hungry a few hours later. This doesn't mean that you need to totally avoid carbohydrates at breakfast. The best carbohydrates for breakfast are slow carbohydrates with a lot of fiber. I recommend eating one or two servings of fruit as part of your breakfast. You can also eat high-fiber, whole-grain carbohydrates like steel-cut oatmeal, whole-grain toast and waffles, and high-fiber breakfast cereals. Although I advise against drinking skim milk, it is okay to have a little milk in your cereal or in coffee. Low-fat dairy products like Greek yogurt or low-fat cottage cheese are a great choice for breakfast because they contain a healthy mix of protein and carbohydrates.

More Breakfast Ideas

Cooked oatmeal and fruit

Fat-free cottage cheese and fruit

Greek yogurt with fruit topped with chopped nuts

High-fiber breakfast cereal with skim milk

Low-fat chicken or turkey sausage

Sandwich on whole-grain bread

Smoked fish, low-fat cream cheese, onion, and tomato on whole-grain toast or a thin bagel

Smoothie

Protein for Breakfast

Many people struggle with finding sources of protein for breakfast. The key is finding a few things you like to eat that sustain you for the day. Try different proteins in the morning. You can eat any healthy protein in the morning, even if it isn't traditionally thought of as a breakfast food.

Beans	High-protein oatmeal
Beef	Lentils
Chicken breast	Low-fat chicken sausage or turkey sausage
Eggs (mostly whites)	
Fat-free cottage cheese	Protein shakes
Fish	Shrimp
Greek yogurt	Turkey breast
High-protein breakfast cereal	

Research from the National Weight Control Registry has found that most people who have successfully lost weight have a habit of eating breakfast every day. A high-protein breakfast lowers levels of appetite-stimulating hormones and raises levels of appetite-reducing hormones. Dr. Daniela Jakubowicz performed a study she called the "Big Breakfast Study," which showed that people who ate a big breakfast lost weight because it helped control hunger and cravings throughout the day.

The Problem with Skipping Breakfast

Have you ever seen a sumo wrestler? These Japanese titans often weigh well over 400 pounds, a handy size to be when you're trying to force your opponent out of the ring—or simply knock him down. But do you know how a sumo wrestler gains all that weight? Sumo wrestlers don't eat breakfast. They wake up, exercise and practice their technique all morning (for big men, sumo wrestlers can be quite nimble), and have a big lunch. The lunch contains some healthy foods—the Japanese have notably healthy diets, high in seafood and low in fat—but it's also loaded with starch in the form of white rice, a high-glycemic

Not Hungry for Breakfast?

Even if you don't feel hungry in the morning, you need to eat breakfast. By shifting your calories earlier in the day, you will have more energy and less hunger. Start off with a small breakfast and slowly increase over time. Within a few days, you won't feel like eating as much at dinner. Continue eating your meals and snacks on a schedule, and eventually your body's hormones will reset your appetite so that it will feel natural to eat a big breakfast.

food. After lunch, they sleep for several hours. As I've noted, metabolism slows after a big meal, and sleep slows metabolism (and digestion) even more. Sumo wrestlers become very fat.

At least during their careers, they're not in terrible shape. They exercise frequently, so the fat tends to be a healthier type of fat. Rates of diabetes and cholesterol are very low among active sumo wrestlers. But once they retire, all those problems hit with a vengeance. Suddenly fat shifts to the belly; cholesterol and blood sugar shoot way up. All the weight they carry around becomes a burden, not an advantage. Studies have linked obesity to skipping breakfast. In fact, the more meals you have per day the less likely you are to be overweight.

Have a Morning Snack If You Need Extra Support

If you are eating a big breakfast and still get hungry before lunch, you should add a morning snack. I also recommend having a morning snack any time you have a busy day or a high-stress day. It is best to plan for this snack when you make your breakfast and keep it close at hand. Try to eat the morning snack a few hours after breakfast.

Cup of Greek yogurt   Whole piece of fruit
Cup of vegetables (cooked or raw)   Smoothie
Hardboiled egg

Lunch Suggestions

Baked potato topped with turkey chili

Grilled or baked fish, chicken, or beef with several servings of vegetables and a potato

Healthy, broth-based soup with vegetables and protein

Leftovers from dinner

Salad with veggies and protein (chicken, salmon, shrimp, lean steak), top with crushed nuts and fat-free feta cheese (use low-calorie dressing)

Sandwich with lean meat, tomato, lettuce, and mustard on whole-grain bread

Many of my patients have told me that they simply aren't hungry for breakfast. I have found that the most common reason for not being hungry for breakfast is overeating the night before. It becomes a vicious cycle. If you start eating breakfast, you will eventually become hungry for breakfast because you won't eat as much at night.

How to Have a Healthy Lunch

It is important to start eating vegetables early in the day. If you haven't eaten any vegetables by lunchtime, you should make sure you get at least two or three servings for lunch. You also need to eat at least 4 ounces of healthy protein at lunch. Make sure your lunch is heavy and filling. This reduces late afternoon

Afternoon Snack Suggestions

Beans	Ham or turkey roll-ups	Protein smoothie
Chicken	Hard-boiled egg	Shrimp
Fat-free cottage cheese with fruit	Protein breakfast cereal	Tuna
	Protein oatmeal	Turkey

Dinner Suggestions

Broiled fish with broccoli, wild rice, and corn

Chili made with beans and any lean protein on top of a baked potato or brown rice

Egg white omelet or quiche with low-fat cheese and packed with vegetables

Grilled lean beef steak with salad, corn, and spinach

Shepherd's pie made with lean custom-ground lamb and extra vegetables on the side

Soup and a salad and an extra plate of vegetables

Turkey meatloaf with boiled red potatoes, carrots, mushrooms, and sliced tomatoes

Whole-grain pasta with vegetables and diced chicken or shrimp

cravings and prevents overeating at dinner. The most important thing you can do to have a healthy lunch is to plan it out in advance. Take the time to make your lunch and bring it with you to work or school every day. One shortcut is to eat a frozen entrée combined with a package of frozen vegetables.

Eat a High-Protein Snack in the Afternoon

Although I usually recommend eating balanced meals and snacks, the afternoon snack is an exception. This is because eating a pure protein snack in the mid- to late afternoon works on hunger hormones to reduce appetite right before dinner. Eat at least 10 grams of protein two or three hours after lunch. Try a few egg whites, some high-protein breakfast cereal, or a few pieces of cut-up chicken breast. A high-volume protein smoothie is also a great afternoon snack.

Eat a Substantial Dinner with Extra Vegetables

Most people are at their hungriest at dinnertime. This is the time of the day that the body craves foods that are substantial and satisfying. A common dieting problem is undereating during the day, then feeling ravenous and overeating at dinner. The key to having a healthy dinner is to eat healthy foods throughout the day. Eat a big protein breakfast, have a healthy lunch, and don't forget a protein snack in the afternoon; then your hunger will be manageable so that eating a healthy dinner is an achievable goal.

At dinner you should eat healthy versions of comfort foods, like turkey meatloaf with potatoes, whole-grain pasta with meat sauce, or hearty chicken soup. Comfort foods are foods that make you feel satisfied and full. Your body needs to feel satisfied, and eating foods that fit this bill

Reward Yourself with a Healthy Dessert
Fruit
Fruit pie (homemade with healthy ingredients)
High-fiber cereal with skim milk
Low-calorie frozen desserts
Muffin (small)
Smoothies
Yogurt

is critical for long-term success. The comfort foods reduce cravings by helping you feel satisfied. This helps you stick with your healthy eating plan.

Always eat low-calorie, filling foods at the beginning of your dinner. Start with a bowl of healthy soup, several servings of vegetables, and a salad. Starting your meal with low-calorie foods fills up your stomach and starts your gut hormones working. You will feel full sooner and will have less room to fill up on higher-calorie foods.

Enjoy a Tasty, Sweet Dessert with Healthy Slow Carbohydrates

A healthy dessert like fruit, yogurt, or a low-calorie frozen treat is both satisfying and beneficial for your hormones. Make dessert a healthy reward that you look forward to instead of an indulgence that you feel guilty about. It is important not to feel deprived. If you feel deprived, you won't be able to continue your healthy eating plan. Having a sweet yet healthy dessert has been shown to be a useful tool to support weight loss. In a clinical study, subjects who ate a sweet, slow-carbohydrate dessert lost more weight than subjects who did not eat dessert. This type of dessert keeps you feeling full at the end of the day. The slowly digested carbohydrates stimulate brain serotonin, which helps you have restful sleep while preventing the sugar and insulin surges that come from fast carbohydrates.

Condiments and Free Foods

In addition to vegetables, fruits, and egg whites, the following foods may be consumed in unlimited quantities.

Cayenne pepper	Lemon or lime juice
Diet shakes (low-calorie)	Mustard
Fat-free sour cream	Salad dressing (fat-free, low-calorie)
Flavoring extracts	Salsa
Garlic	Spices
Herbs, fresh or dried	Vinegar (balsamic, red wine, rice, apple cider, flavored)
Horseradish	
Hot sauce	Worcestershire sauce

Chapter Review

If you want to lose weight permanently, knowing the root cause of your weight gain problem is an important first step. This chapter set the stage to help you determine whether a hormonal imbalance is behind your weight loss difficulties. Along with the information that will be presented in the rest of this book, you should be able to work with your own doctor to build a diet regime to address any potential links between hormonal imbalance and your difficulties maintaining a healthy weight level.

The next chapter provides some practical strategies to help you outsmart your hunger hormones and to ultimately control food craving urges.

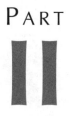

Balancing Your Hormones

5

Outsmart Hunger Hormones to Control Appetite and Cravings

Hunger hormones affect our appetite, cravings, and metabolism. They influence our brain's motivation or lack of motivation to find healthy foods and to exercise. When hormones are unbalanced, you have less motivation to have a healthy lifestyle. A lack or overabundance of certain hormones causes changes in metabolism. Those changes either prompt the body to start putting on weight immediately or start a boomerang effect that will cause it to put on weight soon enough. Either way, the end result is a weight problem, and that weight problem can lead to a host of other problems.

Although many people think an empty stomach is the only thing that causes hunger, such is not the case. Hunger is a brain process driven by hormones that send signals to the brain to turn your appetite on or off. The brain is the master control center for appetite; it senses what nutrients the body needs and sends hormonal signals to the body to act. Hunger originates in a portion of the brain called the *hypothalamus*. As I've noted elsewhere in this book, the hypothalamus is the part of the brain that controls the pituitary gland—the master gland—and thus many of our

In This Chapter

▶ What Makes Us Hungry

▶ Why Most Weight Loss Is Not Permanent

▶ How to Reset Your Natural Hormonal Balance

▶ How Brain and Gut Hormones Control Food Cravings

hormones. Certain things are known about hunger and the hypothalamus. One is the idea of satiety, the concept that you eat until you're satisfied. A sector in the hypothalamus is called the *ventromedial hypothalamus;* it's nicknamed the "satiety center." The *lateral hypothalamus* is the feeding center. Together, these two portions of the hypothalamus balance hunger and satiety.

To an extent, most hormones can influence your appetite. Insulin, thyroid hormone, estrogen, progesterone, and cortisol all have potent effects on appetite, but dozens of other hormones also affect appetite, and unlike traditional hormones, they're not necessarily made by traditional glands. In fact, one of the biggest hormone producers in the body is fat. Yes, the same little piece of the puzzle that collects and reproduces and causes so much of our misery also makes hormones. Until recently, fat was thought of as an innocent bystander in the obesity saga, but now we know better. Fat is one of the biggest hormone producers in the body. The main hormone made by fat is leptin.

Hunger hormones are also produced by parts of the body central to digestion and food storage. The stomach and intestines produce potent hunger hormones, influenced by the foods you eat. These hormones, known as gut peptides, have effects on hunger and satiety. The brain makes hunger hormones as well. Our knowledge of these hormones is still limited but is growing every day.

Dozens of hunger hormones influence appetite, satiety, and metabolism. The list includes the following:

Acyl stimulation protein
Adiponectin
Agouti-related peptide
Amylin
β-endorphin
Bombesin
Cholecystokinin
Ciliary neurotrophic factor
Cocaine- and amphetamine-regulated
    transcript
Corticotrophin releasing hormone
Dopamine
Dynorphin
Endocannabinoids
Enkephalins

Enterostatin
GABA (Gamma-aminobutyric acid)
Galanin
Gastric inhibitory peptide
Ghrelin
Glucagon
Glucagon-like peptide-1
Glutamate
Interleukin 6
Leptin
Melanin concentrating hormone
Melanocyte stimulating hormone
Melatonin
Neuromedin S
Neuropeptide Y

Neurotensin

Norepinephrine

Obestatin

Omentin

Orexin

Oxyntomodulin

Pancreatic polypeptide

Peptide YY

Pituitary adenylate cyclase activating polypeptide

Pro-opiomelanocortin

Relaxin

Resistin

Secretin

Serotonin

Somatostatin

TGF-β

TNF-α

Urocortin

Visfatin

This chapter discusses the most recent breakthroughs in the area of hunger-related hormones; however, as you will see, there is a great deal more to discover. This area of endocrinology is still in its infancy.

Hunger Hormones Protect You from Starving to Death

Our hormone mechanisms are deeply evolved. Hormones and the genes that control them have developed to cope with times of famine, to make the most of the nutrients we consume, and to make sure we respond to food in our vicinity. Today, however, with abundant sources of high-calorie food all around, our antiquated hormone/hunger mechanism works against us. For example, if you are overweight, your body does not need food. Most overweight people could go without eating for weeks to months without starving to death. Your body fights against going without food, though, causing you to be hungry, even after you just ate. Our senses, our organs, our very being demand that we search for—and eat—food. Consider the following:

- **Taste and smell.** Imagine walking down the street, smelling freshly baked bread. Suddenly you are hungry. Smelling or anticipating the taste of delicious food can strongly turn on the hunger centers of the brain, and surprise! If you eat a little good-tasting food (an appetizer, for example) you get hungrier. Similarly, if it smells and tastes bad, you lose your appetite.

- **Mouth feel.** The way food feels inside your mouth contributes to its flavor. High-fat foods have a more appealing mouth feel, contributing to their delicious taste.

- **Appearance of food.** Just looking at good food makes you hungry.

■ **Variety.** Variety makes us hungry, which may be why you get hungry for dessert even though your stomach is bursting. It also explains the success of many fad diets. These diets frequently have very limited food choices. The monotony of the diet reduces the appetite, another reason why meal replacement products such as bars and shakes can be successful.

■ **Stomach distention.** Distention of the stomach sends powerful hormonal signals to the brain, inducing satiety. Foods high in fiber, which distend the stomach without adding a lot of calories, can greatly improve satiety.

■ **Genetics.** For the vast majority of us, both genes and environment control hunger. In some cases, however, severe genetic obesity can be caused by a variety of genetic mutations, so the genes that allowed your great-great-grandfather to be lean are working against you. If you were to adopt the diet and activity level of someone two hundred or three hundred years ago, you would likely lose weight. Genes and environment thrive on one another. Much of evolution has favored fat storage. Evolution is now working against us.

Leptin Is Made by Fat

Leptin is simply one of the most significant discoveries in the science of obesity.

Over the past thirty years, scientists and medical doctors have developed a better understanding of how fat produces hormones that control appetite, cravings, and metabolism. Fat produces many different hormones, but most important, leptin. The main target of leptin is the hypothalamus, where it finds lots of leptin receptors, the place that regulates food intake and body weight. Scientists have linked the hypothalamus to body weight for many years, but the discovery of leptin, a hormone produced by fat, acting directly on the hypothalamus was a huge breakthrough. It quieted skeptics who had claimed that obesity was simply a matter of weak willpower.

A tremendous amount of research on leptin has been done in the past several years, and the more that's discovered, the more complicated leptin is known to be. It turns out that leptin is involved in all aspects of life. As an endocrinologist, I find it amazing that this hormone, with such tremendous importance, was discovered only recently. Given the speed at which news travels in the modern

Fat Mice and Discovery of Leptin

A mutant strain of mice known as *ob/ob* (a genetic term for a double mutation of a gene resulting in obesity) was found to have a syndrome of obesity and related complications very similar to insulin resistance in humans. The ob/ob mouse was hungry all the time and had high insulin levels, increased body fat, high cortisol levels, low thyroid levels, and high blood sugar. In addition, these mice had low body temperature, indicating low metabolism.

Scientists believed that the ob/ob mouse lacked a satiety factor—a hormone, then still undiscovered, they called "leptin." To prove this theory, in the 1970s a scientist named Doug Coleman preformed some odd experiments—animal rights activists would cringe—that are now considered classics of the genre. These studies, known as parabiosis experiments, sought to prove the existence of leptin. Parabiosis is not the kind of thing we perform on humans. Two creatures, in this case the mice, are surgically joined, right down to their circulation, like artificial conjoined twins. Hormones made in one mouse, therefore, could be transferred to the other mouse. When a fat ob/ob mouse was united with a lean mouse, a startling thing happened. The mutant obese mouse lost weight. The theory that obese mice lacked a blood-borne factor that shut off appetite in the brain was strengthened.

It would take many years before the gene for leptin (known as the *ob gene*) would be cloned and its hormone product, leptin, discovered. It finally happened in 1995. The obesity gene was cloned, and leptin made prime time. Researchers demonstrated that they could make the ob/ob mouse lose weight by injecting it with the missing hormone. This critical study was direct evidence that leptin regulates body weight and body fat.

Leptin resistance has parallels in the mouse world. Another strain of obese mice, known as *db/db,* is resistant to leptin, because of a mutation in the receptor for leptin. The db/db mouse is identical to the ob/ob mouse, but instead of low leptin levels, the db/db mouse has very high leptin levels, just like obese humans, and all because the db/db mouse has a dysfunctional, mutated leptin receptor.

scientific world, countless numbers of scientists are now jumping on the leptin bandwagon and doing their own research, and more power to them.

Leptin gives your brain precise information regarding the amount of fat in your body. If you have a normal amount of body fat, leptin signals the brain that everything is okay. Leptin is a long-term weight hormone that is ultimately responsible for the body weight set point. From an evolutionary standpoint, leptin acts as a protector from starvation. Weight loss and low body fat result in low leptin levels. Low leptin stimulates appetite, slows metabolism, and motivates you to find food, so you won't starve to death.

Leptin Controls Your Set Point

The fat cell is a smart cell. It knows and regulates your body weight using leptin as a chemical messenger. The set point is a natural resting point for your body weight. Each of us has a somewhat predetermined body weight. Your body tends to want stability. If your weight drifts above your set point, your appetite tends to go down and you shed a few pounds. If you lose weight, the opposite occurs: your metabolism slows, and hunger increases as your body craves to get back to the set weight. The concept of a set point is not new and not unique to humans. Animals tend to have their own set points; however, like humans, animals gain weight under specific circumstances. Take the family dog, for example. If he gets dog food only, and in the right proportion to his weight, he'll be lean and trim, but add table scraps and high-calorie treats, and Rover plumps up, particularly if he's not getting much exercise.

Don't be a victim of your set point. You can change a set point with a delicious diet. As you achieve a new healthy weight and balance your hormones, you can achieve a new set point.

Leptin Deficiency Is Very Rare

People who have leptin deficiency have a genetic mutation that disallows their fat cells to make leptin. These people are hungry all the time and are extremely obese. They eat and eat because their brain never gets the signal that they have too much fat. They just keep gaining more and more weight. If you have leptin deficiency, you can take leptin injections and lose a lot of weight without dieting or exercising. It is unlikely that you have leptin deficiency, however, because the condition is uncommon. I've never seen one case of leptin deficiency in my career, while treating thousands of overweight and obese patients. For most people, fixing leptin problems is not simple.

Leptin Resistance Is a Major Cause of Hormonal Imbalance

Most people who are overweight make too much leptin, because they have leptin resistance. The resistance to leptin is analogous to insulin resistance, which I discuss in chapter 6. With leptin resistance, leptin doesn't work as it should and causes unsuccessful signaling in brain appetite centers and brain motivation circuits, which leads to augmented appetite, slowed metabolism, and less motivation to maintain healthy behaviors. Leptin resistance causes cravings for junk food and high-calorie foods. In an attempt to overcome leptin resistance, fat produces more and more leptin.

If you have leptin resistance, your brain doesn't get the communication that it is time to stop eating. Even though your leptin level is high, your brain doesn't know it. The extra leptin is still not enough to satisfy your appetite, leaving you feeling hungry, even when you shouldn't be. When you have leptin resistance, your brain thinks it is starving, even when you are overweight. So far, studies on treating leptin resistance by giving leptin injections have been disappointing, but you will continue to hear about new leptin-based treatments for obesity. New types of leptin—medications that mimic leptin and medications that enhance the action of leptin—are under development.

Leptin Resistance Is Caused by Inflammation

Fat tissue is the major culprit that causes leptin resistance, because it produces powerful chemicals called cytokines, which cause inflammation. Cytokines are the mediators of inflammation, which make the brain oblivious to the effects of leptin.

Leptin and Cancer

There is a strong link between obesity and cancer. Scientists believe that leptin is partially responsible for that link. Leptin promotes cancer growth, including breast cancer (see chapter 8). Experts believe that leptin is just one of many hormonal connections between obesity and cancer.

Inflammation is at the root of many complications of obesity. It's well known that inflammation causes problems such as insulin resistance, diabetes, cardiovascular disease, and hypertension. The good news is that these conditions improve when you beat inflammation. The way to alleviate leptin resistance is to reduce the amount of inflammation in your body. Alleviating leptin resistance allows your brain to hear the signal that you're full.

Inflammation

Cytokine substances are the chemical mediators responsible for inflammation. Fat tissue is the body's largest source of cytokines. Cytokines are made by white blood cells known as *macrophages* and were originally noted to help fight infections and cancer. Cytokines are also responsible for causing diseases. The latest research has found that macrophages don't just live in the bloodstream. They are in important part of fat tissue and are the main cells responsible for cytokine production. These macrophages are known as *adipose tissue macrophages*.

Alleviate Leptin Resistance to Lower Your Set Point and Lose Weight Permanently

If you've lost weight on a diet and then gained it back, you probably have leptin resistance. Leptin resistance is the reason why 98 percent of people who lose weight on a diet eventually gain it all back. Even after you lose weight, leptin resistance persists. Metabolism slows, appetite increases, and the motivation for healthy behaviors dwindles, driving the body weight back up to the higher set point. To lose weight permanently, you have to alleviate leptin resistance, which helps your body feel normal at your new healthy weight, resetting the set point back to normal. The following are ways you can naturally lower leptin resistance.

Eat Healthy Fats

Unhealthy fats cause inflammation and leptin resistance. To alleviate leptin resistance, you must eat healthy fats. Unhealthy fats are saturated fats or trans fats in meat, butter, and cheese as well as coconut oil and palm oil. These fats build up in blood vessel walls, causing cardiovascular disease. Processing unsaturated fats creates trans fats. Trans fats are synthetic fats that are extremely unhealthy. Trans fats and saturated fats cause inflammation and leptin resistance, which results in inappropriate appetite and junk food cravings.

Balance Your Nutrients

You should eat roughly equal percentages of carbohydrates, protein, and fat:

40 percent carbohydrate

30 percent protein

30 percent fat

Balance Your Meals

Evenly spread calories throughout the day. You should never skip meals. To eat balanced meals, have half your total calories by lunch and the other half divided among the afternoon snack, supper, and dessert.

Breakfast*	30 percent of calories
Lunch	20 percent of calories
Afternoon snack	10 percent of calories
Supper	30 percent of calories
Dessert	10 percent of calories

*Calories for breakfast can be divided into breakfast and a morning snack.

Fast food and snack foods (especially crunchy snack foods) have an addictive quality that causes cravings for even more unhealthy food. These foods stimulate the brain's dopamine reward system. Replacing unhealthy foods with foods that have healthy fats will break the addictive cycle of cravings for fast food or snack foods.

Hormone-Friendly Substitutions

High-Calorie Food	Hormone-Friendly Food
Chips	Whole-grain, high-fiber crackers
Cheese	Small amount of cheese with a piece of fruit
Candy	Dark chocolate
Chicken wings	Bowl of soup and a salad
Chips and guacamole	Carrot sticks and hummus
Sweet tea	Iced tea with lemon
Dried fruit	Fresh fruit

Boosting Leptin

In addition to alleviating leptin resistance, boosting leptin production is also very important. Here are three ways you can help your body make more leptin:

1. **Sleep six to eight hours every night.** Researchers have found that sleep deficiency and poor-quality sleep cause both leptin resistance and leptin deficiency. Leptin is usually produced at night, during sleep. If sleep is bad, leptin gets a double whammy. Studies have shown that just a couple of nights of poor sleep will lower leptin levels 25 percent. You need to sleep at least six to eight hours every night.

2. **Get enough zinc.** Leptin production is regulated by the mineral zinc, and zinc helps leptin work properly. A 50 milligram zinc supplement is all that is needed if you don't get enough from your diet. Foods high in zinc include oysters, beef, wheat germ, lima beans, and dairy products.

3. **Don't smoke.** Smoking lowers leptin levels, providing yet another reason to quit.

Drink Two Quarts of Water Daily

Dehydration causes leptin resistance and stops you from losing weight even if you are eating healthy foods. Keeping the body hydrated burns fat and decreases inflammation. Drink at least 2 quarts of cold filtered water every day. Some of my patients have told me that they don't feel thirsty or they forget to drink water. We lose our sense of thirst as we get older. Be mindful of drinking enough water, even if you don't feel thirsty.

Move Your Body

To alleviate leptin resistance, exercise as often as possible. Daily exercise gives you the best results. Regular exercise, like a balanced diet, is a great way to keep leptin resistance at a minimum. Research has found that people who exercise consistently are most likely to have permanent weight loss.

Lower Your Cortisol

High cortisol causes leptin resistance and insulin resistance. Follow my advice in chapter 11.

Brain Hormones

Just like other glands, the brain produces many hormones that are important in the regulation of appetite, satiety, and metabolism. Brain hormones, also known as *neurotransmitters,* work differently from other hormones, because they tend to stay within the brain, sending messages to receptors there. Brain hormones, however, have effects throughout the body, not just the brain. The most important brain hormones that control appetite are neuropeptide Y, dopamine, serotonin, and endocannabinoids.

Neuropeptide Y

Neuropeptide Y (NPY) is the most potent stimulator of appetite known to man. NPY can make you feel lazy, making you want to stay on the couch. NPY has effects that go beyond the brain, directly stimulating fat cells to grow and multiply. NPY has a diurnal rhythm, rising during the day and falling at night. In fact, poor sleep results in higher NPY levels. Compulsive overeating is related to overproduction of NPY or being too sensitive to its effects. A high-fat and high-sugar diet increases NPY levels as well. Scientists speculate that people with anorexia nervosa have resistance to NPY. The National Center for Biotechnology Information, U.S. National Library of Medicine, found that that NPY problems cause high cholesterol, higher alcohol use, metabolic syndrome, and cardiovascular disease.

NPY is responsible for making hunger feel uncomfortable, the primitive sensation that drives all living creatures to seek food. Studies in animals have found that NPY injections cause hunger and make animals overeat. Animal studies have also found that repeated stress causes higher NPY levels. Researchers believe high NPY levels are one of the reasons why some people eat more when they are stressed out.

NPY is directly influenced by leptin. Leptin works in the hypothalamus to keep NPY levels low. NPY has complex actions on the hypothalamus and other areas of the brain, promoting accumulation of body fat and slowing metabolism. When you go on a diet, NPY levels skyrocket, working against you. NPY increases production of the hypothalamic hormone corticotrophin-releasing hormone, which stimulates the pituitary gland to make hormones that stimulate the adrenal gland to make too much cortisol.

At least five pharmaceutical companies are working on medications that block NPY as potential weight loss medications. For now, I recommend taking

Your Brain's Internal Clock Affects Your Weight

Your circadian rhythm is the twenty-four-hour clock that drives wakefulness and sleep. Disruptions to this biological clock have profound effects on our bodies and our hormones. New research has identified genes for the biological clock, known as *clock genes,* that may be the basis for metabolic diseases such as obesity, diabetes, and insulin resistance. The biological clock has a powerful influence on metabolism and appetite. When someone's circadian rhythms are out of whack—from dysfunctional genes or from not getting enough sleep, jet lag, or eating at unusual times—metabolism slows down and appetite increases. Research has shown that a high-fat diet is also one of the things that can disrupt the biological clock.

In the past we thought the brain was the main controller of our circadian clock. We now know that organs such as the pancreas, liver, and intestines all have their own circadian rhythms. Each organ produces hormones, enzymes, and other molecules at various times of the day. The brain acts like a conductor of the symphony, coordinating the various organs. Metabolic disorders occur when the brain is not in sync with the organs. Insulin resistance is the classic example of this lack of coordination, when the pancreas is out of sync with the liver and the brain, causing insulin production to be too high or too low.

The discovery of clock genes has led to questions about how disruptions in circadian rhythms can contribute to metabolic disease, and whether fixing dysfunctional rhythms could treat conditions such as diabetes and obesity. For example, studies are under way to determine whether there is an ideal time of day to eat to help with weight loss and blood sugar control.

Researchers have focused on the body's internal clock to look for ways to treat metabolic derangements. The idea is to find out whether a dysfunctional biological clock is the cause

a natural approach to lowering NPY, which means you should do the following things:

- **Don't starve yourself.** Food restriction is a potent stimulator of NPY production.

- **Eat enough protein.** Diets lacking in protein increase NPY production. See chapter 3 for protein guidelines.

or the result of metabolic problems. It's the classic "chicken-or-egg" scenario. What comes first? Do metabolic problems precede a dysfunctional biological clock or vice versa? Dr. Hitoshi Ando, professor at Jichi Medical University in Japan, has set out to answer this question.

It is thought that leptin plays an important role in maintaining circadian rhythms. Dr. Ando is studying mice that are genetically deficient in leptin and are susceptible to obesity and diabetes. It turns out that these mice have defective circadian rhythms. Dr. Ando fed one group of mice a healthy diet and the other group a high-calorie diet for one month. The healthy diet only partially corrected the circadian rhythm problem. Next he tried giving leptin injections to the mice, which also had only a partial effect. The conclusion was that a healthy diet and replacing the missing hormone only partially reversed the defective biological clock, and inherent defects in the biological clock have a detrimental effect on hormones. Dr. Ando concluded that the problems in the biological clock were not caused by metabolic abnormalities, but that treatment with leptin and a healthy diet can partially reverse the abnormality. It is difficult to reverse the effects of metabolic disease once the wheels are set in motion.

The link between metabolic disease, leptin production, and the circadian clock is especially important for people who work at night and sleep during the day. Studies have shown that people who work these hours are at increased risk for metabolic disease such as type 2 diabetes, metabolic syndrome, and obesity. As we learn more about the influence of circadian rhythms and hormones, it becomes clear that a normal sleep-wake cycle is vital for a healthy body and hormonal balance.

- **Don't eat too much fat.** Studies have found that eating too much fat boosts NPY levels.

- **Eat healthy carbohydrates.** Research at Rockefeller University found that a high-carbohydrate diet increases NPY production. We should eat carbohydrates, so choose less starchy ones, such as tomatoes, lettuce, broccoli, squash, and cabbage, rather than starchy ones, such as potatoes, rice, or pasta.

■ **Alleviate leptin resistance.** Eat balanced meals with healthy fats, exercise consistently, and get enough sleep.

Dopamine

Dopamine is responsible for pleasure and rewards. Pleasure from food can entrain dopamine to emphasize food for the pleasurable qualities rather than the nutritional value. Any time you even think about food, dopamine works to make you hungry for foods that taste good. The pleasure from food is similar to that from alcohol and drugs. Studies have found that obese people have fewer receptors for dopamine in their brains. They can't get the normal feelings of pleasure when they eat. Researchers speculate that being obese results in overeating, because it takes more good-tasting food to satisfy the dopamine-reward pathway, similar to the way addicts and alcoholics need more and more drugs or alcohol to satisfy their addiction.

Reward yourself to boost dopamine.

Eating healthy foods takes a lot of self-discipline. Most people call it willpower. It is much easier to eat unhealthy foods, and unhealthy foods usually taste good, so they give us pleasure. Everyone needs rewards. Without any rewards, life would be wretched. If you never reward yourself, you will feel restricted and depressed. This situation is impossible to maintain. The dopamine reward system will eventually win out, and you'll overeat. Without rewards, you will surely get depressed. I have seen that my patients who start an ultra-strict diet sometimes get depressed from being on a diet. They feel like they have lost a friend or a loved one. In this case, the friend was food. When you live a healthy lifestyle, it takes a lot of self-discipline and self-motivation. This is what some people call willpower. You can call it willpower, or something else, but if you reward yourself from time to time, your drive to maintain a healthy lifestyle for a lifetime will be much stronger.

Serotonin

You're probably quite familiar with serotonin, since its discovery has led to a greater understanding of depression and SSRIs (selective serotonin reuptake inhibitors)—antidepressants such as Prozac, Paxil, Celexa, Lexapro, Remeron, and Zoloft. Serotonin is made from the amino acid tryptophan (found in turkey and other foods with protein), and because of serotonin's importance in regulating

Choosing the Right Reward

You can reward yourself with food if you follow my advice. It is better to eat a tasty meal as a reward for a week of healthy eating than to eat unhealthy food as a revolt or a binge. The idea is that eating a special meal or a special food as a reward helps prevent the feelings of deprivation that you get from an ultra-strict diet. You can also reward yourself with nonfood items like a getting car wash, massage, or new clothing item.

hunger and appetite, tryptophan is known as an essential amino acid. Eighty percent of the body's serotonin is produced by the intestines, and serotonin is important for proper gut function. Serotonin also functions as a neurotransmitter that helps regulate hunger and appetite. Bulimia and compulsive eating are related to improper serotonin regulation. Serotonin is also involved with sleep and memory.

Serotonin is responsible for carbohydrate cravings, because serotonin creates the calm feeling that occurs when you eat a high-carb food. Many people "treat" their depression and fatigue problems by eating, and usually eating high-carbohydrate sweets. You feel bad and you have low energy, so you grab some sweets to make the bad feelings go away, and they do, with the initial sugar rush, but the spike subsides, even plunges, and you're back on the rollercoaster, craving more sweets.

SSRI medications have an interesting side effect: they can influence your weight, causing either weight *loss* or weight *gain*. In my clinical practice, I have seen that Prozac and Zoloft commonly cause weight loss (in the first six months only), and Paxil and Remeron usually cause weight gain, but I have also seen the opposite occur with all of them. In addition, these drugs aren't too different from prescription diet pills such as Phen-Fen, diet medications on which some people gained weight. The point is that serotonin has powerful influences on your weight, but it is not the only factor.

Three Fruits to Boost Dopamine

Increase your consumption of apples, bananas, and watermelon. These three fruits are thought to help regulate dopamine levels.

St. John's Wort and 5-HTP are herbal supplements that affect the serotonin system in a way similar to

SSRIs. They have been promoted as an herbal treatment for both depression and obesity. Studies have not been consistent, though. It appears that these products are not very effective for weight loss and can have potentially dangerous side effects.

The antidepressant medications venlafaxine (Effexor), desvenlafaxine (Pristiq), and duloxetine (Cymbalta) work by increasing levels of serotonin, norepinephrine, and dopamine. This combination approach seems to both decrease hunger and cause weight loss. The antidepressant medication bupropion (Wellbutrin) affects both the norepinephrine and dopamine systems and also causes weight loss. Designer serotonin medications are under development. Research shows that the 5-HT_{2C} receptor is the one that is most important when it comes to hunger and appetite. Early reports claim that the medication works better than available medications and with fewer side effects.

You don't need to take medication to raise your serotonin. Here are some ways you can naturally raise your serotonin levels:

- **Eat turkey and foods with protein.** Turkey, meat, low-fat dairy products, and other foods high in protein contain tryptophan, the building block for serotonin.

- **Eat slow carbohydrates.** High-sugar foods and processed carbohydrates cause serotonin crashes. Healthy carbohydrates (see chapter 3) help prevent serotonin crashes that lead to carbohydrate cravings.

- **Maintain a normal sleep/wake cycle.** Disturbances in your sleep and wake cycle can cause decreased serotonin levels. Go to bed on time. Turn on lights in the morning and keep them off at night. Appropriate lighting helps set your biological clock, which raises serotonin levels. Spending more time outdoors during the day can also help maintain normal biological rhythms.

Endocannabinoids

Endocannabinoids are potent appetite stimulators produced by the brain that have properties similar to marijuana. Endocannabinoids work in the hypothalamus to stimulate appetite. Drugs that block endocannabinoids used to be intensively studied as a cure for obesity. Unfortunately, these medications caused depression, and some of the subjects in the clinical trials committed suicide. Leptin resistance causes the brain to overproduce endocannabinoids. Alleviating leptin resistance is your best bet for lowering endocannabinoids naturally, without making you feel depressed.

Gamma-Aminobutyric Acid

Gamma-aminobutyric acid (GABA) is a potent brain chemical that is affected by several prescription medications. Benzodiazepine medications such as Xanax, Valium, and Librium relieve anxiety and make you sleepy by stimulating the receptor for GABA. This class of medications has also been reported to promote weight gain. The medication topiramate (Topamax), indicated for the treatment of epilepsy, has a slightly different effect on the GABA receptor. Unlike benzodiazepines, topiramate causes weight loss. It seems to have particular benefit in reducing binge eating and night-time eating.

Orexin

Orexin is a brain hormone important for controlling appetite. Orexin also activates brown fat (see chapter 2), which helps raise metabolism and burn calories. Researchers have found that mice that were deficient in orexin were obese even though they ate less than normal mice. The mice with orexin deficiency had brown fat that didn't develop properly. The defect in brown fat was even detectable in unborn mice. Without orexin, the mice were permanently destined to become obese. Now researchers are looking for ways to use orexin to prevent humans from becoming obese.

Gut Hormones

The stomach and intestines, known as the *gut,* comprise one of the largest endocrine organs in the body. The first gut hormone to be discovered, secretin, was described by Ernest Starling and William Bayliss in 1902. Since that time, many more gut hormones have been identified. Gut hormones are responsible for proper gut health and motility and have effects in the brain that regulate appetite and satiety. There is a gut-brain connection that regulates food intake through control of appetite, satiety, and gut motility.

Gut Hormones and Satiety

Gut hormones control appetite on a minute-to-minute and hour-to-hour time frame. When food enters your stomach, the distention turns on and off gut hormones, which signal the brain to tell it about the food you just ate. These hormones help you feel satisfied, because they send a "Stop eating" message to your brain. Gut hormones tell your brain that you feel full and have had enough to eat. They make you feel satisfied, so you don't overeat. The best foods for gut hormones are bulky, high-volume foods, including vegetables, fruits, and whole grains, in addition to low-fat dairy products. Foods that are high in fiber and protein, such as beans, broccoli, and eggs, also are very satisfying. High-fat food, junk food, and fast food are not satisfying and disrupt gut hormones.

Ghrelin

The stomach makes the hormone ghrelin, which mainly boosts appetite. I call ghrelin a "gremlin" that makes you hungry. Ghrelin (*Gh* means growth hormone; *relin* means releasing) was initially named because it also is involved in growth hormone (GH) release, but it's now known that ghrelin's major role is in regulating hunger, appetite, and satiety. Weight loss surgical procedures such as gastric bypass surgery work in part by reducing ghrelin levels by up to 85 percent. Ghrelin-blocking medications hold promise for the future. For now, a natural approach to keeping ghrelin low is best.

Get more sleep to control ghrelin surges.

Studies have found that sleep deprivation causes increased appetite in part because it causes increased ghrelin levels.

Eat on a schedule.

Ghrelin peaks, and therefore, so does your appetite, when you haven't eaten, and both ghrelin and appetite fall after a meal. Eating a standard breakfast, lunch, and supper causes variable ghrelin levels throughout the day. To keep ghrelin low, eat more frequent meals and snacks. Gut hormones work best when you eat balanced meals and snacks on a schedule. In chapter 4, I emphasize guidelines that help gut hormones work in your favor. You must eat a big breakfast with protein, eat a healthy lunch, eat an afternoon snack with protein, eat a satisfying healthy dinner, and end the day with a sweet, slow-carbohydrate dessert. (See Figure 5.1.)

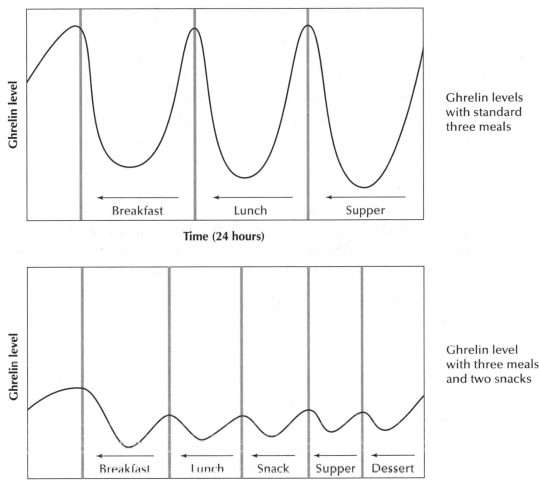

Figure 5.1   Ghrelin Levels

Ghrelin levels peak if you don't eat for three or four hours. Ghrelin is lowest twenty to thirty minutes after a meal. If you eat three meals, ghrelin levels go up before a meal and go down after the meal. If you skip breakfast, your ghrelin levels will soar, which typically leads to overeating at dinner. If you eat every three to four hours, though, you will keep your ghrelin levels lower, which controls appetite throughout the day.

Peptide YY

The intestines make another important gut hormone, peptide YY (PYY), which reduces appetite and increases feelings of satiety. The key to feeling full all the time is keeping ghrelin levels low and PYY high. PYY levels fall before meals and rise after meals. PYY lowers NPY levels. PYY also slows down the gut, which helps you feel full and satisfied. Increasing PYY suppresses appetite and increases satiety. A study found that overweight people don't make enough PYY.

Eat filling foods that are low in calories.

To boost PYY levels, eat heavy foods that are low in calories. Filling foods include high-fiber foods, whole grains, fruits, vegetables, beans, lean meats, lean poultry, seafood, low-fat dairy products, and thick healthy soups. These foods also tend to have high water content and are low in sugar and fat.

Eat 25 to 35 grams of fiber every day.

You must eat 25 to 35 grams of fiber every day. I recommend that you eat fiber in food, but you can get fiber from supplements, in powder or pill form. High-fiber foods, however, are filling and satisfying. High-fiber foods also suppress ghrelin and raise PYY. Fiber distends the stomach to turn off ghrelin and turn on PYY.

Eat slowly.

Slow down your eating to give your gut hormones a chance to work. It takes twenty to thirty minutes for gut hormones to kick in after you start eating. When you eat quickly, you overeat before your gut hormones start working and tell you that you're full.

Glucagon-Like Peptide-1

A cousin of glucagon, glucagon-like peptide-1 (GLP-1) has been gaining lots of attention in the medical community since the FDA approval of the GLP-1 medication exenatide (Byetta). Now there is another GLP medication called liragulatide (Victoza). GLP-1, produced by the gut, controls insulin secretion and feeding behavior. GLP-1 slows the empting of the stomach and reduces hunger. Since GLP-1 is a peptide, it cannot be taken in pill form, or the stomach will simply digest it. It must be injected. For more information on these medications, see chapter 6.

Cholecystokinin

Cholecystokinin (CCK) is a peptide hormone produced by the small intestine. It's sometimes known as the "feel-full protein." It slows stomach emptying and decreases appetite. CCK works in several parts of the body, notably in a circular muscle at the bottom of the stomach known as a sphincter. CCK tightens the sphincter, and with the sphincter tight, food stays in the stomach. Nerves from the stomach transmit the feeling "I've had enough to eat" to the brain. CCK also acts directly on the appetite centers of the brain, regulating appetite and making it another satiety hormone. CCK also slows movement of food out of the stomach and into the intestines, making you feel full longer. You can help your body produce more CCK to help you feel full longer by eating more protein and fewer processed carbohydrates.

Enterostatin

Enterostatin is a hormone made by the stomach and small intestine that decreases appetite. Initial studies are promising for using this hormone as a weight loss agent.

Pancreatic Hormones

The main hormone made by the pancreas is insulin, which I discuss in chapter 6, but insulin is not the only hormone that the pancreas produces. The pancreas is really two organs rolled into one. The *exocrine pancreas* makes digestive enzymes that are secreted into the gut. The *endocrine pancreas* is found in specialized islands of cells, known as the islets of Langerhans, and produces hormones that are secreted into the blood. Different cells in the islets produce different hormones. Three important pancreatic hormones are glucagon, somatostatin, and amylin. Each, like insulin, is closely related to the food you eat, and each affects your appetite.

Glucagon

Glucagon is a digestive hormone that is released when food—particularly protein—leaves the stomach and enters the small intestine. It helps perform a wide variety of tasks: it slows the exit of food from the stomach, making you feel full; acts to raise blood sugar; and tells the liver to pump out glucose. Glucagon is also known as a counter-insulin hormone. People with diabetes who are prone to

hCG

hCG, also known as the "pregnancy hormone," is an injectable medication extracted from the urine of pregnant women and is approved for the treatment of infertility and other uses. hCG injections have been prescribed by doctors for weight loss, but there is little to no evidence that they work. In theory, hCG stimulates the body to produce more testosterone, resulting in a leaner, more toned body.

Patients flood into the offices of weight loss doctors, paying as much as $1,000 a month for hCG injections. hCG has been promoted as a weight loss miracle for more than fifty years, and it has become more popular in recent times. The hCG diet was first promoted in the 1950s by A. T. W. Simeons, a doctor in Italy. Since then, twelve out of fourteen studies have shown that hCG has little to no weight loss effect. Doctors who prescribe hCG say it works, even though the research does not back up this claim.

The hCG diet combines an extremely low-calorie diet with daily injections or drops of hCG and promises that patients can lose up to a pound a day without hunger. Patients are often told that hCG can stimulate the body to burn off fat stored in problem areas such the stomach, thighs, and upper arms. In January 2011, the Food and Drug Administration reiterated its warning from the 1970s that weight loss claims made about hCG are fraudulent and illegal. The FDA requires the following statement on hCG packaging: "It has not been shown to increase weight loss, to cause a more 'attractive' distribution of fat, or to 'decrease hunger and discomfort' from low-calorie diets."

To make matters worse, the side effects of hCG include blood clots, headaches, depression, ovarian stimulation, and breast tenderness.

"Aside from the issue of side effects, the use of hCG as a diet tool was manipulating people to give them the sense that they're receiving something that's powerful and potent and effective, and in fact they're receiving something that's nothing better than a placebo."

—Pieter Cohen, M.D., Harvard Medical School

A Rare Tumor

Rare cases exist of tumors of glucagon-producing cells, known as *glucagonoma*. In these cases, the extremely high glucagon levels created by the tumors cause diabetes. The condition is accompanied by an itchy, red, sandpaper-like rash. Although the condition is very, very rare, I bring it up because it's not rare if you're the one who has it. If you have diabetes and an itchy red rash, visit your endocrinologist and ask to have your glucagon levels tested. He may look at you funny at first, but be persistent.

hypoglycemia carry a syringe of glucagon. If they have severe low blood sugar, a shot of the glucagon will make the blood sugar shoot right up.

Somatostatin

Somatostatin, which is primarily produced by the hypothalamus, is also created in the islets of Langerhans in the pancreas, just like insulin and glucagon. Again it's a hormone that blocks other hormones—in this case, the secretion of its sister pancreatic hormones, insulin and glucagon. It shuts down β-cells, the pancreatic cells responsible for insulin secretion, but in certain situations, somatostatin may also help with weight loss. One of these situations is that of hypothalamic obesity, a condition in which a brain injury or certain brain tumors cause obesity by damaging satiety centers in the ventromedial hypothalamus. Hypothalamic obesity is perhaps the most difficult form of obesity to treat. Insulin levels are very high, but not because of insulin resistance, something known as *primary insulin hypersecretion*. Scientists hypothesize that damage to the hypothalamus may increase nerve signals to the pancreas, boosting insulin levels and causing extreme hunger. Somatostatin injections in these patients dramatically lower insulin levels. Once the insulin levels go down, weight is lost and leptin levels also go down. Carbohydrate cravings are dramatically reduced.

Amylin

Amylin is co-secreted with insulin from the beta cells of the pancreas. Like insulin, amylin is secreted in response to food. Amylin reduces appetite and slows the release of food from the stomach, which reduces the rate of entry of food into the intestines and increases the feeling of being full. The synthetic form of the hormone is available in a medication known as pramlintide (Symlin). It is an injectable medication that is used to treat diabetes, but it also helps with weight loss.

Chapter Review

Willpower has little to do with our ability to resist the urge to consume food. Instead, the primal urge to feel full (satiated) is rooted in a complex interplay of more than two dozen hormones that influence appetite, satiety, and metabolism.

This chapter discussed in detail the role of leptin and its impact on our natural appetite "set point" that helps us balance our urge to eat. Most people with weight issues suffer from an overproduction of leptin, and it is this excess production that leads to leptin resistance. In fact, the chapter points out, leptin resistance is the reason that the vast majority of people (98 percent) on diets eventually gain back all the weight they lose.

The chapter offered a variety of tips and suggestions on what foods help reset your set point back to normal. A number of specific suggestions were offered to encourage lower leptin resistance levels in your body, including eating healthy foods, calorie control, drinking water, and exercising.

Finally, the chapter discussed a variety of brain and gut hormones produced by the stomach, intestines, and the pancreas. A number of these hormones were highlighted, including familiar ones such as dopamine and serotonin as well as the "most potent stimulator of appetite known to man"—neuropeptide Y (NPY)—which directly influences your body's leptin hormone.

The next chapter discusses the importance of insulin and its role in controlling weight. Specifically the chapter addresses the condition known as insulin resistance, which occurs when the body's cells don't "listen" to insulin's messages.

CHAPTER

6

Alleviate Insulin Resistance

More than 90 million Americans have insulin resistance, but most don't know it. It's the most common hormone problem in the world. Insulin resistance occurs when the body's cells don't listen to insulin's messages. The main function of insulin is to take sugar out of the bloodstream and move it into cells so it can be used as fuel. Without insulin, your cells would starve. When you have insulin resistance, your cells struggle to take up enough sugar out of the bloodstream. This means you can't burn as much sugar for energy. The result is feeling tired and hungry and having a slower metabolism.

Insulin resistance causes increased appetite because it blocks appetite centers in the brain so that fullness signals can't get through. If you have insulin resistance, you also have leptin resistance, which I discuss in chapter 5. Leptin and insulin resistance conspire to make you hold on to body fat, especially in the abdomen. Leptin resistance makes the body numb to excess fat, so that you aren't aware of how much being overweight is affecting you day in and day out.

Insulin resistance slows metabolism by damaging the mitochondria of muscle cells. Mitochondria are known

In This Chapter
- Causes, Indicators, and Risks of Insulin Resistance
- Accurate and Reliable Tests
- How to Manage and Control the Condition
- Treatments for Insulin Resistance

> ## Insulin Resistance Causes Carbohydrate Cravings
>
> People with insulin resistance make a lot of insulin, but their cells cannot hear its command. As a result, you crave sugar in the form of sweets or salty, crunchy foods like chips, pretzels, or popcorn. Your body mistakenly thinks that eating unhealthy carbohydrates will fix the problem, but the problem is damaged insulin receptors.

as the powerhouse of the cell because they are responsible for burning fuel and producing energy. Insulin resistance leads to higher levels of unhealthy blood fats, known as *triglycerides*, and free fatty acids caused by dysfunctional fat cells that leak. The liver takes up the excess blood fats and becomes filled with fat. Blood fats make insulin resistance worse, a condition known as *lipotoxicity*. High blood fats interfere with the proper functioning of many hormones, including insulin itself.

Insulin resistance is a hormone disruption that occurs when a hormone is perfectly fine but the body can't respond to it. If you go back to the lock-and-key analogy that I discussed in chapter 2, think about insulin as a key that can't properly open a damaged insulin receptor lock. The body compensates by making more insulin that helps gets sugar into cells, preventing overt diabetes, but this causes other problems. Insulin resistance is a complex disorder that is the root cause of diseases like diabetes, PCOS (polycystic ovary syndrome), sleep apnea, liver disease, high blood pressure, cardiovascular disease, and many other problems. Making more insulin is not the best way to overcome insulin resistance. Alleviating insulin resistance is the better way and is a key part of overall hormonal balance that lowers blood sugar and reduces the risk for these diseases.

Excess Fat, Especially in the Belly, Is a Key Contributor to Insulin Resistance

Being overweight is the most common cause of insulin resistance. Most individuals become insulin resistant when they are even slightly overweight. Being normal weight but having excess body fat can also lead to insulin resistance. Everyone who is overweight has some degree of insulin resistance, and the heavier you are the more insulin resistance you have. People with a body mass index

---

Insulin Spikes and Hypoglycemia

Eating any type of carbohydrate causes blood sugar to rise. This is followed by a release of insulin. Unhealthy carbohydrates like sugary foods or processed foods are digested quickly, causing a lot of sugar to rush into the blood all at once. This is followed by an insulin spike and rapid fall in blood sugar. This typically results in feelings of hunger and tiredness a few hours after eating high-sugar foods. If you eat a slowly digested carbohydrate, like whole grain, vegetables, or fruit, the body releases insulin slowly and is able to manage the carbohydrate load.

(BMI) of 25–27 kilogram per meter squared (kg/m^2) or greater are at high risk for insulin resistance. The heavier you are, the more likely you are to have insulin resistance. For more information on how to calculate body mass index, see "Practical Strategies for Intelligent Weight Loss" at the end of the book.

Increased abdominal fat is a telltale sign of insulin resistance. A person has android obesity or central obesity if he or she is fat in the middle section with skinny arms and legs—"apple-shaped" obesity. A person with gynecoid obesity or peripheral obesity has a large rear end and hips—"pear-shaped" obesity. Think of the two kinds as "gut versus butt." (Fat in the gut is worse than fat in the butt.) People with excess fat in the belly are more likely to have insulin resistance. A man with a waistline of more than 40 inches and a woman with a waistline of more than 35 inches are classified as having central obesity.

Inflammation Fuels Insulin Resistance

Recent studies have determined that inflammation plays a key role in causing insulin resistance. Inflammation is caused by chemicals known as *cytokines*. These substances play a key role in fighting infections and preventing cancer. As I discuss in chapter 5, cytokines produced by fat cells are the major source of inflammation in the body. These substances, known as *adipokines,* are the root cause of insulin resistance and leptin resistance. Chronic infections or illness lead to inflammation and can also be a source of insulin resistance. Illness can cause increased levels of inflammatory cytokines like tumor necrosis factor and interleukin 6, which make tissues in the body more resistant to the actions of insulin.

Insulin Resistance and Your Genes

Genetics determines at what weight you will develop insulin resistance rather than whether you will develop it. If you have a family history of diabetes or obesity, you are more likely to have insulin resistance. People of certain ethnic backgrounds (Native Americans, African Americans, Hispanics, Asians—especially South Asians—and Pacific Islanders) are at increased risk for insulin resistance.

Physical Inactivity Causes Insulin Resistance

Lack of exercise is a major cause of insulin resistance. Studies have shown that as little as three weeks of regular exercise can improve insulin resistance.

Stress Causes Insulin Resistance

Stress causes insulin resistance for many reasons. Two hormones secreted when the body is under stress—cortisol and epinephrine—promote insulin resistance. (See chapter 11 for more on cortisol.) The stress of poor health also increases insulin resistance. A person with diabetes who gets a cold, for example, has a rise in blood sugar levels because his insulin resistance is worse. This is true for any number of ailments, from infections to mental illness.

Kidney or Liver Problems Cause Insulin Resistance

For a number of reasons, kidney or liver problems may cause insulin resistance. Hemochromatosis is a common genetic disorder of iron metabolism that causes liver problems and insulin resistance. (For more on hemochromatosis, see chapter 10.)

Insulin Needs Potassium to Work Properly

Low potassium levels increase insulin resistance. Diuretic medications, which are commonly used to treat high blood pressure, can cause low potassium through excessive loss of potassium in the urine. High levels of the adrenal gland hormones cortisol and aldosterone can cause low potassium.

Hormonal Imbalances Can Cause Insulin Resistance

Disruptions of many different hormones can cause or worsen insulin resistance. I discuss these hormones throughout this book; cortisol (chapter 11), growth hormone (chapter 12), and leptin (chapter 5), in atypical quantities, can make people insulin resistant. These hormones are considered counter-insulin hormones in that they provide checks and balances for insulin.

> ### Another Reason to Quit Smoking
>
> For decades, people have used smoking as a way to keep their weight down. Nicotine acts as a stimulant, after all, and the buzz of a nicotine high can keep away thoughts of eating more food. (Many smokers suffer a great gain in weight when they quit smoking, or even try to quit: the desire to put something, anything, in one's mouth is overwhelming.) But smoking is also a known cause of insulin resistance. For this reason—as well as many others—smoking should be avoided.

Vitamin D Deficiency Is Linked to Insulin Resistance

Vitamin D deficiency has been directly linked to the development of insulin resistance and diabetes, but no one knows why. Vitamin D levels are lower in obese people because fat tissue serves as a depot for vitamin D, sequestering it away where it can't be used. People with low vitamin D have an easier time losing weight once vitamin D is replaced. Vitamin D enhances insulin sensitivity and improves blood sugar levels.

Diseases Caused by Insulin Resistance

Insulin resistance is linked to a variety of medical complications. Treating insulin resistance can treat all of the complications at the same time.

Abnormal Cholesterol and Triglycerides

Insulin resistance causes abnormal blood fats—low "good" cholesterol, high "bad" cholesterol, and high triglycerides. Cholesterol comes in two basic kinds: HDL, high-density lipoproteins or "good cholesterol"; and LDL, low-density lipoproteins or "bad cholesterol." Triglycerides are not cholesterol but rather another type of blood fat that contributes to cardiovascular disease. Most people know that high-LDL cholesterol is a risk factor for cardiovascular disease, but research has shown that low-HDL is an even greater risk factor for developing heart and blood vessel problems. The dyslipidemia of insulin resistance has a classic pattern with low-HDL cholesterol, normal or high-LDL cholesterol, and high triglycerides.

Insulin Resistance throughout Life

Puberty

Adolescents have low levels of insulin resistance, but obese adolescents going through puberty have very high levels of insulin resistance. This would seem to correlate with other effects of puberty: some children lose their baby fat and become strapping young adults, while for others weight problems just get worse. We are now seeing alarming increases in rates of type 2 diabetes in teenagers.

Pregnancy

Pregnancy is a classic insulin-resistant state. The prototypical insulin-resistant person is apple-shaped: big stomach, thin arms. Sound familiar? In a pregnant woman, all her weight—in this case, the baby—is on the stomach, while her arms and legs stay thin. In fact, all pregnant women are tested for gestational diabetes because insulin resistance makes the condition so common. Insulin resistance is associated with an increased risk for gestational diabetes and high blood pressure in pregnancy, known as *preclampsia*.

Getting Older

Does aging make people more insulin resistant? There's some controversy about whether aging causes insulin resistance. Some experts say it's not aging itself as much as our decreased physical activity and weight gain that increase insulin resistance; others maintain aging itself can have these effects. More research needs to be done.

Menopause

The decreased estradiol (healthy estrogen, see chapter 9) levels in menopausal women can promote insulin resistance. The effect of estrogen is small when compared to other factors that contribute to insulin resistance.

HDL cholesterol is considered good cholesterol because it removes harmful cholesterol from blood vessels and brings it to the liver for excretion from the body. HDL cholesterol controls a process known as *reverse cholesterol transport,* moving cholesterol out of the heart and blood vessels, lowering the risk for heart attacks and strokes.

This scavenger action of HDL cholesterol prevents the formation of clogged arteries, a condition is known as *atherosclerosis.* Low HDL is a major risk for cardiovascular disease. Insulin resistance not only causes low-HDL levels but also decreases its quality, making it less protective.

LDL cholesterol is considered bad cholesterol because it penetrates blood vessels, causing atherosclerosis. LDL cholesterol elevations are not always caused

Candida

I have heard some people say they believe that insulin resistance and blood sugar problems are caused by overgrowth of a type of fungus or yeast known as *Candida albicans*. In fact, some books have made the outrageous claims that Candida overgrowth or toxicity is responsible for chronic medical conditions like chronic fatigue syndrome, fibromyalgia, eczema, psoriasis, scleroderma, lupus, arthritis, attention deficit disorder, asthma, headaches, irritable bowel syndrome, multiple sclerosis, autism, food allergies, carbohydrate cravings, insulin resistance, and diabetes. Proponents of this theory blame antibiotics, birth control pills, and high-sugar diets for yeast overgrowth. There's even something they call leaky gut syndrome: they claim that Candida migrates from the bowels into body. The yeast in bread is blamed for causing diabetes (I blame the carbohydrates and calories in the bread).

I have seen patients who take heavy-duty antifungal medications to fight what they believe to be Candida overgrowth. My opinion and the opinion of many of my colleagues is that Candida has nothing to do with these conditions. All human beings have Candida in their intestines and stool as part of what is called the intestinal flora. Medical problems, like AIDS and uncontrolled diabetes, that lower the immune system can lead to infections with Candida, primarily vaginal yeast infections and mouth infections (known as thrush). But a yeast infection is a consequence—not the cause—of high blood sugar. Candida can infect the whole body and get into the bloodstream, but this is only seen in patients who have severe immune system problems like AIDS or in transplant patients. This condition, known as systemic Candidiasis, is a life-threatening condition with severe illness and very high fevers. Although Candida infections can be a real medical problem, there is absolutely no truth to the claims that Candida overgrowth is a cause of insulin resistance.

by insulin resistance. In fact, high-LDL cholesterol is usually a genetic condition. Insulin resistance alters the quality of LDL, making it smaller and denser, which makes it more dangerous and more likely to penetrate blood vessel walls.

Triglycerides are considered a non-cholesterol blood fat. High triglycerides cause atherosclerosis and cardiovascular disease just like cholesterol does. Insulin resistance makes triglyceride levels soar. Triglycerides and HDL cholesterol have a powerful effect on each other. High triglycerides cause lower HDL levels, and the reverse is also true. If HDL increases, triglycerides decline. Triglyceride elevations above 1000 mg/dL (milligrams/deciliter) can cause inflammation of the pancreas known as *pancreatitis.*

Abnormal Testosterone

Men with insulin resistance commonly have low testosterone levels, known as *hypogonadism,* which I discuss in chapter 10. This condition causes muscle loss, fatigue, depression, and sexual dysfunction. Men with insulin resistance find it very difficult to get motivated to exercise. This makes insulin resistance worse.

Women with insulin resistance tend to have high testosterone levels, as I discuss in chapter 8. Insulin resistance is one of the major contributors to polycystic ovary syndrome. Insulin resistance stimulates the ovaries and adrenal glands to produce excess male hormones, resulting in irregular menstrual cycles, fertility problems, acne, hair loss, and facial hair growth.

Cancer

Insulin resistance increases the risk for many cancers, including pancreatic cancer, colon cancer, breast cancer, uterine cancer, and prostate cancer. Many studies have shown a link between cancer and insulin resistance, diabetes, and obesity. It is thought that high insulin levels can mistakenly stimulate the receptor for another hormone, IGF-1. IGF-1 is produced by the liver in response to growth hormone (see chapter 12) and is known to increase cancer risk.

Cardiovascular Disease

Cardiovascular disease is the number one cause of death among people with insulin resistance. Cardiovascular (*cardio* = heart, *vascular* = blood vessels) disease refers to diseases of the heart and blood vessels caused by atherosclerosis, a process in which deposits of cholesterol and fat build up "plaques" in the arteries. High blood pressure, diabetes, and cholesterol problems all contribute to cardiovascular disease. Other factors such as increased blood clotting and inflammation also play a role.

Cardiovascular disease includes heart attacks and strokes, but any organ or any blood vessel can be affected. Insulin resistance and high blood pressure to put strain on the heart. This causes the heart to become overworked, and it enlarges in an abnormal way. Over time the thickened muscle becomes stiff, loses flexibility, and is unable to pump adequate amounts of blood to the body. This is known as *heart failure* or *congestive heart failure.*

There are several major forms of cardiovascular disease:

- **Coronary artery disease,** which leads to heart attacks

- **Carotid artery disease and cerebral vascular disease,** which lead to strokes.

- **Peripheral arterial disease,** which is atherosclerosis in the blood vessels of the legs that can to lead leg pain or an amputation

- **Renal vascular disease,** which can lead to kidney failure and makes high blood pressure very difficult to control

Diabetes and Prediabetes

The number of people with diabetes continues to climb. In 2008, the Centers for Disease Control and Prevention (CDC) reported 23.6 million people had diabetes and 57 million had prediabetes. According to a 2011 report by the CDC, 26 million Americans have diabetes and 79 million have prediabetes. The World Health Organization reported that in 2011 346 million people worldwide had diabetes. By 2050, it is predicted that one in three people will have diabetes. Dr. Paul Jellinger, past president of the American Association of Clinical Endocrinologists has referred to the epidemic of diabetes as a "tsunami."

> *"In a little more than 10 years, the numbers went from nothing to something . . .*
> *and that's something to worry about."*
>
> —Larry Deeb, past president of the
> American Diabetes Association

Twenty-seven percent of people with diabetes, or 7 million people, have not yet been diagnosed. More than one-quarter of Americans over the age of sixty-five have diabetes, and half have prediabetes. Thirty-five percent of Americans over age twenty have prediabetes. At the time of the first edition of *Hormonal Balance,* type 2 diabetes, which used to be called "adult-onset" diabetes, was almost entirely a disease seen in adults. But the childhood obesity epidemic has caused an increase in diabetes in adolescents and young adults. The number of new diabetes diagnoses has increased from practically zero to tens of thousands over the past ten years. When type 2 diabetes occurs at an early age, there are new concerns: Will these children have heart disease in their thirties, need kidney dialysis or go blind in their forties? Because type 2 diabetes in young adults is such a new thing, we don't really know what is going to happen to these patients over the course of their lives.

Endocrinologists don't use the term "borderline diabetes." The earliest stages of blood sugar elevations are termed *impaired fasting glucose* and impaired *glucose tolerance* and are collectively referred to as *prediabetes*. Prediabetes means your pancreas is already starting to show signs of strain, and blood sugar is elevated, but not high enough to qualify for diabetes.

The diagnosis of prediabetes is based on blood sugar levels, not insulin levels. Insulin levels are not reliable for testing for diabetes or insulin resistance. Early on, most people don't have symptoms from elevated blood sugar. If not diagnosed early, blood sugar rises and symptoms set in: excessive thirst, excessive hunger, frequent urination, and blurred vision. Early diagnosis of prediabetes is important because even when blood sugars are minimally elevated, they can cause damage to the heart, blood vessels, eyes, nerves, and kidneys. People with prediabetes can work aggressively on diabetes prevention by losing weight, becoming more active, and getting healthier.

Do You Have Type 1 Diabetes?

Studies have shown that 10 percent of patients who have been diagnosed with type 2 diabetes actually have type 1 diabetes. Originally named juvenile-onset diabetes, type 1 diabetes can occur at any age and is caused by an autoimmune destruction of insulin producing cells in the pancreas. Indicators of type 1 diabetes include rapid progression of the disease and failure of traditional diabetes medications. However, even if you appear to have typical type 2 diabetes, there is a 10 percent chance you might have type 1. Testing for type 1 diabetes includes a fasting insulin level and measurement of glutamic acid decarboxylase (GAD) antibodies.

Fatty Liver Disease

Also known as *nonalcoholic steatohepatosis* or *nonalcoholic fatty liver disease,* this very common but often overlooked condition is caused by excess fat in the liver. It is similar to liver disease seen in alcoholics. Excess fat in the liver can result in inflammation and permanent scaring, known as *cirrhosis* of the liver. Fatty liver disease is also a risk for cancer of the liver.

Gallstones

Insulin resistance and obesity increase the risk for gallstones. This can result in inflammation of the gallbladder and the need for gallbladder removal.

Gout

Gout is a painful disorder caused by deposits of a substance known as *uric acid* in the joints, most commonly the big toe. Insulin resistance causes increased levels of uric acid. Increased uric acid levels have also been associated with an increased risk of cardiovascular disease.

High Blood Pressure

More than half of Americans over the age of fifty have high blood pressure, also known as *hypertension.* Hypertension is known as the "silent killer" because most people don't have any symptoms. Hypertension is a major risk factor for serious medical problems like heart failure, kidney failure, blindness, heart attack, stroke, or even sudden death. Insulin resistance has an effect on blood pressure for several reasons. Inflammation damages the lining of the blood vessels and they become less compliant. Normally blood vessels are like rubber, but insulin resistance makes them more like leather. Insulin causes retention of sodium, or salt, in the bloodstream. This increases the volume of blood, leading to a rise in blood pressure. Insulin resistance causes blood vessels to become stiffer or less compliant, which raises blood pressure.

Increased Blood Clotting

Insulin resistance causes an increased ability for blood to clot. There is also a decreased ability for the body to dissolve blood clots. Increased blood clotting plays a role in worsening cardiovascular disease and contributes to heart attacks and strokes. There can also be blood clots in the legs, known as *deep vein thrombosis,* or a blood clot in the lungs, known as a *pulmonary embolism.*

Aldosterone Contributes to High Blood Pressure

Insulin resistance causes the adrenal gland to produce excessive amounts of aldosterone, a blood pressure hormone. Excess levels of aldosterone cause very high blood pressure and low potassium levels. And because potassium is required for proper insulin function, the low potassium worsens insulin resistance. If you have high blood pressure and low potassium, or high blood pressure that is very difficult to control, you should ask your doctor to check your aldosterone level.

Insomnia

Many people with insulin resistance have difficulty falling asleep or staying asleep. Improving insulin resistance often improves sleep. The reverse is also true; improving sleep also improves insulin resistance.

Kidney Disease

Insulin resistance causes protein leakage from the kidney known as *microalbuminuria*. Insulin resistance, combined with high blood pressure and blood sugar elevations, can result in decreased kidney function known as *chronic renal failure* or *chronic kidney disease.* Chronic kidney disease worsens insulin resistance, creating a vicious cycle.

Skin Problems

Insulin resistance is associated with a host of skin problems, including acanthosis nigricans, skin tags, psoriasis, acne, stretch marks and fungal skin infections.

Acanthosis nigricans is a skin condition that appears as a black velvety skin rash or dark discoloration in a ring around the neck. Acanthosis nigricans also occurs under the arms, around the belly button, under skin folds, or in the groin. It looks like dirt, but it won't wash off. Acanthosis nigricans is caused by insulin resistance and is usually a sign of prediabetes or diabetes. Insulin is a growth factor—and insulin also makes skin grow. In the presence of abnormally high insulin levels, skin grows in very strange ways, making

Metabolic Syndrome

Metabolic syndrome is not a single condition but a clustering of medical problems that are all connected by the common thread of insulin resistance and increase the risk of diabetes, cardiovascular disease, and early death. It's estimated that as many as 40 percent of Americans over the age of fifty have metabolic syndrome. Metabolic syndrome is also known as insulin resistance syndrome or syndrome x. The ailments of metabolic syndrome have a common thread of insulin resistance, but some experts criticize the diagnostic criteria, stating that they are ambiguous or incomplete.

The criteria for metabolic syndrome are if you have three or more of the following:

Elevated blood sugar

Increased belly fat

Elevated blood pressure

High triglycerides

Decreased good cholesterol

it turn dark. If you have acanthosis nigricans, you are virtually guaranteed of having insulin resistance. But it's not an incurable condition: as you lose weight, the acanthosis nigricans disappears as well. One word of warning, however: on rare occasions, acanthosis nigricans is not caused by insulin resistance; it is caused by cancer. If you have this condition under any circumstances, see your doctor.

Psoriasis is a common skin condition that causes redness, irritation, and silver scaly patches usually found on the elbows, knees, stomach, chest, and back. A 2010 study from the *Archives of Dermatology* found that having psoriasis doubles your risk of having insulin resistance.

Sleep Apnea

Sleep apnea is extremely common in people with insulin resistance. Symptoms include sleepiness, snoring, restless legs, difficulty concentrating, and high blood pressure. Ninety percent of people who have sleep apnea are overweight or obese.

Testing for Insulin Resistance

There is no perfect test for diagnosing insulin resistance. The most reliable test for is known as the *hyperinsulinemic euglycemic clamp*. The test is used for medical research only. This test requires simultaneous infusions of glucose and insulin into two different veins (IV catheters are placed in both arms). Blood sugar levels are checked every five minutes for three hours, and the rate of the glucose going in is adjusted to keep blood sugar levels stable. The amount of glucose required to keep blood sugar in the normal range is used to determine the level of insulin resistance. The euglycemic clamp is difficult to perform, and there is a risk of causing low blood sugar levels.

For most people, blood tests to diagnose insulin resistance are not necessary. If you are overweight or if you have metabolic syndrome, you most like likely have insulin resistance.

Fasting Plasma Glucose

The fasting plasma glucose test measures the amount of sugar in the blood after an eight-hour fast. This is a simple yet important test for assessing blood sugar status and diagnosing diabetes or prediabetes. If you have a fasting blood sugar level between 100 and 125 mg/dL, you are classified as having impaired fasting glucose, although most experts believe that a fasting blood sugar above 95 is definitely abnormal. If your level is 126 mg/dL or higher on two separate occasions, you have diabetes.

Random Plasma Glucose

The random plasma glucose test can be done at any time without fasting. For this test, a normal blood sugar level is below 140 mg/dL. A diabetic level is 200 mg/dL or higher. A random glucose level between 141 and 199 mg/dL is considered prediabetes.

Oral Glucose Tolerance Test

The oral glucose tolerance test is like a "stress test" for the pancreas. It determines how quickly and efficiently your body can handle a load of glucose. The test is done after an eight-hour fast. First, a fasting blood glucose level is measured. Then a pure glucose beverage is consumed, and a second glucose level is measured two hours later. The amount of glucose consumed and the time between blood glucose measurements can vary, but the standard version is to drink 75 grams of glucose and to wait two hours to get the second reading. Extension of the testing (for several more hours) will sometimes show a drop in blood sugar levels, which is a result of a delayed but exaggerated response of insulin production. Anyone diagnosed with prediabetes should have a two-hour, 75 gram glucose tolerance test. A version of the oral glucose tolerance test is used to screen pregnant women for gestational diabetes.

Meal Tolerance Test

The meal tolerance test, also known as a *postprandial blood glucose test,* is a real-life version of the oral glucose tolerance test. Instead of drinking a glucose beverage, you eat a big meal, and blood glucose level is measured before and two hours after. The meal tolerance test is not as reliable as other tests but can be used to diagnose diabetes or prediabetes using the same cutoffs as the random glucose level.

Self-Monitored Blood Glucose

The most accurate way to measure glucose levels is from a sample of blood that is processed in a laboratory. Home glucose monitors measure blood sugar from a drop of blood from a prick of the finger but are not as accurate as laboratory testing. A reading from a glucose monitor cannot be used to make a definite diagnosis of diabetes or prediabetes but can help give you a general idea of what

---

Know Your Blood Sugar Level

Fasting Blood Sugar Levels

Normal: Below 95 mg/dL

Impaired fasting glucose
  (prediabetes): 100–125 mg/dL

Diabetes: Above 125 mg/dL

Random Blood Sugar Levels

Normal: Below 140 mg/dL

Prediabetes: 140–199 mg/dL

Diabetes: Above 200 mg/dL

Two-Hour Glucose Level on a 75 Gram Glucose Tolerance Test

Normal: Below 139 mg/dL

Impaired glucose tolerance
  (prediabetes): 140–199 mg/dL

Diabetes: Above 200 mg/dL

your blood sugar is doing during different times of the day. It's best to test at different times throughout the day, because blood sugar can be normal at one time but high at another. The highest blood sugars are usually two hours after a meal, especially a large meal.

A_{1c}

A blood glucose test provides only a snapshot in time of your blood glucose levels and may not give the whole story. The hemoglobin A_{1c} test, also known as A_{1c}, estimates the average blood sugar level over the previous three months. A_{1c} is a protein in red blood cells that bonds with blood sugar. Because red blood cells can live about ninety days, the hemoglobin A_{1c} represents the average blood sugar

A_{1c} and Diabetes

The A_{1c} is now used to diagnose diabetes, not just to assess diabetic control. An A_{1c} less than 5.7 percent is considered normal. An A_{1c} of 5.7 percent to 6.4 percent is in the prediabetic range, and an A_{1c} of 6.5 percent or above is the diagnosis for diabetes.

level for this length of time. A reading above 5.7 percent indicates that blood sugar is higher than normal. In the past, this test was recommended for only those persons with diabetes. More recently, however, A_{1c} has been recognized as an excellent test for assessing long-term blood sugar levels in people with insulin resistance. Elevated A_{1c} is also an independent risk factor for cardiovascular disease.

Insulin Levels

It's logical to think that high insulin levels are the best way to diagnose insulin resistance. However, most experts do not recommend measuring insulin levels for two reasons. First, laboratory testing methods for insulin are still unreliable and can be inaccurate. Each laboratory uses a slightly different testing method, and the results have not been standardized against each other, so no one really knows what normal is. Second, many people with insulin resistance have normal or even low insulin levels because of pancreatic burnout.

Nevertheless, I often measure insulin levels to determine how much insulin a patient's pancreas is producing and what medications may be most effective. If insulin is measured after an eight-hour fast, a level above 10–15 μU/ml (micro unit/milliliter) is considered high. Insulin is sometimes measured in conjunction with the oral glucose tolerance test—referred to as a stimulated insulin level. The

Estimated Average Glucose

There has been a big push to replace the A_{1c} with the estimated average glucose, also known as eAG. The American Diabetes Association and others have been encouraging this because it is easier for people to understand. Many laboratories provide both the A_{1c} and the eAG on their reports. The formula to calculate eAG from the A_{1c} is

$$eAG = (28.7 \times A_{1c}) - 46.7$$

Following is an approximation eAG according to A1c:

A_{1c} (percentage)	eAG (mg/dL)
5	97
6	126
7	154
8	183
9	212
10	240
11	269
12	298

fasting insulin level and the insulin level two hours after consuming a glucose beverage are compared to one another. C-peptide is a byproduct produced when insulin is made by the body. C-peptide is an easy and accurate test that is a good indicator of insulin levels. High C-peptide levels indicate high insulin levels.

Urinary Microalbumin

This test measures microscopic amounts of protein in the urine. The microalbumin test is very sensitive and will detect levels of protein much lower than will a traditional urinalysis. People with insulin resistance, diabetes, and high blood pressure can have increased levels of protein in the urine. It is recommended that everyone at risk for insulin resistance be tested for microalbumin once or twice a year.

Glucose and Insulin Calculations

Researchers have developed ways to estimate insulin resistance based on sophisticated calculations. These calculations have been criticized, however, because they were originally developed as a research tool to look at large groups of people. The critics note that calculations aren't always accurate for an individual person.

The Homeostatic Model Assessment of Insulin Resistance (HOMA-IR) uses the formula:

$$HOMA = \text{insulin } (\mu U/m) \times [\text{glucose (mmol/L)}/22.5]$$

This formula requires that glucose be converted to the units of mmol/L (millimoles/liter), which is different than the standard unit of mg/dL. Patients with a HOMA score of 2.6 or above are considered to have insulin resistance.

The Quantitative Insulin Sensitivity Check Index (QUICKI) uses the formula:

$$QUICKI = 1/\log \text{insulin } (\mu U/m) + \log \text{ fasting glucose (mg/dL)}$$

Patients with a QUICKI score of 0.33 or above are considered to have insulin resistance.

Aldosterone

If you have high blood pressure and insulin resistance, there's about a 10 percent chance that you have elevated aldosterone levels. Aldosterone is a hormone produced by the adrenal glands, and when produced in excessive amounts, causes high blood pressure and low potassium levels. Anyone who has both high blood pressure and low potassium (or is taking potassium supplements to keep her potassium level normal) should be tested for hyperaldosteronism. Diagnosis of the hormonal condition is imperative, because the cause can be a tumor in the adrenal gland that may need to be removed surgically. Even if a tumor is not present, knowing that hyperaldosteronism is present will guide your physician to use more appropriate medications.

Uric Acid

Insulin resistance causes elevations in uric acid, the substance that causes gout. I check a uric acid level in any patient in whom I suspect insulin resistance.

Liver Tests

Fatty liver disease is very common in patients with insulin resistance and can cause abnormal liver enzyme tests. Alanine transaminase (ALT), aspartate aminotransferase (AST), gamma-glutamyl transpeptidase (GGT), alkaline phosphatase, bilirubin, albumin, and prothrombin time are all tests of liver function.

Lipid Profile

A standard lipid profile includes total cholesterol, LDL cholesterol, HDL cholesterol, and triglycerides. The total cholesterol can be misleading because it measures both good and bad cholesterol and does not tell you how much of each. It is better to focus on the LDL and HDL cholesterol levels. Insulin resistance causes a typical pattern of low-HDL cholesterol and high triglycerides. This pattern is also an indication of your risk for cardiovascular disease. A person with an HDL level below 40 mg/dL is likely to have insulin resistance. A fasting triglyceride level above 150 mg/dL puts one at risk for insulin resistance. The ratio of triglycerides to HDL cholesterol is an excellent way to assess for insulin resistance. A ratio above 3 is high risk for insulin resistance.

In a standard lipid profile, the LDL cholesterol is not actually measured but is calculated using the following formula:

LDL cholesterol = Total Cholesterol × [HDL cholesterol + (Triglycerides*/5)]

Direct LDL measurement is available and is routinely done as part of advanced cholesterol testing. This testing gives a more detailed measurement of LDL and HDL cholesterol. There are two types of LDL cholesterol: small dense (known as pattern B) and large fluffy (known as pattern A). Although all LDL cholesterol is bad, the small dense LDL cholesterol is the most dangerous type of LDL cholesterol. Insulin resistance does not always increase LDL cholesterol, but it does cause an increase in the more dangerous small dense LDL particles.

There are two types of HDL cholesterol: HDL_2, and HDL_3. HDL_2 is the most protective from cardiovascular disease. Insulin resistance causes lower HDL_2 levels.

---

*This formula is not accurate when the triglyceride level is above 400 mg/dL.

Lipid Guidelines

Total Cholesterol

Desirable	Below 200 mg/dL
Borderline high	200–239 mg/dL
High	Above 240 mg/dL

HDL Cholesterol

High	60 mg/dL (higher is better)
Normal	40–60 mg/dL
Low	Below 40 mg/dL

LDL Cholesterol

Ideal	Below 70 mg/dL
Normal	70–100 mg/dL
Borderline high	100–130 mg/dL
High	130–160 mg/dL
Very high	Above 160 mg/dL

LDL Subtypes

Pattern A Less Dangerous Type (large fluffy particles)

Pattern A/B Intermediate Type (combination of particles)

Pattern B Most Dangerous Type (small dense particles)

Triglycerides

Ideal	Below 100 mg/dL
Normal	Below 150 mg/dL
High	150–199 mg/dL
Very high	200–499 mg/dL
Extremely high	Above 500 mg/dL
Danger of pancreatitis	Above 1000 mg/dL

Advanced lipid testing can also measure the proteins that carry cholesterol, known as *apolipoproteins*. Apo A or Apolipoprotein A is primarily found in the HDL particle and is a good way of assessing the body's ability to clear cholesterol from the blood. Apo B, also known as Apolipoprotein B, represents LDL cholesterol.

Plasminogen Activator Inhibitor-1

Plasminogen Activator Inhibitor-1 (PAI-1) is a blood clotting test that is often done in conjunction with advanced lipid testing. Insulin resistance is associated with an increased risk for blood clotting and elevations in PAI-1 levels. PAI-1 elevations are associated with an increased risk of cardiovascular disease.

Homocysteine

This is a toxic amino acid that increases the risk of blood clots and cardiovascular disease, even among people who have normal lipid profiles. High homocysteine levels can be the result of a deficiency of vitamin B_9, folic acid, or vitamin B_{12}. People with insulin resistance tend to have high homocysteine levels.

CRP Levels
Low risk: Below 1.0 mg/L (milligram/liter)
Average risk: 1.0–3.0 mg/L
High risk: Above 3.0 mg/L

C-Reactive Protein

The C-reactive protein (CRP) test is a measure of inflammation, which is a major feature of insulin resistance. CRP levels can be high from any type of inflammation—for example, when the body experiences injury, infection, or other stress. The CRP test is a very good test to predict future cardiovascular disease in otherwise healthy individuals.

Sex Hormone Binding Globulin

Sex hormone binding globulin (SHBG) is a blood protein that carries the sex hormones estrogen and testosterone in the bloodstream. For reasons that are not fully known, a decreased level of SHBG is associated with an increased risk for insulin resistance.

Cardiovascular Testing

Because insulin resistance is a major risk factor for cardiovascular disease, it is recommended that testing be done to screen for potential problems. Many tests are available, and the exact tests needed should be determined by your physician. Cardiovascular tests include electrocardiogram, echocardiogram, treadmill stress test, nuclear cardiac testing, cardiac CT (computerized axial tomography) scans, and carotid ultrasound.

Treating Insulin Resistance

Alleviating insulin resistance is a critical step toward achieving hormonal balance. Insulin resistance is not incurable. The solution to insulin resistance is a healthy diet and lifestyle. Even modest diet and lifestyle improvements can improve insulin resistance and dramatically lower your risk of getting complications like diabetes and cardiovascular disease. Although improved nutrition and increased physical activity are the best way to treat insulin resistance, other treatments, including supplements and medications, can improve insulin resistance and can treat many of the complications of insulin resistance, but they should not be a substitute for having a healthy lifestyle.

Lose Weight

Losing weight is the best way to alleviate insulin resistance. Insulin resistance always improves with weight loss. If you get down to a normal body weight, there is a very good chance that insulin resistance can be completely alleviated.

Balance Your Diet

To counter insulin resistance—and, by no coincidence, promote balanced nutrition—the Hormonal Health Diet is a balanced diet consisting of about 40 percent carbohydrates, 30 percent protein, and 30 percent fat. (Exact percentages aren't critical, as long as you're in the ballpark.) You should eat frequently throughout the day. Don't eat too much at one time.

Eat Slow Carbohydrates

Slow carbohydrates are the lower glycemic index/glycemic load foods that I discuss in chapter 3. Slow carbohydrates take a long time to be digested, so there are fewer insulin spikes and the body can absorb the energy from sugar gradually, which has a salutary influence on other body processes.

Eat Foods High in Potassium

Potassium is important for proper insulin action. Foods high in potassium include sweet potatoes, white potatoes, tomatoes, yogurt, clams, fish, carrots, bananas, spinach, watermelon, apricots, cantaloupe, peas, beans, and oranges.

Eat Fish High in Omega-3 Fatty Acids

The omega-3 fatty acids found in fish, eicosapentaenoic acid and docosahexaenoic acid, can help alleviate insulin resistance. Moreover, fish are a terrific source of protein. Eating fish can lower bad cholesterol and raise good cholesterol, and studies have shown that diets high in fish improve insulin resistance. The American Heart Association recommends eating fish twice a week.

Seafood High in Omega-3 Fatty Acids		
Anchovies	Oysters	Trout
Atlantic herring	Salmon	Tuna
Mackerel	Sardines	
Mussels	Snapper	

It's okay to take omega-3 fatty acid supplements, but you won't get the benefit of the protein from fish. Flaxseed contains a different omega-3 fatty acid, alpha-linolenic acid, which does not have the benefits of the omega-3 fatty acids in fish oil. I don't recommend flaxseeds as a substitute for fish.

Physical Activity

Physical activity is one of the best ways to alleviate insulin resistance. Even without weight loss, exercise can have a dramatic effect on lowering your level of insulin resistance. Physical activity reduces insulin resistance in part because it builds muscle. The more muscle you have, the more tissue you have to take up glucose, and the better your sensitivity to insulin.

Physical activity allows your body to handle blood glucose better. When you exercise, the muscles are not only stronger, but metabolically stronger. Exercise allows glucose to enter into the muscle more easily—and your insulin levels drop. Simply put, if you have two people of identical body weight, and one exercises and the other doesn't, the one who exercises will have lower insulin levels and less insulin resistance. Unfortunately, there's no magic pill, no as-seen-on-TV contraption that will take the place of a good solid workout. I recommend that you set a goal of getting 60–90 minutes of moderate-level physical activity every day. It's helpful, but not mandatory, to do a variety of types of physical activity over the course of a week.

Reduce Stress

Part of what makes contemporary Americans so susceptible to insulin resistance is our sedentary, comfortable lifestyle. We don't even get up to change the channel on the TV anymore—we simply click a button on a remote control.

Take One-Minute Walk Breaks

Exercise helps improve insulin resistance. However, it's not just the amount of time we spend exercising that matters. The amount of time we spend sitting down can also affect our health. Prolonged periods of sitting, even by those who exercise regularly, can increase insulin resistance and lower CRP levels. According to researchers from University of Queensland in Australia, taking short (1- to 2-minute) walk breaks during sedentary time has been shown to lower cardiometabolic inflammatory markers like CRP and improve insulin resistance and overall body weight.

Ironically, though, we're probably working harder than ever. In days past, we were allowed to take time to do our work, and if it didn't get done by the end of the day, we would always have tomorrow. Nowadays, with faxes, e-mail, and other forms of instant communication, not only do we not have the end of the day, we don't even have the end of the hour! No wonder we're so stressed: we don't exercise, we're trying to get things done yesterday, and there seems like there's more to do than ever.

When your body is physically or emotionally stressed, cortisol—the stress hormone—is released. Cortisol is a counter-insulin hormone, and thus it can undo much of the positive effects on blood sugar that exercise is having. I discuss stress and cortisol in more detail in chapter 11, but let me leave you with a piece of advice: take a hot bath. Taking a hot bath or sitting in a hot tub has also been shown to improve insulin resistance comparable to exercise training. Why? We don't know. But consider: warm water improves blood flow. Warm water relieves stress. A warm bath at bedtime improves sleep. Perhaps it's not so surprising that with all of these positives, warm water also improves insulin resistance.

Supplements for Insulin Resistance

People with insulin resistance may benefit from supplementation with certain vitamins, minerals, and herbs. The concern, however, is that most of

Daily Doses for Supplements for Insulin Resistance			
Alpha-lipoic acid	400–600 mg	Selenium	50 mcg
Biotin	30–100 mcg (micrograms)	Vanadium	25–50 mg
Calcium	1000–1500 mg	Vitamin B6	25–50 mg
Chromium	500–1000 mcg	Vitamin B12	500–1000 mcg
Folic acid	500–1000 mcg	Vitamin D	1000–5000 IU (International Units)
Iodine	500 mcg		
Omega-3 fish oil	2000–4000 mg	Vitamin E	400–600 IU twice daily

these remedies have not been adequately tested. The quality, purity, and potency of many products may be unreliable, since they are not well regulated by the U.S. Food and Drug Administration (FDA). The most important thing to know is that vitamins, minerals, and herbs are not a substitute for proper nutrition and physical activity and are usually not as potent as medications. Any diet should include a lot of foods high in vitamins, minerals, and antioxidants. Antioxidants are important for reducing inflammation and alleviating insulin resistance. I always recommend trying to get the bulk of your vitamins, minerals, and antioxidants from the foods that you eat, primarily from eating lots of vegetables and fruits. If your diet is lacking, you should add a supplement.

Biotin (Vitamin B₇)

This water-soluble B vitamin is essential for proper carbohydrate metabolism as well as cell growth and replication. Eating foods high in biotin or consuming biotin supplements enhances insulin sensitivity and increases the activity of enzymes necessary for proper carbohydrate metabolism; conversely, a biotin deficiency can cause insulin resistance or diabetes.

Most of us have plenty of biotin in our diets, however. Among the foods that contain biotin are brewer's yeast, egg yolks, whole grains, breads, fish, nuts, beans, meat, dairy products, lentils, peas, peanuts, walnuts, and molasses.

Chromium

This element—yes, the same one from which "chrome" in automobiles is made—is essential to our health. Without chromium, insulin doesn't work properly. Chromium is only required in trace amounts in the diet, but without those small amounts, people can suffer from chromium deficiency, which causes insulin resistance, impaired glucose tolerance, and overt diabetes. Doctors usually don't test for chromium deficiency because testing is unreliable. Maintaining chromium in the body is difficult. For one thing, we don't consume enough chromium-rich food; for another, chromium is easily passed out of the body in urine and sweat—even more easily if a person has high blood sugar or consumes high-glycemic index foods.

Foods high in chromium include brewer's yeast, beef, mushrooms, wheat germ, broccoli, hard cheese, chicken, shellfish—especially clams—corn oil, whole grain, and a variety of fruits. I highly recommend incorporating these foods into a diet, but chromium supplements (500–1000 mcg daily) can also be used. One word of caution: if you do not have chromium deficiency, chromium supplementation is unlikely to help. A 2011 study from Yale University School of Medicine concluded that if your chromium levels are already normal, supplementation does not lessen insulin resistance or reduce diabetes risk.

Moreover, biotin is a natural product of the bacteria in our intestines. The recommended daily allowance of biotin is 30 to 100 micrograms a day, a relatively miniscule amount. Alcohol raises the biotin requirement, as does estrogen. And food-processing techniques, such as canning and cooking, can destroy biotin.

Like the deficiency of any vitamin, a deficiency in biotin can cause a variety of ailments, not just insulin resistance. Symptoms include hair loss, scaly red rash around the nose and mouth, anemia, high cholesterol, loss of appetite, nausea, depression, sleeplessness, and hallucinations.

Cinnamon

Evidence varies as to whether or not cinnamon improves insulin resistance. If you want to try it, I recommend mixing half a teaspoon in yogurt or cottage

---

Vanadium

Another periodic table element, vanadium—ironically—was mistaken for a form of chromium when it was discovered in the early nineteenth century. One of the hardest of all metals, it is never found in a pure state, but always in a compound form with other elements. Scientists still aren't sure about the exact contribution of vanadium to our diet, but they know that vanadium deficiency can cause insulin resistance.

Though bodybuilders and people with diabetes have taken a form of vanadium, vanadyl sulfate, to improve the way insulin works, there isn't proof it does this. What vanadium probably does is mimic the action of insulin by turning on the insulin receptor. However, another form of the element, vanadate, is not recommended because of toxic effects ranging from anemia and green tongue to cataracts and death. Because of those toxic effects, I do not encourage taking vanadium supplements. I do support eating foods high in vanadium. These include beets, black pepper, buckwheat, carrots, dill, eggs, fish, milk, mushrooms, oats, olive oil, radishes, parsley, shellfish, soybeans, sunflower oil, and whole wheat.

---

cheese each day. There is also a product called cassia cinnamon that can be taken in doses of 1–6 grams daily.

Fiber

I recommend that you get at least 25–30 grams of fiber every day. Fiber is improves insulin resistance for several reasons. It adds volume and bulk to food without adding calories. It helps you feel and satisfied and stimulates release of the appetite-suppressing hormone cholecystokinin (see chapter 5). Fiber also lowers the glycemic index and glycemic load of foods, which slows the rate at which sugar hits your blood stream. The best sources of fiber are vegetables, fruits, and whole grains. High-fiber cereals and over-the-counter fiber supplements such as Metamucil, Citrucel, and Benefiber are another way to increase fiber but are not as good as eating a high-fiber diet.

Fish Oil Supplements

Fish oil supplements can be helpful for insulin resistance but are not the ideal source of omega-3 fatty acids. It is better to get omega-3 fatty acids from eating coldwater fish. If supplements are required, I recommend taking Lovaza (see page 139), a prescription formulation that is much more potent and pure than over-the-counter preparations.

Folic Acid (Vitamin B$_9$)

Folic acid helps prevent complications of insulin resistance like heart attacks and strokes by helping the body break down the toxic amino, homocysteine. Folic acid is found in whole grains, green leafy vegetables, nuts, avocados, bananas, and oranges. Many physicians recommend supplementation with up to 1000 micrograms of folic acid every day.

Garlic

Garlic has antioxidant properties and has been promoted to help lower cholesterol and blood pressure. A government study concluded that garlic doesn't do much for cholesterol but may have a modest effect in lowering blood pressure.

Myoinositol

Myoinositol supplementation has been shown to improve insulin resistance, cholesterol, and triglycerides. Patients in one study took 2 grams of myoinositol twice daily to see these improvements.

Niacin (Vitamin B$_3$)

High doses of niacin or a prescription formulation of niacin are used to treat the lipid abnormalities of insulin resistance. Niacin is considered ideal because it simultaneously corrects the three major lipid abnormalities: lowering LDL cholesterol and triglycerides while raising HDL cholesterol. Unfortunately, niacin can raise blood sugar levels and can worsen insulin resistance. Even though niacin is available over the counter, I recommend that you take it only under the supervision of a physician.

Red Yeast Rice

Red yeast rice supplements are used to lower cholesterol. It is not a surprise that they work, because statin medications are made by the same process of fermentation of rice with yeast. Some red yeast supplements have been found to contain up to 5 mg of statin per tablet. Many experts advise against red yeast rice because it can cause all the same side effects as regular statin medications without a reliable effect on cholesterol. I have had some patients who had side effects from statin medications but who were able to tolerate red yeast rice.

Vitamin E

Research from the Women's Health Study has shown that vitamin E appears to be helpful for people with insulin resistance because of its antioxidant effects, especially in those who are genetically deficient in natural antioxidants. About one-third of adults have a gene, known as "haptoglobin 2-2," that means they don't have a healthy effect from this naturally occurring antioxidant. Women in the study who had the haptoglobin 2-2 gene took 600 IU of vitamin E daily for ten years and had a 15 percent decreased risk for heart attacks and strokes. People without the gene did not show this effect. Other studies have shown a similar effect using 400 IU of vitamin E. Testing for the haptoglobin 2-2 gene is not routine, but it can be done if you ask your doctor for the test.

Vitamin E has also been shown to help reduce fat in the liver. Studies have shown that high-dose vitamin E supplementation can increase the risk for prostate cancer, so check with your doctor before taking this supplement.

White Mulberry Leaf

White mulberry leaf has become a popular supplement to treat insulin resistance. It is purported to prevent the digestion of carbohydrates, but there is not much evidence that it works.

Colon Cleansers

Colon cleansers are typically a mixture of herbs and laxatives. They are sometimes combined with probiotics to restore the healthy bacteria of the colon. There is no proof that colon cleansers are beneficial. Those that contain stimulant laxatives like senna or cascara can cause dehydration and mineral depletion.

Liver Cleansers

Liver cleansers usually contain milk thistle and are promoted to help clean out toxins, boost immunity, and help with weight loss. Milk thistle seems to be harmless, but there is no proof that liver cleansers do any good.

Medications to Treat Insulin Resistance and Its Complications

There are no drugs that are approved by the U.S. Food and Drug Administration for the treatment of insulin resistance. Many medications do alleviate insulin resistance as well as treat the manifestations and complications of insulin resistance. There is no perfect medication for insulin resistance. A drug that treats one aspect of insulin resistance may make another feature worse. The best way to have hormonal balance is to achieve a balance between the benefits a medication offers and its risk.

Medications are never a substitute for nutrition and physical activity. I tell my patients that you can out-eat any drug. When doctors use medications for insulin resistance, they have several goals in mind. Some medications can make insulin work more efficiently, lowering blood sugar and insulin levels, and can reduce the risk of diabetes. Medications that have weight loss as a side effect are also used to treat insulin resistance. Other medications prevent or treat cardiovascular disease, high blood pressure, lipid abnormalities, blood clotting, or inflammation. It's also important to treat other hormone problems associated with insulin resistance like PCOS and male hypogonadism.

Because insulin resistance is an underlying cause of type 2 diabetes, it is logical that diabetes medications are first-line treatments.

Types of Medications Used to Treat Insulin Resistance
Diabetes medications
Lipid medications
Blood pressure medications
Antidepressants
Other medications

Metformin (Glucophage, Glucophage XR, Fortamet, Glumetza, Riomet)

Metformin is the most common medication in the world prescribed for diabetes. It works mostly by reducing the liver's ability to make sugar. Metformin has weight loss as a side effect, but without improved nutrition and physical activity this effect is minimal. Metformin reduces the risk of cardiovascular disease and the risk of getting type 2 diabetes by as much as 45 percent. The original, short-acting version of metformin is better for weight loss and treating insulin resistance. The long-acting formulation is good for treating insulin resistance, can be taken once a day, and has fewer side effects. If the pills are too difficult to swallow, a liquid form, called Riomet, is available.

The most common side effects of metformin are nausea, diarrhea, and upset stomach, which occur in about one of four people who take it. These side effects are almost always temporary and subside in seven to ten days, but they can last for several weeks. To minimize side effects, start with the 500 mg tablet once a day with breakfast and gradually increase over several months. A fiber supplement can also be helpful for the side effect of diarrhea. The best dose for alleviating insulin resistance is 850 mg three times a day. It's important to take metformin with a substantial meal to minimize side effects. You should not drink alcohol while taking metformin. Metformin can cause problems in people who have severe infections or kidney or liver disease because of a rare but deadly side effect known as lactic acidosis. For the most part, however, metformin is a very safe drug.

Exenatide (Byetta) and Liraglutide (Victoza)

Exenatide and liraglutide are medications that work by imitating the actions of the incretin hormone, glucagon-like peptide-1 (GLP-1), which is discussed in chapter 5. These medications treat diabetes but also cause very significant weight loss. Nausea is a side effect because it slows down the digestive system, but the nausea is usually temporary. Rare cases of pancreatitis have been reported. There have also been reports of thyroid cancer in animals. Exenatide is taken as an injection twice a day; liraglutide is taken once a day and seems to be slightly more effective. A long-acting version of exenatide (Bydureon) is taken once a week.

Sitagliptin (Januvia), Saxagliptin (Onglyza) and Linagliptin (Tradjenta)

These medications, known as *gliptins* or *DPP-4 inhibitors,* work by prolonging the action of natural incretin hormones. They have a neutral effect on weight.

Pramlintide (Symlin)

Pramlintide was listed as experimental in the first edition of *Hormonal Balance.* Now approved, it works by mimicking amylin, a pancreatic hormone that regulates blood glucose. It is not widely used to treat insulin resistance, but it can help for people who have diabetes. Pramlintide is given as an injection. Nausea, vomiting, low blood sugar, or headache are all possible side effects.

Pioglitazone (Actos)

Pioglitazone is a diabetes medication known as a thiazolidinedione, glitizone, PPAR-gamma agonist, or simply *TZD*. TZDs make cells more sensitive to insulin by turning on and off genes. Pioglitazone improves insulin resistance and lowers blood sugar. Pioglitazone decreases triglycerides, raises good cholesterol levels, and shifts bad cholesterol from a dangerous, small dense type to a less dangerous, large fluffy type. There is still controversy, but it is thought that pioglitazone could reduce the risk of cardiovascular disease. It has also been used as a treatment for fatty liver disease. An interesting effect of pioglitazone is the ability to redistribute body fat, moving it from dangerous areas like the belly and vital organs to safer areas like the hips, buttocks, and under the skin.

Pioglitazone might seem like a perfect drug if it weren't for one pesky side effect: weight gain. Even though the pioglitazone improves insulin resistance, it does so by making your fat cells grow and multiply. This is why I don't recommend pioglitazone for most patients with insulin resistance. Fluid retention is a more serious side effect; it can result in swelling of the legs and can be responsible for some of the weight gain. Heart failure is a contraindication to the use of pioglitazone because there can be a worsening of symptoms due to fluid retention. There have been reports of fractures and bladder cancer caused by pioglitazone. The 15 mg dose of pioglitazone is best for treating insulin resistance because there is less weight gain and less fluid retention. The medication rosiglitazone (Avandia), also a thiazolidinedione, is not recommended because of studies linking it to an increased risk of heart attacks.

Lipid Medications

Lipid problems are a hallmark of insulin resistance, so it's not surprising that many people with insulin resistance take medications.

Statins: Atorvastatin (Lipitor), Pravastatin (Pravachol), Simvastatin (Zocor), Fluvastatin (Lescol, Lescol XL), Lovastatin (Mevacor, Altoprev, and Generics) and Rosuvastatin (Crestor), Pitavastatin (Livalo)

Statin medications are considered the best first choice for lowering cholesterol. That's because they have a proven track record of decreasing heart attacks and strokes as well as prolonging life.

Statins have been on the market since 1987. By 1994 they had been proven to prevent heart attacks in high-risk patients—those who had already had a first

---

How Aggressively Should Diabetes Be Treated?

In 2008, three landmark studies called ACCORD (Action to Control Cardiovascular Risk in Diabetes), ADVANCE (Action in Diabetes and Vascular Disease Controlled Evaluation), and the VADT (Veterans Affairs Diabetes Trial) showed an increased risk of dying in patients who had aggressive diabetes treatments. The results of these three major trials led the American Diabetes Association, the American Heart Association, and the American College of Cardiology to reexamine the recommendations for aggressive blood sugar management for patients with diabetes. Doctors still agree that treating diabetes is important, but we understand that low blood sugars can be just as harmful as high blood sugars. I recommend avoiding both high and low blood sugars and keeping the A_{1c} around 6.5–7 percent.

---

heart attack and those with very high cholesterol. In 2008, a study known as JUPITER showed that statins are also helpful for preventing a heart attack in patients without heart disease or high cholesterol. The patients who had high levels of C-reactive protein, a marker for insulin resistance and inflammation, cut their risk for a heart attack in half when they took a statin medication.

Insulin resistance causes the quality of LDL to shift to the dangerous small dense type. Statins help in insulin resistance because they improve the quality of LDL from the dangerous, small dense type to the less dangerous, large fluffy type. Statins have antioxidant properties that decrease inflammation and blood clotting. Statins dramatically reduce the risk of cardiovascular disease and can even reverse it. This is why statins are being prescribed more and more commonly and in higher doses than ever before.

The most common side effect is muscle problems that can range from mild aches and pains to severe muscle damage. Up to 10 percent of patients who take statin medications may experience some muscle pain or weakness. A test called CK (creatine kinase) can be done to determine whether the drug is causing muscle damage. Because statins have such tremendous health benefits, most physicians now recommend that you continue taking them if they are causing only mild muscle pain.

Pravastatin, rosuvastatin, and fluvastatin have fewer side effects and interactions than other statin medications. Some people use coenzyme Q10 for muscle pain caused by statins. Although there is no proof that it works, some of my patients have noticed an improvement taking 100 mg once or twice a day. Grapefruit and grapefruit juice increased the risk for muscle problems due to decreased metabolism of the statin medication. This is most common with, lovastatin, and simvastatin. Low vitamin D levels can also cause muscle pain. It is important to check your vitamin D levels before blaming a statin for muscle pain. Many of my patients who have been unable to take statins in the past have no side effects once vitamin D is replaced.

Inflammation of the liver is an infrequent side effect. Your doctor will need to monitor liver tests periodically. I have had many patients who were told they had elevated liver tests because of statin medications, when it turned out that fatty liver was the culprit.

Fibrates: Fenofibrate (Tricor, Lofibra, Antara, Triglide), Gemfibrozil (Lopid and Generics), Fenofibric Acid (Trilipix)

Known as *fibric acid derivatives* or *fibrates,* these medications are a good choice for patients with insulin resistance because they lower triglycerides and LDL cholesterol while boosting HDL cholesterol. Side effects are uncommon, but muscle problems or liver problems can occur. Fenofibric acid is an active metabolite of fenofibrate and is the newest medication in this class of drugs. Gemfibrozil, the oldest medication in this class, is the only one that has been shown to prevent heart disease.

Niacin (Niaspan)

Also known as *nicotinic* acid or *vitamin B_3,* niacin in high doses simultaneously treats multiple lipid abnormalities by lowering triglycerides and LDL cholesterol while raising HDL cholesterol. Regular niacin is available as an over-the-counter supplement but is very hard to take because the doses needed (usually 1000–2000 mg per day) almost always cause side effects of flushing, tingling, or redness of the skin. To reduce side effects, start with a low dose and gradually increase the dose over several months. The flushing can also be reduced by taking an aspirin and drinking a full glass of water one hour before taking niacin. The slow-release prescription formulation of niacin known as Niaspan is easier to take because there are fewer side effects, but there can still be significant flushing with this product.

A concern with niacin is that it can worsen insulin resistance and can raise blood sugar levels. For many people, the benefits can outweigh the risks, and niacin can be beneficial for an overall plan for health and wellness. Even though niacin is available without a prescription, it should be taken only under medical supervision.

Omega-3 Fatty Acids (Lovaza)

Lovaza is a prescription formulation of the omega-3 fatty acids approved for the treatment of high triglyceride levels. This substance, found naturally in coldwater fish, also improves insulin resistance. The prescription formulation is better than over-the-counter preparations because it is more potent and more pure.

Bile Acid Sequestrants: Colesevelam (WelChol), Cholestyramine (Questran, Questran Light), and Colestipol (Colestid)

These drugs, known as *bile acid sequestrants* or *bile acid resins,* lower LDL cholesterol by pulling it out of digestive juices, allowing it to pass in the stool. Colesevelam not only lowers cholesterol but can lower blood sugar as well. In 2008, colesevelam was given approval for the treatment of diabetes. Cholestyramine and colestipol come in granular form, in a packets or canisters, and are mixed with water. They are usually taken several times a day. Questran Light is a sugar-free version and is recommended for people with blood sugar problems. WelChol is a tablet taken once or twice a day. Bile acid resins can raise triglyceride levels. The most common side effect is constipation. Fiber supplementation and proper hydration help decrease constipation.

Ezetimibe (Zetia)

Ezetimibe lowers LDL cholesterol by blocking absorption of cholesterol from the intestines. Ezetimibe doesn't do much for triglycerides or HDL cholesterol. Side effects are rare, but there can be abdominal pain or diarrhea.

Blood Pressure Medications

High blood pressure is a major feature of insulin resistance that frequently requires treatment with medications. Some of these drugs can improve insulin resistance and can reduce the risk for diabetes and cardiovascular disease. Other blood pressure medications can slow metabolism and worsen insulin resistance.

The Ezetimibe Controversy

Do you remember those Vytorin ads touting the benefits of combining medications to treat high cholesterol? The commercials displayed an interesting character matched up with a plate of food in the same colors and design as the actor's ensemble. There are benefits, the ad explained, to treating cholesterol by treating the genetics as well as the food. The drug's makers claimed that two drugs were better than one. Important studies called ENHANCE and ARBITER 6-HALTS question the benefits of ezetimibe, one of the components of Vytorin. This was a big shock to physicians and patients. In the ENHANCE study, the combination of ezetimibe and simvastatin (sold as Vytorin) was compared to simvastatin alone. It turned out that cholesterol buildup in the arteries was no different between the two treatments, even though the combination drug was more potent at lowering cholesterol. The ARBITER 6-HALTS study showed that ezetimibe was inferior to niacin at preventing cholesterol accumulation. Researchers are working to under-stand these results and what they really mean. We don't really know if ezetimibe reduces heart attacks or saves lives. However, simvastatin and other statin drugs as well as niacin are proven to do just this.

A 2008 ezetimibe study published in the *New England Journal of Medicine* suggested that it may increase the risk for a variety of cancers including prostate, colon, and skin cancers. Death from cancer was more common in patients who took ezetimibe. We don't know if the increased cancer is truly an effect of ezetemibe or something else. One theory is that ezetemibe increases risk because it not only blocks the absorption of cholesterol but it also blocks the absorption of other cancer-fighting substances.

Most experts, including the American College of Cardiology, recommend that statin drugs are the best first approach for fighting cholesterol; and to use other medications like niacin, fibrates, colesevelam, cholestyramine, and omega-3 fatty acids as the next line of defense. Ezetimibe should be reserved as a last resort.

ACE Inhibitors: Ramapril (Altace), Perindopril (Aceon), Trandolapril (Mavik), Lisinopril (Zestril), Benazepril (Lotensin) and Quinapril (Accupril), Enalapril (Vasotec), Captopril (Capoten)

ACE, or angiotensin-converting enzyme inhibitors slow the production of a hormone that raises blood pressure. ACE inhibitors are good at lowering blood pressure, but the benefits of this class of drugs go far beyond this effect. They have been shown to reduce the risk for diabetes, kidney disease, and cardio-vascular disease. This is why ACE inhibitors are one of the best medications for people with insulin resistance. To get the protective effects from an ACE inhibitor, the maximum dose is needed. One side effect is high potassium levels, so potassium should be monitored a few weeks after starting an ACE inhibitor. Other side effects include dry cough, fatigue, or headache. In rare cases a serious allergic reaction can cause lip and tongue swelling with sudden trouble in swallowing or breathing.

Angiotensin Receptor Blockers (ARBs): Losartan (Cozaar), Valsartan (Diovan), Ibesartan (Avapro), Candesartan (Atacand), Olmesartan (Benicar)

ARBs—angiotensin receptor blockers—work on the same hormone system as ACE inhibitors but work by blocking the receptor for the same blood pressure-raising hormone. These drugs tend to be better at lowering blood pressure than ACE inhibitors. The beneficial effects of ARBs are similar to those of ACE inhibitors. Side effects are rare, but high potassium levels are sometimes seen. There is debate about whether ARBs cause cancer, but many experts feel the potential risk is very small, if it even exists. There is a risk for elevated potassium; however, most patients don't experience any side effects.

Aliskiren (Tekturna)

Aliskiren is a new blood pressure medication known as a *direct renin inhibitor.* It works by blocking the effects of the hormone renin, which is produced by the kidney and activates an important cascade of hormones known as the RAAS (renin-angiotensin-aldosterone system). The ultimate effect of aliskiren is similar to ACE inhibitors and angiotensin receptor blockers. Aliskiren should not be combined with ARBs or with ACE inhibitors.

Carvedilol (Coreg)

This medication is a second-generation beta-blocker medication. Carvedilol is a unique version called an alpha-beta-blocker that tends to improve insulin resistance when other beta-blocker medications make insulin resistance worse. Side effects include fatigue, slow heart beat, or difficulty breathing.

Potassium-Sparing Diuretics: Spironolactone (Aldactone), Amilioride (Midamor) and Triamterine (Dyrenium), Eplerenone (Inspra)

Low potassium causes insulin resistance, so these mild diuretics help by lowering blood pressure and raising potassium levels. Side effects can include liver problems or elevation of potassium levels. Potassium levels and liver tests should be monitored at regular intervals.

Antidepressants

Most antidepressants affect your weight in one way or another. This is because the brain chemicals related to depression—serotonin, norepinephrine, and dopamine—are the same brain chemicals that help regulate appetite. (See chapter 5 for more information.) Although some antidepressants cause weight gain, others cause weight loss. The effect of antidepressants on weight is variable and the effect can differ from one person to another. It is thought that antidepressants that may improve insulin resistance if they make you lose weight. But depression itself raises cortisol levels that can also cause insulin resistance, so treating the depression improves insulin resistance as well.

Venlafaxine (Effexor, Effexor XR), Desvenlafaxine (Pristiq), Duloxetine (Cymbalta), Milnacipran (Savella)

These medications are used to treat depression, anxiety, chronic pain, and fibromyalgia. They work by increasing levels of serotonin and norepinephrine in the brain. The effect is decreased appetite and weight loss. This class of medications usually takes two to three weeks to start working. Desvenlafaxine has less of a weight loss effect than venlafaxine. The brand-name Effexor XR capsules seem to be more effective than the generic venlafaxine extended-release tablets. The most common side effects are high blood pressure, rapid heartbeat, and insomnia. It is recommended that you have your blood pressure monitored regularly while taking these medications. These drugs can also cause "withdrawal" syndrome if discontinued abruptly. I have had many patients who have had a difficult time discontinuing these medications. If you need to stop taking any of these medications, you should taper the drug slowly, under the supervision of your physician.

Bupropion (Wellbutrin, Wellbutrin SR, Wellbutrin XL, Aplenzin)

Bupropion is a unique type of antidepressant that affects several brain chemicals, including dopamine and norepinephrine, and is well known to cause weight loss. Bupropion works by decreasing appetite and increasing metabolism. There have also been reports that bupropion can increase libido. Side effects of bupropion are related to its stimulant actions and include agitation, insomnia, and in rare cases, seizures. Very few of my patients seem to experience side effects from bupropion. Wellbutrin SR (sustained release) is supposed to be taken twice a day. Wellbutrin XL (extended release) and Aplenzin are newer versions, designed for once-daily use. Bupropion is also in Zyban, which is used to help people quit smoking.

Other Medications

Zonisamide (Zonegran) and Topiramate (Topamax)

These medications are used to treat seizures, chronic pain, and migraine headaches and are sometimes prescribed for weight loss because they can decrease appetite and prevent overeating. The exact way these medications work is unknown, but they are thought to have effects on appetite control centers as well as improving insulin and leptin resistance. Topiramate is especially helpful in reducing episodes of binge eating and nighttime eating. A dose of 200 mg or more of topiramate is most effective for weight loss, but it is recommended to start with a low dose and slowly increase the dose over several weeks. My experience is that many patients who have tried these medications never took a high enough dose to get any significant weight loss. Unfortunately, the higher doses that are more effective for weight loss also increase the likelihood of side effects like tingling of the hands, kidney stones, tiredness, and memory problems.

Aspirin

Insulin resistance increases the risk of blood clotting and cardiovascular disease. This is why the current recommendation is that anyone with insulin resistance should take a baby aspirin (81 mg) every day.

Orlistat (Xenical, Alli)

Orlistat works by slowing or blocking the digestion of fat. This results in about a third of the fat from the diet being passed in the stool. The typical weight loss with Orlistat is about 25 pounds in six months. The most common side effect is oily diarrhea. This can be minimized by eating a low-fat diet and by taking a fiber supplement. Orlistat has the risk of blocking the absorption of fat-soluble vitamins A, D, E, and K. I have seen a few patients who had severe vitamin D deficiency from taking Orlistat.

Phentermine (Adipex) and Diethylpropion (Tenuate)

Phentermine is a weight loss medication that was the part of the "Phen-Fen" combination. Phentermine is only approved for short-term use, and people who take it routinely gain back all the weight they lose (or even more) after it is discontinued. Phentermine and diethylpropion can cause agitation, insomnia, and elevated heart rate and blood pressure. For all of these reasons, I do not recommend taking phentermine or diethylproprion.

Medications That Worsen Insulin Resistance

In order to achieve hormonal balance, it's important, whenever possible, to avoid medications that can intensify insulin resistance. Medications can make insulin resistance worse for a variety of reasons.

Growth Hormone

Growth hormone deficiency results in loss of lean body mass, which causes insulin resistance. Growth hormone is considered a counter-insulin hormone because it can raise blood sugar, but the long-term effect is to lower insulin resistance. This is because growth hormone replacement therapy increases lean body mass and decreases fat mass. For more information, see chapter 12.

Corticosteroids

Common medications include prednisone, hydrocortisone, dexamethasone, and methylprednisolone and work by mimicking the action of the hormone cortisol. Excessive cortisol causes severe insulin resistance, massive weight gain, and promotes fat accumulation and muscle loss. Corticosteroids can cause diabetes and can increase the risk of cardiovascular disease and other ailments. For more information, see chapter 11.

Sulfonylureas: Glyburide (DiaBeta), Glipizide (Glucotrol), and Glimepiride (Amaryl)

This class of drugs treats type 2 diabetes by stimulating the pancreas to produce insulin. They work great for blood sugar but make insulin resistance worse. Weight gain is a common side effect of sulfonylureas.

Diuretics: Furosemide (Lasix), Torsemide (Demadex), Bumetanide (Bumex), Indapamide (Lozol), and Hydrochlorothiazide (HCTZ, Microzide, Hydrodiuril), Chlorothiazide (Diuril)

Diuretics cause loss of potassium in the urine. When potassium is deficient from the body, insulin resistance gets worse. If you take diuretics, potassium supplementation is helpful.

Synthetic Progestins: Medroxyprogesterone (Provera), Norethindrone Acetate (Aygestin), Megestrol (Megace), Micronor, Nor-QD, Ovrette, Depo-Provera and Norplant, as well as birth control pills that contain levonorgestrel, norgestrel, or norethindrone

Progestins have high androgenic activity and have side effects like acne and bloating, weight gain, and elevated blood sugars. See chapter 8 for more information.

Beta-Blockers: Propanolol (Inderal), Metoprolol (Toprol), and Atenolol (Tenormin)

Although sometimes necessary to treat other conditions like high blood pressure, congestive heart failure, and abnormal heart rhythms, these medications can slow metabolism and worsen insulin resistance.

HIV Medications: Nelfinavir (Viracept), Ritonavir (Norvir), Saquinavir (Invirase, Fortovase), Tipranavir (Aptivus)

These life-saving drugs, known as *protease inhibitors,* cause severe insulin resistance and diabetes. They also cause a variant of insulin resistance known as HIV lipodystrophy, in which people have many of the physical features seen with cortisol excess.

Antidepressants

Some antidepressants increase appetite and have weight gain as a side effect. The same brain chemicals involved in depression also regulate appetite (see chapter 5 for more information). Older antidepressants, such as amitriptyline and nortriptyline, frequently cause massive weight gain. Mirtazapine (Remeron) is also notorious for increasing appetite and causing weight gain. Antidepressants like as Fluoxetine (Prozac), Sertraline (Zoloft), Paroxetine (Paxil, Paxil CR), Citolopram (Celexa), and Escitalopram (Lexipro) have variable effects on weight.

Antiseizure Medications: Carbamazepine (Tegretol), Lamotrigine (Lamictal), Lacosamide (Vimpat), and Gabapentin (Neurontin), Pregabalin (Lyrica), Valproate (Depakote)

Many antiseizure medications can increase insulin resistance and cause weight gain and sedation. The medications are sometimes used to treat chronic pain, migraine headaches, psychiatric disorders, or other conditions. Researchers from Innsbruck Medical University found that women are more susceptible to gain weight, possibly due to increased carbohydrate cravings and leptin resistance. Oftentimes an alternative medication can be substituted if weight gain is experienced. Topiramate (Topamax) and zonisamide (Zonegran) are best for weight loss. Felbamate (Felbatol), levetricetam (Keppra), oxcarbazepine (Trileptal), and phenytoin (Dilantin) tend to have a neutral effect on weight. I've had many patients who have an atypical response to these medications, gaining or losing weight where the opposite would be expected.

Typical Weight Effects of Antiseizure Medications		
Weight Gain	**Weight Neutral**	**Weight Loss**
Carbamazepine	Felbamate	Topiramate
Gabapentin	Levetiracetam	Zonisamide
Lamotrigine	Oxcarbazepine	
Lacosamide	Phenytoin	
Pregabalin		
Valproate		

Antipsychotic Medications: Olanzapine (Zyprexa), Risperidone (Risperdal), Paliperidone (Invega), Clozapine (Clozaril), Iloperidone (Fanapt), Paliperidone (Invega), and Quetiapine (Seroquel)

These drugs can cause massive weight gain, insulin resistance, and diabetes and have been devastating for people with mental illness. Aripiprazole (Abilify) and ziprasidone (Geodon) are similar medications that have a smaller effect on blood sugar and body weight.

Antihistamines

Older antihistamines like diphenhydramine and other antihistamines that make you sleepy can also worsen insulin resistance and cause weight gain. These antihistamines are a common ingredient in many over-the-counter allergy medications and sleep aids.

Chapter Review

Insulin resistance is one of the major complications of obesity and occurs when your body is not able to listen to insulin's signals to take sugar out of the blood. The condition is also associated with leptin resistance, discussed in chapter 5.

Insulin resistance is a complex disorder and is the root cause of diseases such as diabetes, PCOS, sleep apnea, liver disease, high blood pressure, cardiovascular disease, and many other health problems. Since your body makes more insulin to overcome insulin resistance, alleviating insulin resistance is the best way to establish hormonal balance that will lower blood sugar and ultimately reduce the risk for the many diseases associated with insulin resistance.

In addition to the lifestyle factors related to insulin resistance—including the lack of exercise and stress—the chapter discussed the condition's link to a family history of diabetes and obesity as well as the risks associated with certain ethnic backgrounds. Moreover, the chapter pointed out a number of other factors related to insulin resistance, including vitamin deficiencies, causes related to life stages (puberty, menopause), as well as medical conditions such as high blood pressure and cardiovascular disease. The chapter noted that cardiovascular disease is the number one cause of death among people with insulin resistance.

While no perfect, widely available insulin resistance test is available, a number of reliable indicator tests were discussed, such as tests that measure the amount of protein in the urine or tests for elevated levels of uric acid in the bloodstream.

Insulin resistance is most effectively controlled through diet and changes in lifestyle. The chapter detailed some key ways to control the condition, including eating slow carbohydrates, eating foods high in potassium such as bananas and spinach, and consuming fish and some specific dairy products. Increasing exercise and reducing stress, taking certain vitamin supplements, and increasing fiber in the diet also help with controlling the condition.

Finally, the chapter discussed potential treatments for insulin resistance and noted that no FDA-approved treatments exist. However, some medications are helpful to those with insulin resistance and include a number of lipid medications that are usually taken to lower cholesterol. Some blood pressure and antidepressant medications were also noted to have a positive impact on managing and controlling appetite and weight.

The next chapter discusses the potential weight gain issues associated with the thyroid gland and potential treatments.

CHAPTER

7

Boost Metabolism
with Thyroid Hormone

It is a small, butterfly-shaped, brownish-red organ located at the base of the neck. It weighs only about an ounce and produces relatively small amounts of two potent hormones. This small structure, the thyroid gland, and the hormones it produces have a wide-ranging impact on your health and your weight—an impact that is often misunderstood or ignored. The thyroid controls metabolism and therefore plays a major role in body weight regulation. Low thyroid, or hypothyroidism, causes weight gain or makes it difficult to lose weight, even with vigorous exercise and the right diet.

The thyroid helps maintain organ function, brain function, body temperature, sleep, energy level, sex drive, mood, and much more. Many people struggle with a wide variety of symptoms and don't know the symptoms are caused by their thyroid. It is easy to overlook the effects of a dysfunctional thyroid gland because the symptoms can come on slowly and are often blamed on old age, stress, or depression.

The Facts about Thyroid Disease

Thyroid disease is the third most common disease in America. According to the American Association of Clinical Endocrinologists, thyroid disease

In This Chapter

- ▶ How Thyroid Health and Weight Gain Are Linked
- ▶ Diagnosing and Treating Abnormal Thyroid Hormone Levels
- ▶ Diseases That Affect the Thyroid
- ▶ Healthy Thyroid Lifestyle Choices

affects one in ten people—more than 30 million Americans. Roughly half are undiagnosed. Thyroid disease can affect anyone at any age, but it is more likely to develop as you get older. Women are ten times more likely to get thyroid disease than men. It is also more common during pregnancy or in the year after having a baby. The immune system, stress, nutritional deficiencies, medications, and exposure to radiation and toxins can damage the thyroid gland.

When weight problems begin, many people suspect that the thyroid gland may be at fault. They may have noticed other symptoms, such as fatigue, diminished sex drive, mood swings, constipation, dry skin, hair loss, or feeling cold, but even the best doctors can have a hard time diagnosing thyroid disease. The doctor may perform the standard thyroid stimulating hormone (TSH) test and proclaim the thyroid is normal. As an endocrinologist, I see this result all the time. Many of my patients have been told that their thyroid was not causing their weight problem because their blood tests were normal, but I've seen cases where the thyroid still was the culprit. Once treated, some of these patients lost a lot of weight without a major change in their diets or exercise routines.

Forty percent of overweight Americans have thyroid dysfunction. Many people suffer for years before getting diagnosed. Without a diagnosis and treatment that addresses the thyroid, many patients—who otherwise could have been well on their way to better health—may have painfully slow metabolisms, and slow metabolism is something no diet can cure. In my experience as an endocrinologist, I have seen several situations when the thyroid hinders weight loss. These include the following:

- Undiagnosed thyroid disease

- Improperly treated or undertreated thyroid disease

- Unaddressed issues affecting the thyroid gland

- Mistakenly blaming the thyroid when the thyroid is normal and other issues are the problem

This chapter will help you figure out whether a thyroid problem is affecting your weight, and if so what you can do about it.

Important Thyroid Terms

Central hypothyroidism: Condition in which pituitary or brain problems result in diminished thyroid hormone production because of inadequate production of TSH

Graves' disease: Most common cause of hyperthyroidism, caused by the immune system mistakenly stimulating the thyroid gland

Hashimoto's thyroiditis: Most common cause of hypothyroidism, caused when the immune system mistakenly attacks the thyroid gland

Hyperthyroidism: Condition in which the thyroid gland produces excess thyroid hormone

Hypothyroidism: Condition in which the thyroid gland produces inadequate amounts of thyroid hormone

Iodide: The activated form of iodine when processed by thyroid peroxidase

Iodine: Trace element used by the body to make thyroid hormones

Myxedema: Long-standing untreated hypothyroidism that results in the swelling of organs and tissues throughout the body

Myxedema coma: End stage thyroid failure with 50 percent fatality rate

Reverse T3 (rT3) Inactive form of thyroid hormone overproduced during stress

Thyroglobulin: Protein that provides tyrosine to make thyroid hormones and is frequently the source of attack in autoimmune thyroid disease

Thyroid gland: Organ in the neck that produces thyroid hormones

Thyroid hormone receptor: On/off switch responding to T3, located on cells throughout the body

Thyroid peroxidase (TPO): Enzyme that converts iodine to iodide and is frequently the source of attack in autoimmune thyroid disease

Thyroid stimulating hormone: Thyroid-controlling hormone produced by the pituitary gland

Thyroxine (T4): Inactive form of thyroid hormone

Triiodothyronine (T3): Active form of thyroid hormone

Tyrosine: Amino acid that forms the backbone of thyroid hormones

Your Weight Doesn't Need to Be Held Captive by Your Thyroid

Many of my patients have been told they don't have thyroid problems, or they are taking thyroid medications yet they still can't lose weight. Many of these patients have undiagnosed or improperly treated thyroid problems. Undiagnosed thyroid dysfunction or improperly treated hypothyroidism can be related to:

Diagnosis and dosing that relies too heavily on the TSH blood test

Subclinical thyroid disease

Taking an incorrect dosage of thyroid medication

Taking the wrong type of thyroid medication

Needing to take a combination of thyroid medications

Taking the medication incorrectly or occasionally forgetting

Gluten intolerance

Bowel problems impairing medication absorption

Low-quality medication, fluctuating hormone levels

Stress, inflammation, or immune system issues

Health issues impairing thyroid hormone activation (T4:T3 conversion)

Nutrient deficiencies

Thyroid toxins

How the Body Makes Thyroid Hormones

The thyroid gland does only one thing: it makes thyroid hormones. There two types of thyroid hormones: triiodothyronine (T3) and thyroxine (T4). (See Figure 7.1.) The 3 and the 4 refer to the number of iodine molecules attached to the hormone. T4 is considered a storage hormone. T3 is the active form of thyroid hormone and is primarily responsible for the vast array of biological processes attributed to the thyroid gland. A healthy balance is about 80 percent T4 and 20 percent T3.

Iodine is the key ingredient of thyroid hormones and makes the thyroid unique. The thyroid gland is the only organ in the body that uses iodine. Iodine, element 53 on the periodic table, is a dark gray to purple-black solid that is used

What Can Go Wrong with the Thyroid?

The rate of thyroid disease is expected to double over the next twenty years because of increased toxins and radiation in our environment.

Autoimmune attack of thyroid peroxidase (prevents iodine activation)

Autoimmune attack of thyroglobulin (provides tyrosine for hormone backbone)

Iodine deficiency

Iodine excess

Pituitary or hypothalamic disease

Thyroid injury from toxins or radiation

T4:T3 conversion problems (illness, inflammation, selenium deficiency, zinc deficiency)

Thyroid hormone resistance

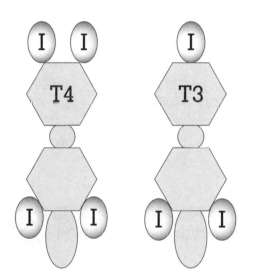

Figure 7.1   T4 and T3

T4 is the main hormone produced by the thyroid gland and is an inactive storage hormone. T4 is converted to the active form, T3, when iodine is removed from the top ring. T3 binds to thyroid hormone receptors located throughout the body, like a key that opens a lock to activate organ systems, boost metabolism, and energize cells.

Testing for Iodine Deficiency

Testing for iodine deficiency is very difficult, rarely necessary, and rarely done. The best test is the twenty-four-hour urine iodine test, which requires collecting urine in a container that is sent to a specialized laboratory. Some practitioners advocate applying topical povidone-iodine to the skin and observing the absorption into the skin as a method of assessing iodine status. This method is not considered accurate and is not recommended.

in a wide variety of products, including preservatives, food coloring, antiseptics, medications, and even photographic chemicals. The thyroid needs just the right amount of iodine, 150-500 micrograms (mcg) each day. Too much or too little iodine can cause thyroid problems. Iodine deficiency results in a goiter—swelling of the thyroid—along with decreased thyroid hormone production and increased risk for thyroid nodules and thyroid cancer.

If the thyroid gland gets too much iodine, it shuts down, resulting in low thyroid hormone levels. I've seen this situation with patients who take iodine supplements for more than a few weeks. The ironic part is that most people take these supplements for thyroid health.

Sometimes a different consequence of iodine overload—iodide-induced hyperthyroidism—occurs. The effect is like spraying a fire with gasoline: huge

Iodine around the World

Most industrialized countries have plenty of iodine, but the same is not necessarily true for the rest of the world. Millions of people worldwide are iodine deficient, resulting in widespread thyroid dysfunction and birth defects. Since 1990, the World Health Organization has focused on reducing iodine deficiency in underdeveloped nations.

> ### Too Little or Too Much Iodine
> ### Can Make Your Thyroid and Your Body Sick
>
> *Iodine toxicity* is a severe reaction from exposure to very high amounts of iodine.
>
> *Jode-Basedow disease* occurs when excessive iodine results in increased thyroid hormone production (hyperthyroidism).
>
> *Wolff-Chaikoff disease* occurs when excessive iodine results in decreased thyroid hormone production (hypothyroidism).

amounts of thyroid hormone are produced, resulting in hyperthyroidism. If the body is exposed to massive amounts of iodine, a person can develop headaches, vomiting, mouth sores, a metallic taste in the mouth, swollen salivary glands, or a rash.

Iodine is processed in the thyroid gland by a chemical, thyroid peroxidase, converting it into a bioactive form that binds with an amino acid, tyrosine. Tyrosine is found in many sorts of protein, such as turkey, soy, dairy products, pumpkin seeds, and almonds. It is important to get enough tyrosine in your diet, but tyrosine supplements are not necessary.

Two tyrosines link to form the double-ring structure of all thyroid hormones. A specialized protein known as thyroglobulin provides the tyrosine for this process. (See Figure 7.2.)

A Misdirected Immune System

Thyroid disease is often caused by a dysfunctional immune system that mistakenly attacks the thyroid gland. This condition, known as Hashimoto's thyroiditis, is the number one cause of thyroid disease. Autoimmune diseases include a wide range of disorders in which a body's immune system attacks its own healthy tissue. A combination of genes and environmental factors (such as stress, excess body weight, or exposure to certain viruses or environmental toxins) determines who is susceptible to developing an autoimmune disease.

People with thyroid disease are at risk for other immune system problems, too, such as type 1 diabetes, pernicious anemia, Addison's disease, or premature

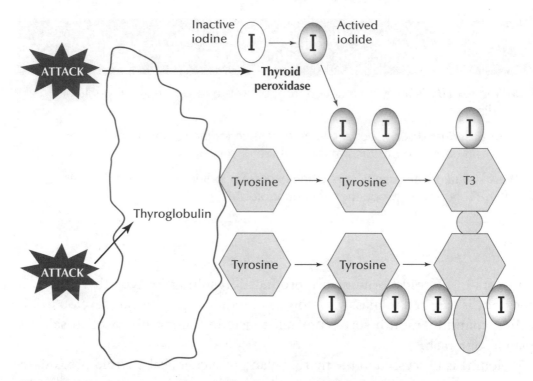

Figure 7.2 Autoimmune Attack of Key Thyroid Components

Thyroid peroxidase and thyroglobulin are extremely susceptible to attack by the immune system. Ninety percent of patients with thyroid dysfunction have thyroid peroxidase and/or thyroglobulin antibodies in their blood. When thyroid peroxidase and thyroglobulin aren't working at full capacity, iodine and tyrosine can't be used to make thyroid hormones.

ovarian failure. More than sixty autoimmune disorders have been described. The following are the most common autoimmune disorders seen in patients with autoimmune thyroid disease:

Addison's disease (see chapter 11)	Crohn's disease
Alopecia areata	Goodpasture's syndrome
Autoimmune hepatitis	Hypoparathyroidism
Celiac disease	Idiopathic pulmonary fibrosis

Being Overweight Can Trigger a Thyroid Problem

Everyone knows that having a low thyroid can make you gain weight, but did you know that the reverse is also true? Studies have shown a link between being overweight and lower thyroid hormone levels. When you are overweight, the thyroid gets a double whammy. This one-two punch decreases both the production and activation of thyroid hormones and can lead to permanent thyroid dysfunction.

First, excess fat in the body produces chemicals that fuel inflammation and stimulate the immune system to attack the thyroid mistakenly. In fact, being overweight can overstimulate the immune system, resulting in a variety of medical problems. When the immune system attacks the thyroid gland, the damage is usually permanent, so losing weight may not fix the problem.

In addition, inflammation chemicals produced by fat cells impair T4:T3 conversion, which prevents proper thyroid hormone activation, so losing weight and becoming healthier can help the body process thyroid hormones more efficiently.

Male hypogonadism (see chapter 10)

Multiple sclerosis

Myasthenia gravis

Pernicious anemia

Premature ovarian failure (see chapter 8)

Primary biliary sclerosis

Raynaud's syndrome

Rheumatoid arthritis

Scleroderma

Systemic lupus erythematosus (also known as *lupus*)

Temporal arteritis /Giant cell arteritis

Thrombocytopenic purpura

Type 1 diabetes

Urticaria

Vasculitis

Vitiligo

Wegener's granulomatosis

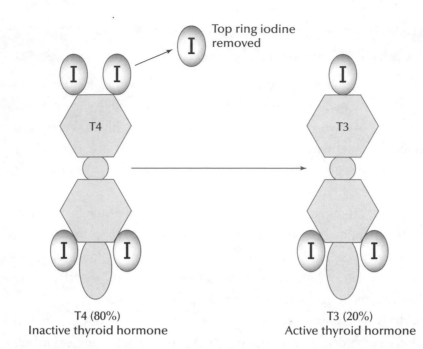

Figure 7.3   **Active Thryoid Hormone Is Produced by Removal of the Top Ring Iodine**

Most of the T4:T3 conversion is done throughout the body, so you don't need a working thyroid gland to convert T4 to T3. You do, however, need a healthy body. Many people have problems converting their T4 into active T3, which can result in lingering symptoms and difficulty losing weight. The body can produce an inactive form of thyroid hormone, known as reverse T3, when the wrong iodine molecule is removed from T4.

Creating Active Thyroid Hormones—T4:T3 Conversion

The thyroid gland produces mostly T4, which is an inactive storage hormone. T4 is also the main form of thyroid hormone replacement, given as the medication levothyroxine, because the body naturally converts T4 into T3—known as *T4 to T3 (T4:T3) conversion*—at a rate that is most appropriate for the body's health. If the body is healthy, it produces T3 efficiently, but if the body is sick, T3 conversion is impaired.

For T4 to become properly activated, an iodine molecule must be

Autoimmune Thyroid Disease

If the immune system causes an underactive thyroid, it is known as Hashimoto's disease. If it causes an overactive thyroid, it is known as Graves' disease.

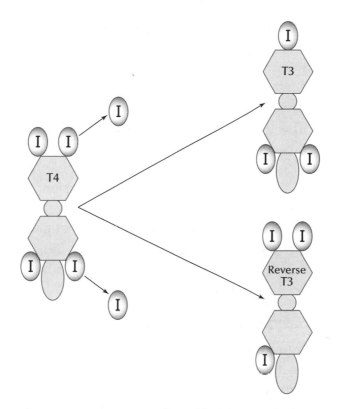

Figure 7.4 Inactive Reverse T3 Is Produced by Removal of the Bottom Ring Iodine

removed from the top tyrosine ring. This process is vital to optimal thyroid hormone balance. The three-iodine version, triiodothyronine, or T3, is the active form of thyroid hormone that must be maintained at a specific level in balance with T4. (See Figures 7.3 and 7.4.)

Stress and inflammation cause the most common T4:T3 conversion problems. Stress, whether psychological or physical, increases inflammation hormones known as *cytokines,* and cytokines impair the iodine removal process and cause T4:T3 conversion problems. Physical illness of any type can inhibit T4:T3 conversion. In chapter 5, I explain how being overweight makes fat cells overproduce a variety of hormones, including inflammatory cytokines.

Healthy Body = Healthy Thyroid

T4:T3 conversion problems with removing iodine or removing the wrong iodine molecule from T4 can lead to thyroid hormone imbalance.

The chemical responsible for removing iodine from T4 requires the elements selenium and zinc. A deficiency of either of these minerals can cause problems converting inactive T4 to active T3. Too much copper in the diet can also block the conver-

> **Minerals Important for Thyroid Hormone Conversion**
>
> Selenium, zinc, and copper are important minerals for T4 to T3 conversion.

sion process. Beta-blocker medications (propanolol, atenolol, and others) and the medication amiodarone can inhibit the T4 to T3 conversion process as well.

Thyroid hormones stimulate virtually every biological process in the body, increasing metabolism, stabilizing body temperature, supporting neurotransmitters, and assisting in organ, muscle, and brain function. Just like other hormones, active thyroid hormone stimulates a receptor, which then goes on to give a cell a message. When it comes to thyroid hormone, the message is *activate!*

Do You Have Hypothyroidism?

Hypothyroidism, or low thyroid, can result in a long list of symptoms, from hair loss to painful joints to dry skin as well as dozens of others. These symptoms usually start subtly and are mild. They may not concentrate in a specific part of the body. Symptoms may be disregarded or attributed to other causes, such as old age, fibromyalgia, menopause, depression, or life stress. The symptoms of hypothyroidism occur because of the body's effort to compensate for a lack of thyroid hormone—too little fuel to run the body's metabolism. As time goes on, symptoms become more and more obvious. Symptoms of hypothyroidism can vary tremendously, depending on the characteristics of the person who has it. One common feature of hypothyroidism, however, is weight gain.

About 2 to 4 percent of the population has severe hypothyroidism, but 7 to 15 percent of the population—and maybe more—suffers from mild or moderate hypothyroidism. Early stage hypothyroidism is known as *mild thyroid failure* or *subclinical hypothyroidism.* During this phase, the symptoms may be mild or nonexistent but are sometimes more severe. In my experience, if a patient is generally healthy, symptoms tend to be milder than those of patients who have other health problems.

The decision about precisely when to start thyroid hormone replacement remains controversial. Most endocrinologists advocate starting low-dose thyroid hormone replacement therapy during the early phase of hypothyroidism, because it reduces symptoms, lowers cholesterol and blood pressure, and reduces the risk of cardiovascular disease.

Risk Factors

Your risk for thyroid disease is increased if

You are female.

You are over forty.

You are overweight.

You are pregnant or recently had a baby.

You are infertile or have had a miscarriage.

You are menopausal or perimenopausal.

You have diabetes.

You have polycystic ovary syndrome (PCOS).

You have a pituitary gland problem.

You had a head injury in the past.

You have mitral valve prolapse.

You have carpal tunnel syndrome or plantar fasciitis.

You have celiac disease or gluten intolerance.

You have depression.

You have chronic fatigue syndrome.

You have fibromyalgia.

You have too much or too little iodine in your system.

Someone in your family has thyroid disease.

You or someone in your family has an autoimmune disease.*

You have had surgery or an injury to your thyroid gland.

You take medications that affect the thyroid gland.**

You have been exposed to radioactive substances or received radiation treatments.

You have been exposed to chemicals toxic to the thyroid.***

You have ongoing medical problems.

You have excessive stress in your life.

* Autoimmune diseases include rheumatoid arthritis, psoriasis, Crohn's disease, vitiligo, lupus, multiple sclerosis, type 1 diabetes, and other conditions.

** Medications that affect the thyroid gland include lithium, amiodarone, interferon, and others.

*** Chemicals toxic to the thyroid include carbon tetrachloride, bisphenol A (BPA), pesticides that contain polychlorinated biphenyl (PCBs), weed killers that contain glyphosate, cadmium, nitrates, and antibacterial products that contain triclosan.

The natural course of hypothyroidism is eventual total thyroid fail-ure, which is almost certain to occur with time, requiring larger doses of thy-roid hormone replacement. Long-standing untreated hypothyroidism is called *myxedema,* a term that refers to the swelling of organs and tissues throughout the body. With myxedema, serious difficulties eventually arise in all major, life-sustaining systems, leading to coma known as *myxedema coma.*

Symptoms of Hypothyroidism

The list of signs and symptoms of hypothyroidism is long, because thyroid hor-mone affects every aspect of the body. Let's look at a few of the symptoms.

Weight Gain

Low thyroid plunges the body into a vicious cycle. Chief among this cycle's in-dicators is weight gain. The lack of thyroid hormone prompts the body to slow its metabolism, so the body burns calories more slowly. As metabolism slows and cells need less energy, the body stores extra calories as fat. Most people with hypothyroidism say they are gaining weight even though they are eating less. As people gain weight, other hormone problems, such as insulin and leptin resis-tance, kick in, which worsen weight gain.

Trouble Losing Weight after Pregnancy

Women who have trouble losing weight after giving birth may have a form of hypothyroidism known as *postpartum thyroiditis.* The condition may be misdiag-nosed as postpartum depression and may never be properly treated. Most of the time, the hypothyroidism improves by itself and is forgotten, but the afflicted woman by that time has been miserable for about a year and likely has gained tremendous amounts of weight. This condition occurs in as many as 5 percent of women.

Loss of Appetite

Even though weight gain is an inevitable part of having hypothyroidism, most people experience decreased appetite, because thyroid hormone regulates ap-petite centers in the brain.

Fatigue, Exhaustion, Drowsiness, and Yawning

Fatigue is one of the most common symptoms in people with hypothyroid-ism. Reduced metabolism leads to low energy levels. People with low thyroid levels are tired all the time. They simply have no energy. Many report sleeping twelve to fourteen hours each night. If left untreated, sleepiness becomes a major symptom, and some patients have even gone into an irreversible coma.

Premature Aging

Cosmetically, hypothyroidism causes people to look older. One need not look any farther than the case of Boris Yeltsin, the former president of Russia. In 1991, when he took over the country, Yeltsin was the very picture of vigor: you may remember the then-youthful sixty-year-old rallying people in the streets of Moscow after an aborted takeover by Soviet hardliners?

Within five years, though, Yeltsin appeared old, tired, and out of touch. He slurred his speech; his face was bloated. In 1996, prior to a heart bypass operation, he was diagnosed with hypothyroidism. The diagnosis was almost certainly overdue, since the disease had probably started much earlier—perhaps brought on by the stress of his job and exacerbated by his alcoholism. Once Yeltsin's thyroid was treated, his heart problems got worse, which is not uncommon. Thyroid hormone accelerates metabolism throughout the body, including the heart. The accelerated metabolism increased the amount of oxygen his heart demanded, and because of his coronary artery disease, not enough blood could get to the heart muscle.

Menopausal Symptoms

Twenty percent of menopausal women have an underactive thyroid gland. Symptoms of weight gain, mood swings, depression, hair loss, and dry skin attributed to menopause could be caused by undiagnosed thyroid disease.

Do You Have a Goiter?

Having a goiter means having an enlarged thyroid gland. Symptoms include:

Swelling in the neck

Feeling tightness in the throat

Difficulty swallowing

Hoarseness

Feeling of food stuck in the throat

Lump in the throat

Difficulty Swallowing, Hoarseness, or Feeling of Fullness in the Neck

An enlarged thyroid gland, known as a *goiter,* can cause a feeling of fullness in the neck. Some people report a choking sensation, hoarseness, or difficulty swallowing. An underactive or overactive thyroid, iodine deficiency, cysts, or noncancerous and cancerous tumors can cause a goiter.

Joint and Muscle Aches or Muscle Cramps

Hypothyroidism causes your joints and muscles to feel stiff, painful, and sore, —all symptoms that can be misdiagnosed as arthritis.

Carpal Tunnel Syndrome or Plantar Fasciitis

Carpal tunnel syndrome is a condition in which pressure on a nerve in the wrist causes pain in the hands and fingers. Plantar fasciitis causes pain in the soles of the feet. Low thyroid levels cause tissue swelling and inflammation, leading to these conditions.

Feeling Cold or Being Cold

Many people with hypothyroidism say they feel cold when others think the temperature is normal. Body temperature is a function of metabolism, so as metabolism slows, less body heat is generated. Hypothyroidism also causes blood vessels in the skin to constrict, making it feel cool to the touch. Basal body temperature measurements have been touted as an early indicator of thyroid dysfunction. Most thyroid experts do not recommend taking your temperature, however, because it is not a reliable test of low thyroid activity.

> **Basal Body Temperature?**
>
> Taking your temperature is not a reliable way to determine whether your thyroid is low.

Decreased Sweating

Lowered metabolism means less body heat, which leads to decreased sweating.

Constipation

Hypothyroidism causes a general slowing of bowel function. Hard, painful bowel movements or abdominal bloating are signs of hypothyroidism, but, like many other symptoms on this list, these signs are often dismissed as something else.

Loss of Memory, Inability to Concentrate, Brain Fog, or Fuzzy Thinking

Given the relationship among hypothyroidism, slowed metabolism, and fatigue, the memory is often sacrificed in favor of other brain functions. The body becomes obsessed with its drives, most notably sleeping and eating. Concentrating and remembering take a back seat. Hypothyroidism is associated with forgetfulness, inability to concentrate, and diminished intellectual function, speech capability, energy, libido, and motivation. Mild hypothyroidism causes forgetfulness and difficulty concentrating. More severe hypothyroidism causes problems that can be mistaken for Alzheimer's disease, especially in older people.

Depression

Ten to 15 percent of people with depression have hypothyroidism. Hypothyroidism causes a generalized slowing of bodily function, including that of the brain. Hypothyroidism also injures brain cells that produce serotonin, a brain chemical that, when low, has been linked to depression. Reduced serotonin levels lead to negative moods, pessimism, feelings of inadequacy and doom, and an inability to enjoy pleasure.

Depression is one of the most common misdiagnoses of hypothyroidism. Nowadays, it's easy to blame depression for many things. We all have moments when we're feeling down, and for a sizable minority of Americans, full-blown depression is a real threat and illness. Although it's as important to look at the physiological roots of depression as it is the psychological roots, many physicians don't look in the physiological direction, and one of the indicators of depression can be hypothyroidism.

Skin Problems

Skin becomes dry, itchy, and develops cracks. In more severe cases of hypothyroidism, the skin takes on a yellow tinge because of a buildup of carotene. Skin may also be cool to the touch, because of the constriction of blood vessels. Hypothyroidism can also cause the skin to bruise easily.

Hair, Eyebrow, and Fingernail Problems

A lowered metabolic rate brought on by thyroid hormone underproduction can slow the growth of hair and cause it to become dry, coarse, brittle, and tangled. Hypothyroidism also causes hair to fall out, sometimes in clumps. People with hypothyroidism frequently lose the hair in the outer third of their eyebrows. Fingernails become brittle and grow slowly.

Fluid Retention

Hypothyroidism causes fluid retention, resulting in puffiness in the face or around the eyes, thickened lips, and swelling of the hands, feet, or legs (known as *myxedema*). Swelling of the tissues in the belly can lead to a bloated sensation.

High Cholesterol

Because of a general slowdown of bodily functions, hypothyroidism causes cholesterol to rise. The lower the thyroid levels, the higher the cholesterol. Anyone with high cholesterol should be tested for thyroid problems.

High Blood Pressure

Abnormal thyroid levels, either high or low, can cause high blood pressure. Everyone who has been diagnosed with high blood pressure should have his or her thyroid checked.

Slow Heart Rate

Hypothyroidism has profound effects on the heart. A slow heart rate is a result of the total body slowdown.

Cardiovascular Disease

Studies have linked hypothyroidism to atherosclerosis and premature cardiovascular disease. An underactive thyroid lets the body's cholesterol levels climb, particularly so-called LDL (low-density lipoprotein cholesterol), also referred to as bad cholesterol. In combination with high blood pressure, this situation puts a person at increased risk for a heart attack or a stroke. Thyroid hormone has direct effects on the heart. Underproduction of thyroid hormone prompts the heart to beat less strongly, more slowly, and may cause fluid to build up around it.

Menstrual Problems and Infertility

Hypothyroidism can cause havoc with the female reproductive system. Periods may be longer, heavier, further apart, or irregular. Increased blood flow is common; the thyroid controls muscle contraction in the uterus. Without the proper contracting of the muscle, the uterus cannot clamp off the bleeding blood vessels. Hypothyroidism can also prompt a situation in which the ovary does not release an egg at all.

Some women with hypothyroidism have reduced menstrual flow or lose their periods altogether. Loss of menstrual cycle with symptoms of low thyroid could mean pituitary gland problems, causing low thyroid hormone production.

Decreased Sex Drive

Lowered sex drive is a common symptom in patients with hypothyroidism.

Gruff or Hoarse Voice

Many people with hypothyroidism report that their voices become hoarse, husky, gravelly, or simply sound deeper, the result of thickening and swelling of the vocal cords.

Anemia

Anemia means low levels of red blood cells. The most common symptom of anemia is fatigue. Hypothyroidism commonly causes a low-grade anemia that is often dismissed by physicians.

Anemia may also be caused by an autoimmune disorder called *pernicious anemia*. Pernicious anemia is caused by problems absorbing vitamin B_{12}. Symptoms of vitamin B_{12} deficiency include weakness, nervous system problems, and gastrointestinal problems, in addition to low levels of red blood cells. It is treated with regular injections of vitamin B_{12}.

Slow Reflexes

Endocrinologists examine reflexes very carefully when determining whether a patient may have thyroid disease, because slow reflexes can be a key to diagnosing hypothyroidism. In hypothyroidism, the *relaxation phase* of the reflex is slowed. For example, in the standard knee-jerk reflex, a doctor hits a knee with a reflex hammer and the knee kicks out. In a patient with hypothyroidism, the return of the knee to a resting position is delayed. The delay may not be apparent to the untrained eye, but an experienced endocrinologist knows how to spot a delay, the most sensitive way of determining subtle thyroid deficiencies during an exam. Through its effects on the nervous system, hypothyroidism can also cause problems such as muscle cramps, numbness or tingling in the hands and feet, or even carpal tunnel syndrome.

Snoring or Sleep Apnea

Sleep apnea is a situation that occurs when excess tissue in the neck cuts off breathing during the night, leading to snoring, poor sleep, daytime sleepiness, high blood pressure, and—if left untreated—eventual heart and lung failure. Sleep apnea is not uncommon among overweight people, and the slowing of metabolism caused by hypothyroidism can contribute to this condition.

Allergies or Hives

Many people with thyroid problems notice worsening of their allergies. Treating the thyroid often reduces a person's allergic reactions. Some people with normal thyroid hormone levels, but with evidence of immune system attack on the thyroid (known as euthyroid Hashimoto's disease), have been known to experience dramatic improvement in their allergies when treated with low doses of thyroid hormone. Hypothyroidism has also been known to cause an increased sensitivity to medications in some people.

Frequent Colds and Sinus Infections

Patients with hypothyroidism are more susceptible to colds and sinus infections, and the symptoms tend to be worse and last longer.

Breast Milk Production

As the brain vigorously tries to produce more TSH, the body can produce more of another hormone, prolactin. Prolactin stimulates breast milk production and can cause menstrual abnormalities. It is a rare event, but it does happen. In some cases, this situation is misdiagnosed as a brain tumor, and patients have been known to have an unnecessary removal of the pituitary gland when all that was needed was a thyroid hormone replacement.

Testing for Thyroid Disease

Experts debate about the testing protocols for thyroid disease. Most doctors rely on a simple blood test, the TSH test, to assess thyroid status. The TSH test is 80–90 percent accurate most of the time, but it can be unreliable in a variety of situations.

The TSH Test

Thyroid experts recognize the TSH test as the test of choice when a doctor suspects thyroid disease. An elevated TSH test diagnoses hypothyroidism. TSH is more sensitive than other thyroid tests, because TSH begins to rise *before* thyroid hormones drop. (See Figure 7.5.) As such, it's a better indicator of early thyroid dysfunction.

TSH values above the normal range indicate hypothyroidism, and the higher the number, the more severe the hypothyroidism. (See Figure 7.6.) Low

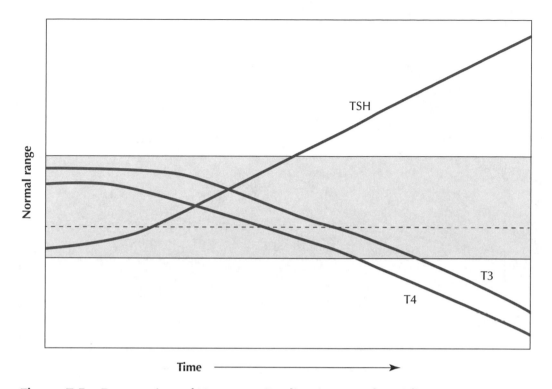

Figure 7.5   Progression of Hormone Decline in Hypothyroidism

In the progression of hypothyroidism, the brain and pituitary gland sense subtle deficiencies in thyroid hormone levels. The result is a rise in TSH levels, which is usually detectable *before* thyroid hormone levels fall below the normal range. During this phase, symptoms are generally mild. As T4 and T3 levels fall, symptoms worsen.

TSH values usually indicate an overactive thyroid (hyperthyroidism). Although the normal range for the TSH test can vary from lab to lab, it is considered a very reliable test. In the past, the normal range for TSH was thought to be 0.5–5.5 μU/ml μ(microunits/milliliter); however, in 2002, some experts came to a consensus to lower the normal range to 0.5–4.5 μU/ml. Many experts feel the normal range should be revised to 0.5–2.5 μU/ml. With these new standards, many people who were previously told they were normal now may be considered to have hypothyroidism.

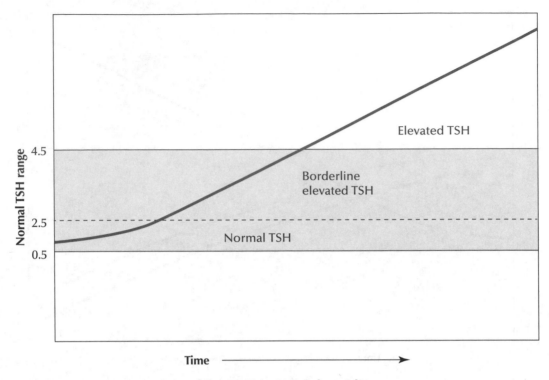

Figure 7.6   Progression of the TSH in Hypothyroidism

TSH is the hormone that comes from the pituitary gland and communicates with the thyroid gland, stimulating it to make and release thyroid hormones. Early in hypothyroidism, TSH levels increase, trying to coax the thyroid to do its job. After a while, the thyroid gland gives up, and T3 and T4 levels drop below normal, but by that time, hypothyroidism has already progressed to a moderate to severe stage.

I've seen several trends in my patients. Women in their twenties and thirties who are generally healthy can have extremely high TSH levels with relatively few symptoms. Women with PCOS and in menopause can have TSH levels that are only slightly elevated and have more severe symptoms. In most people, the higher the TSH level, the more severe the symptoms. Early hypothyroidism, when TSH is high, but thyroid hormone (T3 and T4) levels are normal, is known as subclinical hypothyroidism or mild thyroid failure. Many physicians are reluctant to treat this condition; however, mild thyroid failure is increasingly being recognized as a disease and is being treated.

Most of the time, if the TSH is elevated, it indicates hypothyroidism. There are exceptions, however, to this rule. All these exceptions are possible causes of an elevated TSH.

- **Children and adolescents.** It is normal for children and adolescents to have TSH levels that are higher than adults. TSH levels change substantially during childhood, so that adult TSH levels are not always applicable to children. TSH is highest during the first month of life, followed by a decline as we get older. In newborn babies, the normal TSH range is 1.3–16 μU/ml. After the first month of life, a normal TSH range is 0.9–7.7 μU/ml. From age one until age twenty, the normal TSH range is 0.6–6.4 μU/ml. Many endocrinologists, however, use the standard adult range for all children once they hit puberty. Testing free T4 is can be helpful to confirm a borderline TSH in adolescents and young adults, because it directly reflects hormone production by the thyroid gland.

- **Pituitary tumor.** If the pituitary gland has a tumor, it may overproduce TSH on its own. Patients with this problem usually have symptoms of an overactive thyroid, such as nervousness and rapid heart rate.

- **Medications.** Antinausea medication (that is, promethazine or metoclopramide) and antipsychotic medications (that is, haloperidol or fluphenazine) can elevate the TSH test.

- **Timing.** TSH should always be tested during the day. TSH levels often surge at night, and testing at night can result in an indication of high TSH levels when in fact they're normal.

- **Immune problems.** In rare cases, TSH antibodies can give false readings in the lab test, making a normal test appear extremely high.

Total Thyroxine (TT4)

This test measures the level of all thyroxine (T4) in the blood. More than 99 percent of thyroid hormone is bound to the blood protein thyroid binding globulin (TBG). This bound hormone is inactive. Problems with TBG can invalidate this test. Estrogen-containing medications, such as those used in hormone replacement therapy (sometimes called HRT) or birth control pills, increase TBG levels, making the TT4 test of limited usefulness in women who take these medications.

Free Thyroxine (FT4)

This test measures only the one percent of thyroid hormone that is unbound. This "free hormone" is the active hormone. Bound hormone has no biological activity. Testing for free thyroxine eliminates the possibility of being misled by a protein problem. In general, *free* hormone levels are more accurate than *total* hormone levels.

Total Triiodothyronine (TT3)

As with total thyroxine, this test measures both bound and unbound T3 levels. TBG problems can lead to problems with this test.

Free Triiodothyronine (FT3)

This test measures only the unbound portion of T3 and is not subject to protein problems. It is an important test for people who have problems converting T4 to T3.

Thyroid Binding Globulin

This test measures actual levels of binding proteins in the blood. TBG problems cause false readings for total, but not for free, hormone levels. One cause of elevated TBG, incidentally, is a high estrogen level, which can be caused by pregnancy, birth control pills, estrogen replacement therapy, and high consumption of soy products.

Antithyroid Antibodies

Tests for thyroid antibodies can diagnose autoimmune thyroid disease, the most common cause of hypothyroidism. Antithyroid antibodies attack the critical machinery required for thyroid hormone production. There are two types of thyroid antibodies: *anti-thyroglobulin antibodies* and *anti-thyroid peroxidase antibodies*. Thyroid peroxidase activates iodine, so that it can be incorporated into thyroid hormones. Thyroglobulin provides the tyrosine backbone of all thyroid hormones. If the immune system attacks either thyroid peroxidase or thyroglobulin, the thyroid gland can't make thyroid hormones. Laboratories use a variety of methods for measuring antibodies. I frequently see patients who had positive antibodies at one lab and negative at another.

Making Sense of Antibody Tests

A test result of positive thyroid antibodies and low thyroid hormone means that a person has Hashimoto's thyroiditis.

If thyroid antibody testing is negative, it can still mean the person has Hashimoto's thyroiditis. Antibody testing is not the end-all and be-all of assessing the thyroid. Most people with hypothyroidism have Hashimoto's (autoimmune) thyroiditis regardless of antibody status.

If thyroid levels are normal and thyroid antibodies are positive, there is a 20–30 percent lifetime risk of developing hypothyroidism.

Thyroid antibody testing is most useful for borderline cases when a doctor is trying to make a decision to treat or not to treat. If you have positive antibodies, your doctor will be more likely to start thyroid hormone replacement sooner rather than later.

A large percentage of the general population has antithyroid antibodies in their blood, but only a fraction of them will go on to develop hypothyroidism. Thyroid antibodies may be a clue to thyroid disease; however, they do not guarantee it. Studies have shown that if the TSH is less than 2 μU/ml and antibodies are positive, there is about a 20–30 percent risk of developing hypothyroidism, so having antibodies alone does not guarantee that you will develop hypothyroidism. Researchers believe that stress, genetics, and body weight all play a role in determining the amount of damage antibodies cause and the likelihood of progression to hypothyroidism.

Thyroid antibody tests are reported as a level, but the truth is that you want to know if they are positive or negative, not how high they are. If thyroid antibodies are elevated, it doesn't matter how high. There is no reason to monitor thyroid antibodies. Once you know they are positive, this information is all you need. Repeatedly testing thyroid antibodies is not recommended and will not reveal any additional information.

Thyroid antibodies are a very good test for patients with borderline thyroid testing who need more information to decide whether or not to start thyroid replacement therapy, but the test doesn't tell you whether you are taking the right

Thyroid Antibody Testing Is Not Always Necessary

Determining the presence of thyroid antibodies is helpful in deciding whether to start thyroid medications, but the information won't tell you any of the following:

Whether you are on the right dose of thyroid medication

Whether immune system attack is waxing or waning

Also,

If you have already been diagnosed with hypothyroidism, testing for thyroid antibodies is not necessary, because the decision has already been made to treat.

If your thyroid antibody status is already known, repeat testing is not necessary (unless confirming at a different laboratory).

If you have a strong family history of thyroid disease or personal history of other autoimmune problems, you already have such a high likelihood of having thyroid autoimmunity that blood tests are unlikely to alter management.

If there is no other explanation (surgery, radiation, and so on) for hypothyroidism, an autoimmune cause is presumed, even if thyroid antibody testing is negative.

medication or the right dose. If you are already diagnosed with autoimmune thyroid disease, there is absolutely no reason to test thyroid antibody levels.

Testing for Autoimmune Disorders

Thyroid problems are frequently caused by immune system problems. Having one autoimmune disorder puts you at risk for others. If you have been diagnosed with autoimmune thyroid disease (Hashimoto's or Graves') you should be evaluated for other autoimmune problems. Testing depends on your symptoms but may include blood sugar, cortisol, calcium, parathyroid hormone, vitamin B_{12}, rheumatoid factor, celiac antibodies, antinuclear antibody (ANA), platelets, and blood counts.

Thyroid Ultrasound

A thyroid ultrasound gives information about the size and shape of the thyroid, as well as the presence of nodules or cysts. Fine needle aspiration (FNA) or biopsy is recommended for a nodule or cyst larger than one centimeter. If your thyroid gland is enlarged, it is a good idea to get an ultrasound. Patients with autoimmune thyroid disease commonly show thyroid abnormalities, including nodules, cysts, and a multinodular appearance sometimes referred to as *pseudonodules,* on ultrasound. The thyroid ultrasound is very helpful for patients with borderline TSH levels who are trying to decide whether to start thyroid hormone replacement.

MRI Scan

If pituitary or hypothalamic problems are suspected as a cause for hypothyroidism, your doctor may order an MRI scan of the pituitary gland to look for a tumor or cyst.

TRH Stimulation Test

This test measures the ability of the pituitary gland to respond to an injection of TRH (thyrotropin releasing hormone). TSH is measured, TRH is injected, and TSH is measured again thirty minutes later. If the TSH does not increase, a pituitary gland problem is suspected. If the TSH rises to a level greater than expected, it can indicate hypothyroidism. TRH is difficult to obtain in the United States, but it is available from compounding pharmacies.

Reverse T3

This test measures levels of an inactive hormone produced when T4 is improperly processed. Thyroid experts rarely order this test, but other doctors frequently do. I've heard some doctors say that reverse T3 blocks the thyroid hormone receptor so that active T3 doesn't work properly, but there is no evidence that this is true. Reverse T3 testing not only is expensive, but it is usually not helpful in determining whether there are problems converting T4 to T3. I do not recommend this test.

Saliva Tests

Salivary measurements of thyroid hormones are not reliable. Salivary testing is not accurate enough, and the normal range has not been clearly defined. Salivary hormone measurements hold promise, though, and in the future, they may be more reliable.

Wilson's Temperature Syndrome

In the early 1990s, Florida physician Dr. E. Denis Wilson theorized that many of the symptoms of hypothyroidism were caused by low levels of thyroid hormone despite normal thyroid tests. He claimed that patients with low thyroid have low body temperature, and he recommended taking a morning temperature to determine whether you have low thyroid. Although many websites and books imply that basal body temperature is a good way to assess thyroid status, there is no medical evidence that it is a reliable indicator of thyroid status. The Endocrine Society website states, "Wilson's syndrome is not an accepted medical diagnosis based on scientific facts."

Dr. Wilson popularized his theory with an expensive advertising campaign. The Florida medical licensing board subsequently received complaints about Wilson and forced him to pay a $10,000 fine and stop practicing medicine for six months.

Basal Body Temperature

Basal body temperature measurements are not reliable for detecting thyroid problems and can be misleading. Normal body temperature can be variable and change throughout the day, so a temperature less than 98.6 degrees is not necessarily abnormal.

Why Is the TSH Test So Important?

Why do doctors rely so heavily on the TSH when diagnosing and treating thyroid disease? An elevated TSH accurately diagnoses hypothyroidism 80–90 percent of the time. TSH, or thyroid stimulating hormone, is produced by the pituitary gland and has the primary function of telling the thyroid gland to make hormones. Because the TSH is so reliable, doctors frequently overlook the 10–20 percent of patients who can have a low thyroid function and still have a normal TSH.

The pituitary gland, buried deep inside the brain, works to balance hormone levels. (See Figure 7.7.) The hypothalamus, which is located roughly behind the eyes, is hardwired to nearly the entire nervous system and directs the pituitary gland. To get to the thyroid, the hypothalamus sends a message to the pituitary gland in the form of a hormone, TRH, or thyrotropin releasing hormone. The pituitary gland reacts to the influx of TRH by releasing TSH (TSH is also known as

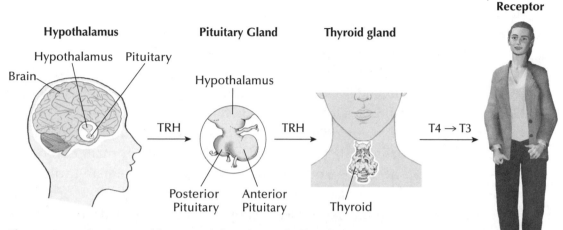

Figure 7.7 Brain Regulation of the Thyroid Gland

The hypothalamus produces TRH, which stimulates the thyroid gland to make TSH. TSH stimulates the thyroid gland to make T3 and T4, which act throughout the body.

Central hypothyroidism happens when the pituitary gland or other parts of the brain are sick and cannot produce TSH properly. (See Figure 7.8.) It is not as rare as many people believe and is frequently overlooked. I've seen a great many patients with central hypothyroidism who were originally misdiagnosed as having normal thyroid function. If the body can't make TSH, the TSH test is less reliable and must be interpreted in conjunction with symptoms along with T3 and T4 levels.

thyrotropin). TSH travels through the bloodstream to direct the thyroid gland to produce thyroid hormones. The pituitary is responsible for making sure the level of thyroid hormones in the blood remains constant, so if thyroid hormone levels fall, the pituitary gland increases its production of TSH. If the pituitary gland is not working properly, it can't increase TSH when thyroid levels drop. In other cases, the TSH production can be so low that low TSH itself causes hypothyroidism.

Borderline Thyroid Tests: When Should You Take Thyroid Medication?

"In the clinical practice of endocrinology, one of the most common clinical challenges is the management of patients with subclinical hypothyroidism."

—Irwin Klein, M.D., Professor of Medicine, NYU School of Medicine

When the TSH test is "high normal," in the range of 2.5–4.5 μU/ml, deciding to take thyroid medication can be a difficult decision. I've seen many patients with this situation. Frequently thyroid tests in this range will normalize within a few months; other times, they progress to overt hypothyroidism. The first step is to repeat the TSH test. I never make a treatment decision based on a single blood test. Experts recommend waiting three months to repeat a borderline abnormal TSH test, but if you have a lot of symptoms, it is better to do it sooner.

In my opinion, many doctors take the easy way out and prescribe a low dose of thyroid medication when the thyroid is actually normal. If you take low-dose thyroid hormone and your thyroid is normal, the gland will make fewer hormones to maintain normal levels, so taking a low dose of thyroid hormone may not do much. I've seen many patients who tried this approach and then came to me still complaining of symptoms. Some of these patients stopped thyroid hormone replacement and felt better. Others feel better while taking low-dose thyroid hormone replacement, but I have always wondered how much of it was a placebo effect. A study was done to determine whether treatment with thyroid hormone could improve the symptoms of hypothyroidism in people with normal thyroid function tests. The results, published in the *British Medical Journal,* showed that thyroid hormone was no more effective than a placebo for relieving symptoms.

However, some people with borderline tests have early thyroid disease that is certain to progress. Diagnosing hypothyroidism in the early stages can be tricky, because when the thyroid starts to fail, tests can remain in the normal range for a period of time. The first thing that indicates low thyroid is an elevated TSH level. A change from a low normal TSH to a high normal TSH over a period of a few months may mean early thyroid failure. If thyroid antibodies are positive or if the thyroid gland is enlarged, the risk for thyroid failure is extremely high. If the thyroid antibodies are normal and the thyroid is not enlarged, the risk is much lower. A thyroid ultrasound can also be helpful. If the ultrasound shows nodules or cysts in the thyroid gland, low-dose thyroid medication may be beneficial.

Several other factors can be important in the decision-making process. Low thyroid can raise blood pressure and cholesterol. Hypothyroidism has also been shown to cause heart problems, which can be seen on a standard electrocardiogram (EKG). The most common problem seen on an EKG is a prolonged Q-T interval, which is basically a problem with the electrical timing of the heart and can lead to more serious heart rhythm problems. Treating low thyroid can

Why Do Some Doctors Refuse to Treat Borderline Thyroid Levels?

Determining the presence of thyroid antibodies is helpful in deciding whether to start thyroid medications, but the information won't tell you any of the following:

It is difficult to assess a true response versus the placebo effect.

Many patients with borderline thyroid tests will never develop hypothyroidism.

Waiting a few months and monitoring closely does no serious harm.

Severity of symptoms corresponds with severity of testing.

Treating a patient who doesn't need treatment could cause harm.

Symptoms of hypothyroidism overlap with symptoms of many other conditions, so it is always prudent to rule out all possible cause of symptoms.

Continued observation, careful monitoring with blood tests, and lifestyle changes alone can be a form of treatment, even if medications are not prescribed.

Patients with genuine hypothyroidism will progress, making diagnosis more obvious and treatment justified.

---

correct this electrical phenomenon. A blood test known as "CK" (for creatine kinase) can also show elevated levels, the result of damage to muscle cells. Low thyroid has also been linked to bleeding and bruising.

Often there is no clear-cut answer. Many of my patients have taken a wait-and-see approach. I've been surprised to see how many patients never take thyroid medications and maintain normal hormone levels over the years and feel perfectly fine or find other causes for symptoms once blamed on the thyroid. Some patients, however, do go on to have low thyroid and require lifelong thyroid hormone replacement.

Causes of Hypothyroidism

Hashimoto's Thyroiditis

Hashimoto's thyroiditis is also known as autoimmune hypothyroidism, Hashimoto's disease, Hashimoto's hypothyroidism, autoimmune thyroiditis, or chronic lymphocytic thyroiditis. It's the number one cause of hypothyroidism and is estimated to affect 15 to 20 million people in the United States. Hashimoto's thyroiditis may begin with a short period of thyroid overactivity lasting anywhere from a few weeks to several months. This condition, known as *Hashitoxicosis* or *silent thyroiditis,* is caused by the release of thyroid hormones because the gland is being destroyed by the immune system. The immune system can cause the thyroid to become and stay overactive; this condition is called *Graves' disease.* Hashimoto's thyroiditis is hereditary, and it affects women seven times more often than it does men. It is frequently triggered by a stressful event.

Postpartum Thyroiditis

Postpartum thyroiditis is a condition that up to 10 percent of new mothers develop. It is an inflammation of the thyroid gland three to twelve months after giving birth. Most of the time, the condition is temporary, but about 30 percent of the time, the condition is permanent and requires lifelong thyroid hormone replacement. Postpartum thyroiditis is a common reason why women have problems losing weight after pregnancy.

Central Hypothyroidism

When hypothyroidism begins in the brain instead of in the thyroid gland, it is called *central hypothyroidism,* referring to the central nervous system. It develops when something such as tumors, infections, or injury damaging or destroying either the hypothalamus or the pituitary gland. Central hypothyroidism is frequently accompanied by deficiencies of other pituitary gland hormones, including the hormones that regulate the menstrual cycle. Women with central hypothyroidism may complain of having an irregular menstrual cycle or absence of the menstrual cycle in conjunction with weight gain.

Central hypothyroidism is a problem frequently missed by doctors who rely too heavily on the TSH as the end-all and be-all of diagnosing hypothyroidism. Unlike most cases of hypothyroidism, TSH levels are typically normal or low in cases of central hypothyroidism.

Causes of Central Hypothyroidism
Elevated prolactin levels
Hemochromatosis
Head injuries
Pituitary tumors and cysts

Reidel's Thyroiditis

Reidel's thyroiditis is a very rare cause of hypothyroidism. For unknown reasons, rigid, fibrous tissue invades normal thyroid tissue and destroys thyroid function.

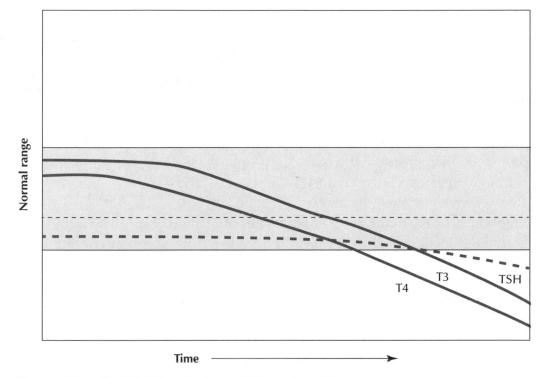

Figure 7.8 The TSH Test in Central Hypothyroidism

In central hypothyroidism, the brain or pituitary gland is unable to make adequate amounts of TSH, resulting in low thyroid levels. Unlike primary thyroid gland failure, which presents with an elevated TSH level, the TSH remains normal or low.

Congenital Hypothyroidism

Some people are born with a defect in the key machinery necessary for thyroid hormone production. In the United States, all newborn infants are tested for this condition, because normal thyroid hormone levels are necessary for growth and development.

Treatment for Hyperthyroidism, Goiter, or Thyroid Cancer

Low thyroid can occur when more than 40–50 percent of the thyroid is surgically removed. Hypothyroidism is also a frequent outcome of radioactive iodine treatment for hyperthyroidism or thyroid cancer and is known as *postablative hypothyroidism.* Drugs used to treat an overactive thyroid, PTU and methiamazole, may result in hypothyroidism.

Medications

The medication lithium is well known to cause hypothyroidism. Drugs used for epilepsy, including phenytoin and carbamazepine, reduce thyroid levels. Medications that contain iodine have properties that affect the thyroid, although their effects are almost always reversible when the medi-

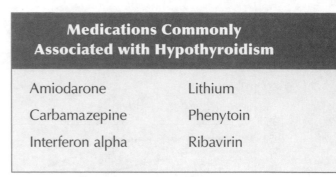

Medications Commonly Associated with Hypothyroidism	
Amiodarone	Lithium
Carbamazepine	Phenytoin
Interferon alpha	Ribavirin

cation is stopped. Some drugs used in cancer chemotherapy or to fight infections (interleukins, sulfamethoxazole and other sulfa drugs, interferon alpha, and ribavirin) can cause hypothyroidism.

Excess Iodine

If the thyroid gland is overwhelmed with iodine, it shuts down, inhibiting production of thyroid hormone. Thyroid support formulas that contain kelp, bugleweed, or bladderwrack often contain megadoses of iodine in a single dose. Thyroid formulas that contain iodine are intended to boost thyroid function but may interfere with its function.

Radiation Exposure

Radiation treatments for cancers or acne in the head and neck area increase the risk for hypothyroidism as well as thyroid nodules and thyroid cancer. People who live (or used to live) in locations where nuclear bombs were tested or there was leakage of nuclear waste are at risk for thyroid problems. I have seen many patients who lived or visited the area near Chernobyl who now have thyroid problems.

Hyperthyroidism: Gaining Weight with an Overactive Thyroid

Hyperthyroidism is the opposite of hypothyroidism: instead of the body producing too little thyroid hormone, it produces too much. Its symptoms are usually the reverse of hypothyroidism: instead of metabolism slowing, it speeds up, so hyperthyroidism usually produces weight loss, not weight gain.

But there's a twist. One of hyperthyroidism's major effects is increasing appetite. If appetite increases faster than metabolism, guess what: weight gain.

The primary symptom of hyperthyroidism is uncontrollable appetite. Patients complain of never eating enough, always being hungry, of waking up ravenous and going to sleep the same way, even if they've eaten far more than recommended during the day.

You might recognize other symptoms as the reverse images of hypothyroid symptoms. They include feeling hot, hyperactivity, increased sweating, irritability, nervousness, tremor, heart palpitations, insomnia, brittle nails, diarrhea, or increased frequency of bowel movements. Fatigue is a symptom of both hypo- and hyperthyroidism.

One extreme form of hyperthyroidism is called *thyroid storm.* Patients can have vomiting, fever, liver problems, mental confusion, and—sometimes—seizures. A thyroid storm requires hospitalization for treatment.

Like hypothyroidism, hyperthyroidism is frequently caused by an attack of an overactive immune system on the thyroid gland. The most common cause of hyperthyroidism is Graves' disease. Graves' disease is an attack on the thyroid gland by the immune system, usually kicked off by stress. The most famous case in recent years occurred in 1991, when President George Bush came down with Graves' disease in the aftermath of the Persian Gulf War, when the president had been under extreme stress for several months. The disease caused heart fibrillations, forcing the president into the hospital. Eventually, after observation and tests, President Bush's Graves' disease was treated with medication. Treatments for hyperthyroidism include radioactive iodine, antithyroid drugs such as methimazole or propylthiouracil (PTU), and—in some cases—surgical removal of the thyroid.

Is Your Doctor Missing Your Thyroid Problem?

Do you have symptoms of hypothyroidism but have been told that your thyroid test is normal? Several conditions may result in low thyroid function despite normal thyroid tests, including the following.

Pituitary or Hypothalamic Disease

In some cases, hypothyroidism is not caused by failure of the thyroid gland but by failure of the pituitary gland or hypothalamus. The most common cause is a pituitary gland tumor. Other causes of central hypothyroidism include head trauma, brain tumors, problems with blood flow to the pituitary gland, tuberculosis, syphilis and other infections, and other diseases, such as hemochromatosis and sarcoidosis. Sometimes a tumor in the pituitary gland causes an abnormal and nonfunctional form of TSH to be made. Through all this, TSH level may be normal, while free T4 is low normal or obviously low. Though central hypothyroidism is rare, the diagnosis should not be overlooked, particularly since it may involve a brain tumor. Early in the disease, all test results may be normal. The first indication may be something as simple as weight gain.

Thyroiditis

Thyroiditis is a temporary inflammation of the thyroid gland caused by antibodies or infection. Symptoms, and abnormal blood tests, can come and go. Sometimes the flow of antibodies and the autoimmune attack on the thyroid is unpredictable. Antibody levels can wax and wane, resulting in alternating periods of hyper- and hypothyroidism. This antibody flux is related to stress in your life, so relieving the stress tends to make the problem better. Thyroiditis can be caused by a virus. Some patients report a flu-like illness that occurred a few weeks prior to the onset of symptoms.

The catch: the thyroid tests are only abnormal if you measure them at the right time. At other times, the testing is normal, but the hormones are only transiently in the normal range, on their way to being higher or lower. Thyroiditis can make your neck swollen or tender, but this symptom doesn't always occur. Because of the effects hypo- and hyperthyroidism have on mental health, patients with thyroiditis are commonly misdiagnosed as having bipolar disorder, popularly known as manic depression.

T4:T3 Conversion Problems

When the body is under stress—and stress can be caused by major life-cycle events such as a death in the family, or seemingly innocuous physical changes such as being overweight or obese—there can be problems producing active thyroid hormones. The name given to this cycle is *sick euthyroid syndrome*. The *eu-* prefix to thyroid is from the Greek for "good" or "well," so sick euthyroid syndrome implies that the thyroid is well but the rest of the body is sick. Low thyroid levels are thought to put the body at a lower level of metabolism to protect it from whatever illness or stress it is experiencing. It's all a natural biological adaptation to stress. Being overweight may not seem like a stressful situation on the surface, certainly not compared to being wounded in battle or undergoing the breakup of a long-term relationship, but the upshot is the same: all the body knows is that something is wrong.

Conversion problems often happen in conjunction with mild thyroid failure. I see this combination all the time among my patients. The person has mild thyroid failure, but the TSH test, pushed and pulled in opposite directions, ends up normal. The result: normal thyroid hormone levels and normal TSH, with symptoms of hypothyroidism. It is a situation frequently missed by doctors. Patients are severely symptomatic but are told nothing is wrong.

The standard requirement of hypothyroidism is a high production of TSH. In the case of sick euthyroid syndrome and its related conversion problems, the opposite happens: TSH production is low or nonexistent. Let me emphasize: you don't have to be sick to have these conditions. Stress of any type, including mental stress, physical illness, or being overweight or obese can produce these problems, though to a lesser degree than the conditions suffered by critically ill patients.

T3 conversion problems

T3 conversion problems can be caused by:

Medical illness

Being overweight

Medications

Inflammation

Stress

Selenium deficiency

Zinc deficiency

Copper overload

Toxins

Thyroid Hormone Resistance

Complete thyroid hormone resistance is an extremely rare condition; there have only been about 600 cases reported to date. In thyroid hormone resistance, the thyroid gland is perfectly normal. The problem is in every cell of the body, each of which contains the thyroid hormone receptor and binding sites for the hormone receptor complex to bind to DNA and turn genes on and off. The condition is described as reduced tissue responsiveness to thyroid hormone. The problem is caused by a genetic defect in the gene that makes a component of the thyroid hormone receptor, so proper binding cannot occur.

Individuals with thyroid hormone resistance typically have mild symptoms of hypothyroidism and an enlarged thyroid gland. In reality, the TSH test is normal, but T4 and T3 levels may be elevated. The reason: there is enough thyroid hormone around, but it is not working properly. Thyroid hormone resistance typically runs in families. It is rarely diagnosed, and cases of partial thyroid hormone resistance may escape diagnosis altogether. One tipoff to thyroid hormone resistance may be a failure to lose weight or improve when treated for low thyroid, despite increasing dosages of medication.

If It's Not Your Thyroid

Most of the time, if thyroid tests are normal, especially the TSH level, thyroid function is adequate. If thyroid testing is repeatedly normal and there is no evidence of central hypothyroidism, then I usually think that thyroid is probably not the cause of a person's symptoms. It's important to rule in or rule out thyroid disease as a cause of symptoms, but if I determine that thyroid function is normal, I then recommend looking for other causes. Many medical conditions have symptoms that overlap with hypothyroidism.

Anemia	Infections
Celiac disease	Kidney disease
Chronic fatigue syndrome	Liver disease
Chronic sinusitis	Menopause
Depression	Multiple sclerosis
Diabetes	Narcolepsy
Food allergies	Pituitary gland failure
Growth hormone deficiency	Sleep apnea
Heart failure	Vitamin B_{12} deficiency
Hypogonadism	Vitamin D deficiency

Treatment of Hypothyroidism with Levothyroxine

If there's a positive aspect about hypothyroidism, it is that for most people, it is easily treatable. The main goal of therapy is to restore thyroid hormone levels to normal, which means that you must have periodic blood tests to make sure all your levels remain in the proper range. Most people who need thyroid hormone replacement have permanent hypothyroidism and need to take thyroid hormone replacement medication for the rest of their lives.

> ## Natural Thyroid Conversion
>
> A healthy thyroid gland produces mostly T4, which is naturally converted by the body to the active form, T3. The medication levothyroxine most closely reproduces this cycle by providing a pure source of T4, enabling T3 conversion to occur naturally.
>
> The average dose of levothyroxine needed is about 0.75 mcg per pound of body weight, so a 150-pound person usually needs to take the 112 mcg tablet. This calculation is just an estimate. The dose must also be adjusted according to a person's symptoms and TSH level.

Despite its effectiveness in the vast majority of patients, levothyroxine has been much maligned. Critics claim that levothyroxine is not ideal because it is not a natural product or because it contains T4 but not T3.

Eighty to 90 percent of patients with hypothyroidism have the best results using pure levothyroxine for thyroid hormone replacement. One pill daily essentially cures hypothyroidism. Levothyroxine is a synthetic form of T4 that is chemically identical to the natural form produced by the body and is available as a generic or as the brands Synthroid, Levoxyl, Levothroid, and Tirosint. Levothyroxine is naturally converted by the body to the active form, T3, and provides the base of the thyroid cycle.

Are You Still Having Symptoms While Taking Levothyroxine?

Ten to 20 percent of patients have persistent symptoms despite treatment with adequate doses of levothyroxine. Many doctors dismiss these symptoms; however, the following suggestions may be helpful.

Get healthy

Health problems of any kind can magnify symptoms of hypothyroidism and impair the body's ability to convert levothyroxine to the active form.

Stress less

Stressful situations, chronic stress, and even the stress of being overweight can be major catalysts in disrupting the normal performance of the thyroid. When under stress, the body sends messages triggering responses from many hormones. Many of these responses are short lived and beneficial. The production of adrenaline, for example, provides people with the extra shot of energy and excitement often needed to get through a stressful situation. (Think of how you feel when making a public speech: the palms sweat, the heart beats faster, you feel afraid and very alive—all part of the "fight-or-flight" instinct developed over millions of years.)

If the stress lasts for a long time, though, such as the kind of stress felt after surviving a tragedy or losing a loved one, your endocrine system and your immune system become overburdened. Naturally, this can lead to health problems. In particular, the immune system becomes dysfunctional, because your brain—using the flood of stress-inspired chemicals as a guide—is focusing its responses elsewhere. With the immune system out of whack, the body is helpless against viruses and other toxins that attack the thyroid. The immune system can become overactive, attacking and destroying the thyroid gland or stimulating it to produces excessive amounts of thyroid hormone. Autoimmune problems are the most common cause of both an underactive and overactive thyroid gland.

When the body is under stress, T4:T3 conversion problems can also occur. In one scenario, the wrong iodine—the inner-ring iodine—can be removed from the thyroid hormone, which creates an inactive form of the hormone called *reverse T3* (see Figure 7.4 on page 159) Given the inert state of reverse T3, metabolism slows to a crawl.

Change the dose of levothyroxine

Precise thyroid hormone levels are necessary for optimal hormonal balance. If you are taking levothyroxine and still have symptoms, adjusting the dose may help. The reference range for TSH varies among labs but is usually 0.5–4.5 μU/ml. The reference range is not the same as the *therapeutic target* for thyroid hormone replacement therapy, which is a TSH level near 1 μU/ml, because most people feel best when the TSH is at the lower end of the reference range. Increasing the dose of levothyroxine by a tiny amount (sometimes just an extra half-tablet once a week) is often enough to bring the TSH closer to the therapeutic target of 1 μU/ml.

Some patients have symptoms of an overactive thyroid if the TSH is treated to reach this range. For these patients, I recommend decreasing the dose to maintain the TSH in the mid-normal range.

Try branded levothyroxine or try a different brand

Brand-name levothyroxine—Synthroid, Levothroid, Tirosint, or Levoxyl—may offer an advantage over generics. The quality control for the branded versions is much better than generics, although generics have improved somewhat in recent years. Differences in the inert ingredients or fillers that make up the tablet lead to differences in absorption of the medication, which can affect blood levels. The cost between brand name and generic levothyroxine is only a few dollars each month.

Check your other medications

Several medications, vitamins, and minerals interfere with the absorption of levothyroxine from the bowels. Among them are serataline, cholestyramine, iron supplements or vitamins with iron, calcium supplements, Maalox, Mylanta, and other aluminum-containing antacids. It is recommended that patients avoid taking other medications for four hours after taking thyroid medications. Drugs that reduce stomach acid, known as proton pump inhibitors, including omeprazole (Prilosec), lansoprazole (Prevacid), rabeprazole (Aciphex), pantoprazole (Protonix), and esomeprazole (Nexium), can inhibit the absorption of thyroid medications.

Estrogen-containing medications, including birth control pills and hormone replacement, will also affect thyroid dosing. When women start taking estrogen medications, most of them need a 20–40 percent increase in their dose of thyroid medication. The reverse is also true when estrogen medications are discontinued.

Are You Pregnant?

Pregnancy can increase thyroid hormone requirements as early as four weeks into pregnancy. Hypothyroidism in pregnancy is a serious issue. It is estimated that 2.5 percent of pregnant women have some form of hypothyroidism; however, the symptoms of hypothyroidism may overlap those of simply being pregnant and the diagnosis may be missed. Hypothyroidism is associated with an increased risk of pregnancy complications. A study published in the *New England Journal of Medicine* showed that women with mild thyroid deficiency during their pregnancies had children with subsequent developmental and intelligence defects. All pregnant women should have their thyroids tested. If you are pregnant and have hypothyroidism, you should have your levels tested every four weeks. Most women need a 40–50 percent increase in their thyroid medication dose by the end of the second trimester. Having thyroid peroxidase antibodies or thyroglobulin antibodies will increase the risk of a miscarriage even if thyroid hormone levels are normal throughout pregnancy. Current guidelines recommend keeping the TSH less than 2.5 μU/ml during pregnancy.

Take thyroid medication on an empty stomach

Take thyroid medication at least one hour before or after food and two hours from soy and peanuts. Food, especially soy products and peanuts, can decrease the absorption of thyroid medications.

Take thyroid medication properly

For best results, take thyroid medication every day. If you forget to take a pill, you can take a double dose the next day to maintain adequate thyroid levels.

Take thyroid medication at night

Studies have also shown higher blood levels when thyroid medication is taken at night. Taking thyroid medication at night will not cause sleep problems.

Are your pills damaged or expired?

Always check the expiration date, which can be particularly short with some thyroid medications. Thyroid medication can be damaged by heat if left in a hot car or over the stove.

Cut back on gluten

Many thyroid patients have gluten intolerance. Reducing gluten may improve bowel function, allowing better absorption of thyroid medications.

See a gastroenterologist

Thyroid patients are at increased risk for autoimmune bowel disease. Bowel problems can impair the ability to absorb mediations. Celiac disease, irritable bowel syndrome, and Crohn's disease are more common in patients who have hypothyroidism.

Tip to Ensure an Accurate Dosage of Thyroid Medication

Even forgetting one pill a month can lead to less than optimal thyroid levels. Because levothyroxine is so long acting, if you forget a pill or two, you can take a double or triple dose to make up the difference. Here is a suggestion to make sure you get the right dose.

Place seven levothyroxine tablets in a separate pill bottle once a week. Each day, take your medication from this bottle. At the end of the week, if there are any leftover pills, take them all. This method ensures that you take seven tablets every week.

Check your vitamin B$_{12}$

Thyroid patients tend to have lower vitamin B$_{12}$ levels. Supplementation with vitamin B$_{12}$ pills, injections, or nasal spray is sometimes necessary to replace a deficiency.

Celiac Disease and Gluten Intolerance

Celiac disease, an autoimmune disease resulting in damage to the small intestine, is one of several causes of gluten intolerance. Symptoms can be exacerbated when a person ingests gluten and other proteins found in wheat, rye, and barley. If you have thyroid disease, you are at increased risk for having problems with gluten. Symptoms of gluten intolerance include:

- Abdominal pain, distention, bloating, gas, or indigestion
- Anemia
- Bone loss (osteoporosis or osteopenia)
- Bone pain
- Constipation or diarrhea
- Depression
- Easy bruising
- Fatigue
- Hair loss
- Infertility and miscarriage
- Irritability and behavioral changes
- Lactose intolerance
- Mouth ulcers
- Muscle cramps
- Nausea and vomiting
- Rash
- Seizures
- Stools that float
- Tooth discoloration
- Vitamin or mineral deficiencies (vitamin D, vitamin B$_{12}$, vitamin C, iron, zinc, selenium, chromium, or others)

Testing for gluten intolerance includes liver tests, vitamin and mineral tests, and genetic and blood tests for special antibodies. Upper endoscopy is usually performed to biopsy the small intestine. The treatment involves eliminating gluten from the diet. Supermarkets and restaurants finally are catching on and offering gluten-free options, although at restaurants you may have to request a gluten-free menu.

Many patients with hypothyroidism are intolerant of gluten but test negative for celiac disease. Eliminating or reducing gluten from the diet can also help patients with symptoms but who test negative for celiac.

Get a full hormone evaluation

If you have thyroid problems, you are at risk for other hormonal problems. Even if you are on the right dose of thyroid medication, you won't feel right unless all your hormone problems have been addressed.

Look for other issues

Many symptoms can have more than one cause. If thyroid levels are optimized and symptoms persist, there could be another cause.

Be patient

Levothyroxine is a very long-acting medication. When you start taking it, it takes five to six weeks to achieve stable blood levels, but because it takes even longer to achieve stable tissue levels, the resolution of symptoms may take longer. Every time your dose is changed, it will take another five to six weeks for levels to stabilize.

What to do when levothyroxine doesn't work

For some patients, despite valiant efforts, levothyroxine alone is not enough to restore optimal hormone balance. Adding T3 or taking a T3-combination product can sometimes be helpful in these circumstances. The use of T3 is still controversial, however, because the vast majority of clinical studies, including a major study published in the *Journal of the American Medical Association,* have failed to show a benefit of taking T3 compared to a placebo. Other studies from the Netherlands, China, and from Spain showed that T3 did not improve mood, fatigue, well-being, neurocognitive function, or any other objective measurements compared to taking T4 alone; however, patients still reported that they preferred taking it.

Liothyronine (Cytomel)

Liothyronine is a synthetic form of T3. T3 supplementation with Cytomel has helped many patients but is still controversial among endocrinologists because studies have failed to show a definite benefit. Despite the research, many patients say they prefer to take a low dose of T3 in addition to levothyroxine.

The dose of T3 varies among individuals. The body needs about 20 percent T3 and 80 percent T4; however, the body will make some T3 from T4, even if the process is impaired. I recommend that the dose of T3 not exceed 10 percent of your total thyroid hormone dosage. Many patients do well with 2.5–5 mcg of liothyronine once in the morning. Some people prefer to take a second dose around 2:00 P.M. to prevent an afternoon slump. Liothyronine can be taken three times a day, but it can cause insomnia if taken too close to bedtime. Unlike levothyroxine, if you forget a dose, you cannot double up on liothyronine.

One of the main problems with liothyronine is that it can cause thyroid levels to go too high. If you take liothyronine, your physician will need to check your blood tests more frequently. If thyroid levels are too high or the TSH is too low, your doctor can reduce the dose of levothyroxine or liothyronine to bring tests back into the normal range.

Sustained release T3

Sustained release T3, custom-made by compounding pharmacists, has shown promise as the ideal method of taking T3, because the T3 that is in liothyronine, Thyrolar, and Armour Thyroid is very short acting. The majority of the T3 from these products is out of your system after a few hours. Sustained release T3 is in special capsules that provide a slower release of the hormone into your system over a period of twelve hours. The problem with sustained release T3 is that the release is not that slow. Pharmacists are still trying to perfect the process of making a better sustained release T3 tablet.

In March 2001, officials from the Georgia Drugs and Narcotics Agency became concerned when several patients who had their T3 filled at a Georgia compounding pharmacy were hospitalized for life-threatening high thyroid levels. It was discovered that pills were made incorrectly and contained one hundred times the prescribed dose of T3. Since that time, reputable compounding pharmacies have become ultra-vigilant in the way they make T3.

Liotrix (Thyrolar)

Liotrix is a mixture of liothyronine (T3) and levothyroxine (T4) available in a single tablet. Available in different strengths, the ratio of T3 to T4 in this fixed combination tablet is 1:4 (one mcg of T3 for every four mcg of T4). This combination tends to have too much T3 for most people. Despite this fact, many doctors believe that the percentage of T3 is too high. Another disadvantage with Thyrolar is that it requires refrigeration.

Desiccated Thyroid (Armour Thyroid, Nature-Throid, Westhroid, and Thyroid USP)

Some patients prefer desiccated thyroid, which is produced from pig (porcine) thyroid glands. Because it comes from a pig, it is considered natural. Desiccated thyroid contains about 25 percent T3 and 75 percent T4, which is different from the normal T4:T3 ratio for humans, who need 20 percent T3. Some people feel better with the higher T3 level; some don't. Some of my patients have done very well taking a low dose of desiccated thyroid (15–30 mg) in addition to their standard dose of levothyroxine.

The quality and potency of desiccated thyroid has improved in recent years. Despite the higher T3 levels and past availability issues, many of my patients feel great and have perfect thyroid levels on desiccated thyroid. Thyroid USP offers an advantage because the dose of the pills can be customized.

One problem with desiccated thyroid is that the T3 part tends to wear off early in the day. A solution is to take a second dose around 2:00 P.M.

Custom T3/T4 combination products

Compounding pharmacies can make just about any dose combination of T3 (usually in sustained release form) and levothyroxine. Compounded thyroid hormone products are difficult to make correctly. It is important to choose a reputable compounding pharmacist that has rigid protocols and regularly tests its products at an independent laboratory.

Thyroid Hormone Abuse

Some people adhere to the philosophy that "if a little is good for me, then more must be better." Maybe that's the case with some things, but with thyroid hormone, it is a prescription for disaster. Unfortunately, since thyroid hormone is usually recommended for people suffering from weight gain caused by hypothyroidism (and that's key—it's not simply weight gain), some patients will increase their dosage on their own, thinking that taking more hormone will speed their metabolism and help them lose weight even faster. Let me emphasize: increasing your thyroid hormone dose is extremely dangerous.

First of all, the "benefits" (if you want to call them that) are short term at best: yes, metabolism may pick up. Yes, it may help shed a few pounds, but the body is as ill equipped to handle what becomes "forced hyperthyroidism" as it is to handle hypothyroidism. Increased dosages blow blood pressure sky high, cause the heart to fibrillate and function poorly, weaken muscle tissues, and bring on thinning of the bones (osteoporosis).

Thyroid hormone is a serious matter. Endocrinologists painstakingly work to find exactly the right dosage for their patients, tweaking the daily regimen by as little as 12 micrograms (that's twelve millionths of a gram, or .000012 grams). They also make patients come in regularly for blood tests to make sure the dosage is still correct. Like any other drug, thyroid hormone is not to be abused. The results can be calamitous.

Diet and Lifestyle for a Healthy Thyroid

"Approximately half of patients ask whether they can change their diet or do something else to treat the condition instead of taking the synthetic hormone."

—Elise M. Brett, M.D., F.A.C.E., Associate Clinical
Professor of Medicine, Mount Sinai School of Medicine

The Hormonal Health Diet is ideal for people with thyroid problems. This diet not only helps you lose weight, it also promotes optimal thyroid balance, psychological well-being, and physical health.

Eat Lots of Fruits and Vegetables

Fruits and vegetables act as antioxidants. Among the best-known antioxidants are beta-carotene, vitamin A, and vitamin C. Antioxidants promote the binding of what are called *free radicals*—oxygen-rich substances in the body that damage cells and hinder the immune system. Immune system attack is the main cause of hypothyroidism. Antioxidants clear toxins from the body and are even thought to help ward off cancer.

Get the Right Amount of Iodine

The recommended daily allowance (RDA) for iodine is 150 micrograms; however, in the United States, the usual consumption ranges between 300 and 700 micrograms a day—a testament to our love of salt and salty products—because most of the salt used in the United States is iodized. (One teaspoon of iodized salt contains more than 300 mcg of iodine.) Iodine has nothing to do with sodium; it's just added to the salt. Non-iodized salt (known as *free running*) and kosher salt do not contain iodine. Iodine also comes from seafood and sea vegetables, and it is found in preservatives and in red dye #3 (red dye #40 does not contain iodine). Many red, orange, or brown processed foods, pills, and capsules contain red dye #3. Iodine is in many medications, such as amiodarone, levothyroxine, liothyronine, cough syrups (expectorants), povidone-iodine topical antiseptics, and IV contrast dye. When reading labels, the words *iodate, iopodate, iodide, potassium iodide,* or *sodium iodide* mean the product contains iodine.

Most multivitamin and mineral supplements contain 150 mcg of iodine. Sources of dietary iodine include seaweed sushi wraps, seafood, commercial baked goods and snack foods, egg yolks, chocolate, molasses, soy products, rhubarb, potato skins, and fruits and vegetables grown in iodine-rich soil (usually near a coast). Dairy products once contained high amounts of iodine because farmers used it as a disinfectant, but new iodine-free products are being used by some manufacturers. Too much or too little iodine can cause thyroid dysfunction, so it is important for you to get the right amount.

Eat Foods High in Selenium and Zinc

Selenium and zinc function as antioxidants. Moreover, selenium has a dual role—besides its antioxidizing properties, it helps convert T4 to T3. Lack of selenium and zinc can reduce levels of active T3 by preventing its conversion from T4. Although selenium and zinc supplements are available from most health food stores, I recommend that you increase your consumption of these vital minerals by eating the proper foods. Foods high in selenium include whole grains, tuna, halibut, mushrooms, oatmeal, wheat germ, and sunflower seeds.

Because selenium is also needed for survival of bacteria, persons infected with a bacterial illness often find themselves with a selenium deficiency and get a double whammy, because the bacteria, growing fat and happy off all the selenium they're diverting, also produce substances detrimental to the production of thyroid hormone.

Foods High in Selenium	
Brazil nuts	Meats
Cod	Tuna
Cereals	Vegetables and fruits
Eggs	

Too much selenium can be as damaging as too little. Among the side effects of too much selenium: abdominal pain, nerve damage, and diarrhea. It is estimated that 50 mcg a day is enough to keep your thyroid healthy and provide a decent amount of antioxidant activity.

A diet low in zinc has been found to cause damage to the thyroid gland. Down's syndrome children are usually low in zinc, and many are hypothyroid as well. Obese people have the same problem. A diet featuring a proper level of this trace mineral can help assuage the problems caused by thyroid

Foods High in Zinc	
Beef	Sunflower seeds
Herring	Turkey
Maple syrup	Wheat bran

dysfunction. Foods high in zinc include beef, herring, maple syrup, turkey, wheat bran, and sunflower seeds.

Take Vitamin A

Take vitamin A in dosages of 3000–5000 IU (International Units) daily. Vitamin A deficiency causes thyroid problems. Vitamin A is involved in T4:T3 conversion and thyroid hormone metabolism throughout the body.

Eat Less Gluten

Having a thyroid problem increases your risk for celiac disease and other forms of gluten intolerance. If you have full-blown celiac disease, you need to be ultra-strict about staying gluten free. Many thyroid patients have mild gluten intolerance and normal testing for celiac disease. Reducing gluten in the diet can sometimes improve absorption of thyroid medications and the symptoms of hypothyroidism.

Spice Up Your Foods

Low metabolism is the hallmark of thyroid problems. Adding chili peppers and other hot spices to your foods can give your metabolism a little boost.

Don't Eat Too Many Raw Goitrogens

Cruciferous vegetables from the *Brassica* family, such as cabbage, broccoli, Brussels sprouts, turnips, rutabaga, mustard, kohlrabi, radishes, cauliflower, cassava, millet, and kale are called goitrogens and are listed as foods to avoid in many thyroid-related books and websites, but read on, because you may not yet have all the facts. These vegetables contain naturally occurring substances known as isothiocyanates that interfere with the function of the thyroid gland, but the reality is that these vegetables won't hurt your thyroid unless you eat huge amounts of them raw. Once cooked, these foods have many health benefits. The key is not to eliminate these foods. Cooking these vegetables is recommended, but you can eat up to two cups of raw cabbage, broccoli, and cauliflower weekly without doing any harm to your thyroid. Peaches, peanuts, pine nuts, spinach, and strawberries also may inhibit thyroid function if consumed in large amounts.

Don't Eat Too Much Soy

Limit your consumption of soy products to four to five servings a week. Although soy products have many health benefits, soy can also increase the risk of thyroid problems. Soy has been shown to interfere with the thyroid peroxidase, which is an enzyme responsible for an important step in the production of thyroid hormone. The National Center for Toxicological Research reports that soy isoflavones have a number of anti-thyroid effects that result in soy toxicity. A study from the University of Belgrade showed that soy isoflavones cause destructive changes in the thyroid tissue, leading to hypothyroidism. Another study from England found that soy products increased the risk threefold for an underactive thyroid.

Soy also contains natural estrogen-like compounds. These compounds have been thought to affect the thyroid, but the truth is the effect is very small. If you take thyroid medication, to allow for adequate absorption, you should take it at least two hours away from eating soy.

Work Out

Regular physical activity is a critical element in maintaining a hormonal balance and a healthy metabolism. Hypothyroidism makes people tired, less energetic, and less motivated to exercise. Try to exercise during a time in the day when your energy levels are at their peak.

Don't Take Thyroid Supplements

There are two types of thyroid supplements: iodine supplements and glandular supplements.

Iodine supplements promise to supply the nutritional needs of the thyroid and contain iodine (in the form of kelp, bugleweed, or bladderwrack), vitamins, minerals, and tyrosine. The high iodine content can cause the thyroid to become underactive or overactive and do more harm than good.

Glandular thyroid supplements are products that are similar to desiccated thyroid but are available without a prescription. These products have no quality control and may contain much less or much more than the dose listed on the label. If you want to take a glandular thyroid supplement, work with a qualified physician who will prescribe a high-quality supplement.

Get the Toxins Out

Toxins and pollutants can cause thyroid problems. Known as *environmental endocrine disruptors,* these substances slow thyroid function and disrupt hormonal balance. The chemical carbon tetrachloride is known to cause thyroid dysfunction and has been found in samples of drinking water.

Pesticides have a chronic mineral-depleting effect that can lead to thyroid problems. Polychlorinated biphenyl (PCB) exposure has been associated with impaired intellectual functioning, memory problems, and learning problems thought in part caused by thyroid dysfunction.

The weed killer Roundup, which contains the chemical glyphosate, has been blamed for thyroid problems.

Smoking may contribute to thyroid disease, because of several toxins, including cadmium, that are contained in tobacco leaves. Cadmium has been linked to thyroid dysfunction. Dried fruits (which are often dried on galvanized chicken wire) can contain high amounts of cadmium as well.

Nitrates and mercury have also been linked to thyroid problems.

Antibacterial products, from dishwashing liquids to bar soap and toothpaste, have become very popular in the last few years, promising cleaner skin and less risk of infection, but many of these products contain a chemical called triclosan, which is thought to interfere with thyroid hormone metabolism. My recommendation is to avoid antibacterial products. The regular versions of the products do an excellent job of killing microbes, without any potential risk to your thyroid.

Chapter Review

The thyroid controls metabolism and plays a big role in weight regulation. The small organ at the base of the neck is also connected to other important functions such as body temperature regulation, sleep, and sex drive. About 40 per cent of overweight Americans have some type of thyroid dysfunction; however, not all weight issues are directly related to thyroid problems. That's why it is important to rule out thyroid problems early when diagnosing the root causes of weight gain.

The chapter presented an extensive review of the many ways the thyroid affects both weight control and overall health.

In addition to information about the direct impact of the thyroid on weight control, the chapter discussed dozens of other health issues related to thyroid functioning, including a number of autoimmune diseases that attack the thyroid and lead to diseases such as Addison's and Crohn's diseases, lupus, and type 1 diabetes.

Diagnosing low thyroid is difficult and often attributed to other causes. Risk factors for low thyroid include age, weight, diabetes, depression, family history, chemical exposure, and stress. Those who suffer from low thyroid weight gain issues may still gain weight even while dieting; the associated weight gain triggers even more problems that are linked to leptin resistance (chapter 5).

Many ways exist to test for and treat both hypothyroidism and hyperthyroidism. For example, rising levels of a specific hormone or the presence of certain antibodies in the bloodstream are both related to hypothyroidism.

A number of avenues are offered in the chapter to diagnose and treat the issues associated with a low-producing or overactive thyroid. Treatments include both the introduction of drugs specifically designed to replace the missing thyroid hormone needed to restore normal functioning and a change in lifestyle (reducing stress and eating foods that enhance thyroid health).

The next chapter discusses the need for women's balanced supply of male and female hormones, including a class of male hormones that are essential for female health throughout life.

8

Women's Hormones I
Thrive in Your Reproductive Years

A woman's reproductive years begin with puberty and end with menopause. For many women, the reproductive years constitute a time when hormones can wreak havoc on metabolism, causing increased appetite, slowed metabolism, and weight gain. During the reproductive years, the hormones estrogen and progesterone follow a monthly cycle, rising and falling in a predictable pattern that controls the menstrual cycle. Many hormonal disorders can ultimately affect female hormones and not only show up as problems with the menstrual cycle but may also result in weight gain. The terms *female hormones* or *women's hormones* refer to estrogen, progesterone, and prolactin, but these terms are very loose. The truth is that both men and women have both male and female hormones. In this chapter, I also discuss men's hormones, or androgens such as testosterone, androstenedione, and dehydroepiandrosterone (DHEA). These hormones work together to play an important role in female hormonal balance.

Balancing female hormones during the reproductive years is imperative for managing your weight. Female hormones are intimately linked to appetite, cravings,

In This Chapter
- ▶ The Importance of Female and Male Hormone Balance
- ▶ What Causes Premenstrual Syndrome and How to Treat It
- ▶ The Most Common Hormonal Condition in Women
- ▶ Testing and Treating Hormonal Imbalances

metabolism, body fat composition, and body fat distribution. If your female hormones aren't in balance, losing weight and keeping it off will be a challenge.

The best-known female hormone is estrogen, which takes its name from the Greek for "mad with desire." It is estrogen, after all, that helps mold a girl into a woman during puberty. The breasts form; the hips, thighs, and buttocks take their adult shape; and vaginal lubrication increases. Estrogen is responsible for the female body shape—weight gain goes to the hips and buttocks. Estrogen is responsible for bone health, one of the reasons men need estrogen too.

Progesterone is known for fluid retention, bloating, weight gain, and PMS. The name pro*gesterone* comes from *gestation,* preparation for pregnancy. Progesterone works together with estrogen to regulate the menstrual cycle and fertility. Progesterone can raise blood sugar and increase appetite.

The pituitary gland makes hormones that control female hormones. Luteinizing hormone (LH) and follicle stimulating hormone (FSH) are known as *gonado*tropin hormones because they stimulate the ovaries, also known as the *gonads.* Prolactin is another pituitary gland hormone; it is important for breast health and breast milk production. Pituitary hormones work together to regulate many of the basic female biological functions, such as puberty, the menstrual cycle, pregnancy, and menopause.

Testosterone, androstenedione, and dehydroepiandrosterone are thought of as male hormones, but they are important in female hormonal balance as well. These hormones are known as *androgen* hormones. Like estrogen, testosterone and androstenedione are produced by the ovaries. DHEA is produced by the adrenal gland. Androgens help build lean body mass, but too much androgen can lead to problems such as weight gain, insulin resistance, irregular menstrual cycles, and facial hair growth. The main cause of androgen problems in women is androgen hormone excess. Testosterone is the primary androgen hormone in men, but in women, the DHEA-S and androstenedione play equally important roles.

Women's Hormones
Estrogen
Progesterone
Prolactin
Testosterone
Androstenedione
Dehydroepiandrosterone

The most common imbalances of female hormones during a woman's reproductive years are

1. Early puberty
2. Premenstrual weight gain
3. Elevated male hormones
4. Premature menopause

Hormone Imbalance: Early Puberty

For the past few decades, doctors have been noticing that girls are going into puberty at younger ages. No one knows exactly why it is happening, but researchers speculate that several factors play a role, including obesity and environmental chemicals. Excess body fat boosts estrogen levels. Environmental chemicals imitate estrogen. Most of the patients I see with early puberty also tend to be overweight or obese.

Most girls start puberty between ages eight and thirteen (boys start around nine to fourteen years of age). Doctors report that as many as 25 percent of girls show signs of puberty by the age of seven, though. A decade ago, only 5 to 10 percent of girls started puberty early. Although the timing of puberty is largely controlled by our genetics, the latest trends may a result from a combination of increasing obesity rates, along with environmental chemicals that mimic estrogen, a subject I discuss in chapter 2. Endocrine-disrupting chemicals such as BPA (bisphenol A), phthalates, parabens, perfluorocarbons, and DDT wreak havoc on hormones, and young girls are especially sensitive to the effects.

Early puberty increases the risk of breast and uterine cancer. A 2007 report from the Breast Cancer Fund indicates that delaying puberty in girls by one or two years can cut lifetime estrogen exposure and reduce the future risk of breast cancer up to 20 percent.

Hormone Imbalance: Gaining Weight with PMS

It's no secret that the menstrual cycle, with its ebb and flow of estrogen and progesterone, has a great effect on the rest of the body, including appetite, cravings, energy level, and mood. Four out of ten women experience problematic symptoms related to premenstrual syndrome (PMS) or premenstrual dysphoric disorder (PMDD), which have been blamed for unpredictable, unpleasant, and unwanted symptoms that can contribute to weight gain.

PMS symptoms can begin one or two days before the menstrual cycle, but for some women they can occur and last up to fourteen days before a cycle. For some women, the symptoms can be mild, but for others, symptoms can be debilitating. PMS has several common symptoms: food cravings, food binges, increased hunger, weight gain, bloating and fluid retention, back pain, breast tenderness, insomnia, depression, crying spells, anger, anxiety, panic attacks, decreased concentration, fatigue, and headaches.

The following can help slow down puberty in girls:

Breast-feed the babies. Babies who are breast-fed are less likely to become overweight. Breast milk contains substances that regulate growth and development that may have an influence on the timing of puberty. In addition, breast-feeding teaches babies to stop eating when they are full instead of stopping when the bottle is empty. Later, breast-fed babies tend to be better at regulating how much they eat.

Avoid obesity in the children. Fat cells produce estrogen, so when the body is fat, it has more estrogen. Many studies have linked obesity with early puberty. Eating a healthy diet and getting regular exercise can help girls maintain normal estrogen levels.

Reduce exposure to BPA and phthalates. These chemicals are hormonal disruptors that imitate estrogen.

Use organic or hormone-free dairy products and meats. Dairy products and meat may contain hormones and chemicals that can affect hormones.

See a doctor. Early puberty can be caused by a number of hormonal disorders. A pediatric endocrinologist is uniquely qualified to evaluate early puberty.

Many women know about the intense craving for food—particularly chocolate and sweets—that hits during the second half of the menstrual cycle, the time before menstruation. No one knows the exact cause of PMS, but researchers believe it is related to fluctuations in female hormones, including progesterone, estrogen, pituitary hormones, and brain hormones like serotonin. The normal hormonal fluctuations of menstruation are perhaps the most elegant hormonal systems in the entire human body. The timing of the signals from the hypothalamus and pituitary gland controls female hormones like a conductor of a symphony. Even these normal hormonal fluctuations can result in symptoms of PMS.

Ten to twelve days before a menstrual cycle, estrogen levels drop slightly and progesterone levels rise markedly. Progesterone is the one of the hormone culprits responsible for the hunger, cravings, and fluid retention that comes during the second half of the menstrual cycle. Progesterone is also responsible

---

Eat Dark Chocolate to Kill PMS Cravings

No matter what you are craving, eating chocolate can reduce or eliminate PMS cravings. Eat a few squares of dark chocolate that is 60–70 percent cocoa when you have a PMS craving and watch the craving melt away like the chocolate. Why chocolate? Dark chocolate contains chemicals such as phenethylmine and theobromine, which have the same effect on the brain as antidepressants, offering a rush of serotonin and a calming and satisfying effect. Part of the calm feeling you get from eating chocolate is also a result of acylethanolamines, chemicals that may have an effect on the brain similar to that of marijuana. Chocolate is high in antioxidants and other nutrients, too. Chocolate is also rich in substances called phenolics, the same beneficial chemicals found in red wine, and may decrease the risk of heart disease as wine does.

---

for preparing a woman's body for pregnancy. The same factors are responsible for stimulating appetite. After all, pregnant women need to gain weight. Progesterone also makes you sleepy and less likely to want to exercise. Progesterone causes insulin resistance and makes blood sugar levels rise, which can add to weight gain, especially during the second half of the menstrual cycle.

"The only cure for PMS is menopause"

—Donnica Moore, M.D.

Hormone Imbalance: Elevated Male Hormones

Androgen excess is the most common hormonal disorder in young women. Polycystic ovary syndrome (PCOS), also known as Stein-Leventhal syndrome, is the most common cause of androgen excess. Other conditions, such as congenital adrenal hyperplasia, pituitary gland tumors, ovarian cancer, adrenal gland cancer, Cushing's syndrome (see chapter 11), and acromegaly (chapter 12) can cause androgen excess and result in the same symptoms as PCOS. Premature menopause, symptomatic menopause, hypothyroidism, and exposure to male hormone gels can

Beat PMS Symptoms

There is no cure for PMS. The good news is that there is a lot you can do to lessen the symptoms and the impact on your weight.

Eat healthy food. Studies have shown that PMS symptoms are worse in women who eat unhealthy diets.

Eat foods rich in B vitamins. B vitamins boost brain serotonin and help reduce the PMS symptoms of moodiness, irritability, and carbohydrate cravings. A study from the University of Massachusetts found that eating spinach, pistachio nuts, almonds, beans, tomatoes, fish, fortified cereals, and other foods high in the B vitamins thiamine and riboflavin decreased women's risk of PMS by 25 percent. The study also found that unlike B vitamin-rich food, vitamin B supplements did not decrease the symptoms of PMS.

Exercise. Lack of exercise is known to exacerbate the symptoms of PMS.

Reduce stress. Many of the symptoms of PMS are undoubtedly made worse by stress. Several studies have found a link between stress and the symptoms of PMS. In a study published in the *Journal of Women's Health,* researchers from the National Institute of Child Health and Development found that women with the highest level of stress were twice as likely to experience anger, anxiety, and irritability and three times more likely to feel sad or depressed or have crying spells. Researchers speculate that stress makes PMS worse because it causes hormonal changes, including raising cortisol levels, which make women more susceptible to PMS. No matter how it works, relaxation is a great way to decrease your PMS symptoms.

Do not smoke. Studies show that women who smoke report worse PMS symptoms than those who do not.

---

also imitate the symptoms of PCOS. The first step to getting the right treatment is to get an accurate diagnosis. I have seen many patients who were initially told they had PCOS but who ended up having entirely different diagnoses. The treatment depends on the cause of hyperandrogenism, so getting the right diagnosis is vital.

The three main androgens are testosterone, androstenedione, and dehydroepiandrosterone. Elevations in any one can cause symptoms that correspond to having excess male hormones. Insights into the causes and treatments of androgen excess have increased significantly in the past fifteen years.

Avoid triggers. Minimize intake of caffeine, alcohol, salt, red meat, or high-sugar foods, all of which can make PMS symptoms worse.

Get plenty of sleep. Poor sleep or lack of sleep makes PMS symptoms worse. Studies have shown that improving the duration and quality of your sleep can alleviate symptoms.

Satisfy your cravings. Eat a little bit of the food you are craving combined with a larger portion of a healthy food. This combination allows you to satisfy your cravings without overeating.

Take calcium supplements. Symptoms of PMS are reduced by calcium. I recommend taking 500 milligrams (mg) twice a day.

Take vitamin C. Fruits and vegetables are an excellent source of vitamin C. For an extra boost, take vitamin C 500–1000 mg daily.

Take vitamin E. A study in Brazil showed that women who took 1000–2000 mg of vitamin E daily had fewer symptoms of PMS.

Remember to consume essential fatty acids. A study published in the journal *Reproductive Health* showed that women who took a combination of gamma linolenic acid, oleic acid, and linoleic acid had decreased symptoms of PMS compared to those who took a placebo. Essential fatty acids decrease levels of inflammation chemicals known as prostaglandins, which have been linked to PMS symptoms.

Consider taking SSRI antidepressants. Antidepressants such as Prozac (also marketed as Sarafem, specifically for PMS), Celexa, Lexapro, Paxil, and Zoloft are commonly used to treat PMS.

The latest research has found that androgen excess can have serious metabolic consequences. Androgen excess and excess weight are linked; the more weight gained, the higher the androgen levels. Gaining weight raises androgen levels, and higher androgens cause insulin resistance and more weight gain, a vicious cycle. Elevated androgens are linked to health problems like high blood pressure, lipid abnormalities, insulin resistance, diabetes, obstructive sleep apnea, cardiovascular disease, and an increased risk for a variety of cancers. Losing weight helps lower androgen levels.

Reduce Fluid Retention and Bloating during PMS

The root of the word *menses,* as in menstrual cycle, comes from *month*—which, in turn, comes from *moon*. The moon has a twenty-nine-day cycle; more or less; the menstrual cycle is twenty-eight days. In ancient times, the body was considered a miniature universe, and from what we know now, the ancients weren't far wrong: after all, life began with water and the chemical reactions of a developing planet, including the cycles of the moon and the tides. Today we carry around that history in our DNA. Unfortunately for many women, water and the menstrual cycle are still closely related. Many women suffer from fluid retention and bloating, conditions that occur right before menses. Not coincidentally, this is a time of high progesterone levels.

Surges of progesterone during PMS causes muscle relaxation, particularly in the smooth muscle—the type of muscle found in the uterus and bowels. During the second half of the menstrual cycle, when progesterone levels are high, the smooth muscle relaxation causes the bowels to expand, stretching the belly and causing the sensation of bloating. The belly sticks out because the muscle tone of the bowels is not as good and the muscles cannot keep everything tight. Bloating is rarely associated with serious disease, incidentally—it is an uncomfortable symptom but is usually not a concern of a serious hormonal disorder. Nevertheless, it is a common complaint during PMS.

To minimize symptoms of bloating, follow these suggestions:

Avoid salt and prepared foods. Salt makes your body retain water, and many prepared foods contain high levels of salt. Do not reduce your water intake, though, which will not help and can make you dehydrated. In fact, drinking more water than usual helps flush your body and reduce swelling.

Avoid foods high in fat, especially high in animal fat. Fat slows the movement of the intestinal tract and makes bloating worse.

Avoid too much fiber. Although normally I recommend eating 25–35 grams of fiber

Signs and Symptoms of Elevated Male Hormones

Androgen excess can cause many problems, ranging from minor cosmetic concerns to significant medical issues. The severity of symptoms usually correlates with the degree of androgen excess.

daily, if you have bloating, fiber consumption should be reduced to 15 grams a day for four or five days. Fiber swells in the intestines and worsens the sensation of bloating. Beans in particular are high in fiber and also cause gas, which could also worsen bloating.

Eat small, frequent meals. Following my meal plan prevents overdistension of the stomach.

Eliminate—or at least moderate—caffeine and alcohol. Both have diuretic effects, and both function as stimulants that artificially raise the body's levels of various hormones, only to send them crashing when the effect wears off.

Exercise. Progesterone tends to make you sleepy, reducing your activity level. Muscle activity is important for reducing fluid retention. As muscles are worked, they force blood into the heart. Swimming can be very good, because the pressure of the water in the pool forces tissue fluid back into the general circulation, where it can be eliminated by the kidneys.

Use a heating pad. Yes, heating pads may reduce bloating, and they're not expensive.

Lose weight. All these practices should help you lose weight, but don't do these things only during "that time of the month." Obesity contributes to fluid retention by increasing pressure inside the abdomen, making it harder for blood to return to the heart.

Avoid diuretics. Diuretic medications should be used only under the careful supervision of a physician.

Get checked by your physician. Incidentally, fluid retention may not be from progesterone. Idiopathic cyclic edema is an extreme form of menstrual fluid retention. (*Idiopathic* is medical jargon for "We don't know what's causing this.") Severe edema can be a sign of more serious diseases, such as heart failure, blood clots, or kidney or liver disease.

Abnormal Lipids (Cholesterol and Triglycerides)

Women with hyperandrogenism have lipid problems typically seen with insulin resistance, which I discuss in chapter 6, with high triglycerides, low HDL (good) cholesterol, and normal or high LDL (bad) cholesterol.

Could It Be Cancer?

If symptoms of excess male hormones arise suddenly or are severe, don't even think of hesitating; get right to a doctor. A sudden onset of an androgen disorder is a warning sign for an androgen-producing cancer of the adrenal gland or ovary. Severe androgen excess is also known as *virilism*.

Warning signs for cancer include:

Cessation of the menstrual cycle

Deepening of the voice

Enlargement of the clitoris

Excessive facial or body hair growth

Excessive body odor

Increased musculature

Loss of breast tissue

Low potassium level

Male-pattern balding

Severe cystic acne

Sudden onset of symptoms

Acanthosis Nigricans

A darkening of the skin, usually on the neck and armpits, is a very common condition that occurs in women with androgen excess and insulin resistance (see chapter 6).

Acne

Up to 50 percent of teenagers have acne, so having acne doesn't necessarily mean that you have hyperandrogenism. Persistence of acne into the late teens or twenties, however—known as *adult acne*—is not normal. Adult acne is usually a sign of androgen excess. Adult acne can be hard to treat with traditional acne medications, but treatments for androgen excess and insulin resistance make these medications more effective.

Anxiety, Depression, Mood Swings, and Anger

Androgens have powerful effects on the brain. Androgen excess has been associated with anxiety and depression. Excess androgens can increase irritability, anger, and aggression. Husbands of women with androgen excess may claim that their wives have "short fuses."

Cardiovascular Disease

Androgen excess increases the risk for cardiovascular disease (heart attacks and strokes). Insulin resistance, abnormal blood glucose, abnormal lipids, and high blood pressure contribute to the risk.

Decreased Libido

Most women with excess androgens experience decreased or low sex drive, which is a paradox, because androgens have been thought to increase libido. No one knows why women with high androgens have a low libido. Many women with androgen excess also have problems with poor body image that can lead to feelings of low self-worth and social isolation, all of which can decrease libido.

Deepening of the Voice

Androgens can cause a thickening of the vocal cords that may cause the voice to deepen. This condition is considered a serious sign of hyperandrogenism. Any woman who experiences deepening of the voice should be evaluated for adrenal gland cancer or cancer of the ovary.

Elevated Blood Sugar, Prediabetes, or Diabetes

Blood sugar problems related to insulin resistance are extremely common in women with hyperandrogenism. For more information on blood sugar problems, see chapter 6.

Enlargement of the Clitoris

On rare occasions, high androgen levels can cause the clitoris to become enlarged. An enlarged clitoris is defined as being longer than one centimeter. It may even begin to take on the appearance of a small penis. This condition is considered a severe manifestation of androgen excess and always warrants an evaluation for cancer of the adrenal gland or ovary.

Excessive Body Odor

Hyperandrogenism increases production of foul-smelling sweat, especially in the armpits. Elevated growth hormone (see chapter 12) can also cause this symptom.

Facial Hair (Hirsutism) or Excess Body Hair

Androgen excess causes hair growth on the upper lip, chin, sideburns, neck, chest, arms, nipples, back, buttocks, stomach, shoulders, arms, legs, and inner thighs. Excessive hair growth is not always a sign of an androgen problem. If your menstrual cycle is perfectly normal, excess hair growth is usually benign and less likely caused by PCOS or other serious medical problems. Facial and body hair can be normal, especially for women of Mediterranean or Middle Eastern heritage, and is known as *benign familial hirsutism*. Hair on the lower back, chest, stomach, shoulders, buttocks, and inner thighs, however, is usually considered abnormal and should be evaluated, even if the menstrual cycle is normal.

Hair Loss (Androgenic Alopecia)

Although excess androgen causes hair to grow on the face and body, it can also cause hair loss from the scalp, a condition known as *androgenic alopecia*. Higher androgen levels cause hair loss in a "male pattern," as a receding hairline or loss of hair on the top of the scalp. Sometimes the pattern of hair loss is thinning hair across the entire scalp. Some women don't have visible hair loss but notice a lot of shedding. This type of hair loss can be caused by excess androgens but can have many other causes as well. Severe male-pattern hair loss may be a warning sign of cancer of the adrenal gland or ovary.

High Blood Pressure

High blood pressure is usually seen with high androgen levels as a consequence of the underlying condition. Insulin resistance (see chapter 6), Cushing's syndrome (see chapter 11), and acromegaly (see chapter 12) are causes of elevated androgens and elevated blood pressure.

Irregular Periods

Irregular periods are a sign that the body's hormones and metabolism have gone off track. Androgen excess almost always affects the menstrual cycle in one way or another. Androgen excess can lead to many problems, including infrequent cycles or irregular cycles, light cycles, or heavy flow. Oligomenorrhea—fewer than nine cycles a year—is typical for many women with androgen excess. In general, doctors correlate the menstrual cycle with ovulation, so it is assumed that abnormal menstrual cycles means a woman is not ovulating properly. Some women with androgen excess have stopped having menstrual cycles entirely. Severe premenstrual cycle syndrome or excessive cramping with the menstrual cycle may also be symptoms. Excessive blood loss, also referred to as dysfunctional uterine bleeding, can cause anemia, which makes you feel tired.

Having fewer than four periods a year is a risk factor for cancer of the uterus. A study from Jewish Hospital in Cincinnati found that teenage girls who have irregular menstrual cycles are more likely to be overweight or obese and have warning signs for diabetes and heart disease by their mid-twenties.

Infertility

Primarily because of ovulation problems, women with hyperandrogenism can have difficulty getting pregnant.

Polycystic Ovary Syndrome

PCOS is the most common hormonal disorder in women. One in ten women has it. Although first described by Stein and Leventhal in 1935, this condition had been largely ignored by doctors until the past decade or so. PCOS is a combination of two hormonal aberrations: insulin resistance and androgen excess. The primary cause is still debated—it is the classic chicken-and-egg situation. High androgens cause insulin resistance, and insulin resistance causes high androgens.

> *"BPA may be more harmful to women with hormone and fertility imbalances like those found in PCOS."*
>
> —Evanthia Diamanti-Kandarakis, M.D., Ph.D.,
> University of Athens Medical School, Greece

Most women who have PCOS are overweight or obese, but as many as 25 percent of women who have PCOS are not overweight. PCOS is a genetic disorder, but a single PCOS gene has not been identified. Several genes are thought to be responsible for the various features of PCOS. It's not unusual to have a sister, mother, or aunt with symptoms of insulin resistance or androgen excess. PCOS can also be transmitted through the father's side. If anyone in your family has insulin resistance or type 2 diabetes, you may have the genetics for PCOS.

Obesity itself is not considered a cause of PCOS, but it is considered a factor that makes the symptoms worse, and it's a cycle. Excess weight goes right to the belly, increasing insulin resistance, leading to even more weight gain. Weight loss breaks the cycle and lessens the symptoms of insulin resistance and androgen excess.

Women with PCOS start developing symptoms not long after puberty, but they usually aren't diagnosed for five or more years. The heavier you are, the

Even Worse Than PCOS

Androgens Out of Control: Ovarian Hyperthecosis

Most women with ovarian hyperthecosis are overweight or obese and have more severe facial hair growth or other symptoms of androgen excess. Unlike PCOS, which occurs during the reproductive years, hyperthecosis can occur in women of any age. Some doctors recommend surgical removal of the ovaries because of the associated risk of ovarian cancer.

Severe Insulin Resistance: HAIRAN Syndrome

HAIRAN is an acronym for hyperandrogenic insulin resistant acanthosis nigricans. It is a mouthful to say, but it refers to a malignant form of PCOS. It's everything bad about PCOS magnified, and it's very destructive to the body. Women with HAIRAN syndrome usually are overweight or obese and have diabetes or prediabetes, high blood pressure, cholesterol problems, and are at high risk for cardiovascular disease.

more likely symptoms will develop at an early age. Every attempt should be made to diagnose and treat PCOS as early as possible. PCOS has serious health consequences that go beyond excess weight and excess androgens. Excessive androgen can cause a girl to go into puberty earlier. Women with the disorder are at high risk for diabetes, high blood pressure, cholesterol problems, sleep apnea, cardiovascular disease, cancer of the uterus, and cardiovascular disease. The symptoms of androgen excess tend to get better when a woman goes into menopause. Insulin resistance and the risk for medical problems get worse with menopause.

The name PCOS is misleading, because it implies multiple cysts are in the ovaries. Although true for some, up to 30 percent of women with PCOS do not have cysts in their ovaries. Women who have cysts in their ovaries but do not have PCOS have subtle signs of insulin resistance and glucose abnormalities when they are carefully tested. Another misnomer is the implication of the ovary as the primary source of androgen excess. Women who have had their ovaries removed can still have PCOS, because the ovary and adrenal gland are equally responsible for elevated androgen levels. High insulin levels stimulate the production of androgens, primarily DHEA, by the adrenal glands.

> ## Obstructive Sleep Apnea
>
> Women with PCOS are at increased risk for sleep apnea. The risk for sleep apnea increases as a woman gains weight; however, studies have shown that when you compare equal-weight women, those with androgen excess have an even greater risk for sleep apnea.. A person with sleep apnea may not be aware that he or she has it, except for vague symptoms such as fatigue and brain fog. The main symptoms of sleep apnea are sleepiness, headache, restless legs, waking up gasping, memory problems, and snoring. Sleep apnea is linked to high blood pressure, heart rhythm disturbances, heart attack, stroke, and sudden death. Sleep apnea is diagnosed using an overnight sleep study also known as polysomnography. For more information, see chapter 3.

PCOS is among the most common causes of infertility. The hallmark of PCOS is a problem releasing eggs from the ovary. Insulin resistance causes the walls of the ovary to become thickened and form cysts, and eggs cannot be released at their normal time of the month. This condition, known as anovulation, is also one of the reasons women with PCOS have menstrual cycle problems and infertility.

Diagnosing PCOS is challenging. The symptoms of PCOS are different for different women and can vary with time. An exact definition of PCOS has still not been clearly developed, but experts agree that to diagnose a woman with PCOS all other types of androgen excess must be ruled out.

An international committee has proposed that a woman have at least two of the following features to be diagnosed with PCOS:

1. **Ovulation problems** (usually manifested as menstrual cycle problems)

2. **Hyperandrogenism,** defined as either skin manifestations of androgen excess (facial hair, body hair, adult acne, male-pattern hair loss) or high androgen levels (in blood tests)

3. **Polycystic ovaries.** Polycystic ovaries do not need to be present to make a diagnosis of PCOS, and polycystic ovaries alone do not establish the diagnosis.

Rule Out Other Androgen Disorders to Rule In PCOS

Cancer

If the symptoms of an androgen disorder come on suddenly or are severe, it could be an indication of ovarian or adrenal cancer. See a doctor right away.

Congenital Adrenal Hyperplasia

Endocrinologists refer to the adult variety of this genetic condition as nonclassical congenital adrenal hyperplasia, or NCAH. The classical form of this disorder (CAH) presents at birth and causes ambiguous genitalia, where little girls are born with a clitoris so enlarged that it looks like a penis. The milder form of CAH is responsible for 1 to 2 percent of the cases of androgen excess in adult women. CAH is particularly common in people of Mediterranean descent and the Ashkenazi Jewish population. The source of the excess androgens comes from the adrenal gland.

Doctors (even endocrinologists) commonly miss NCAH, because they don't usually test for it. Standard androgen testing can appear identical to PCOS. I recommend testing for CAH in any woman with an androgen excess problem. The treatment for CAH is markedly different from the treatment for PCOS. Ask your doctor for the 17-hydroxyprogesterone blood test. In rare forms of CAH, however, even the 17-hydroxyprogesterone level can be normal. Having a high DHEA level can be a clue to having CAH, because DHEA comes from the adrenal gland.

If the symptoms are mild, treatment of NCAH is not mandatory. Sometimes women shave, use creams, or undergo electrolysis to control hair growth. In more severe cases, steroid medications such as dexamethasone or hydrocortisone can be helpful. Because CAH is a genetic

In recent years, the primary treatments for PCOS have shifted from treating androgen excess to treating insulin resistance or using a combination approach. Treatments for insulin resistance almost always improve androgen levels and symptoms of androgen excess but rarely provide a complete cure. If you have PCOS, special attention should also be given to the prevention of diabetes, cancer of the uterus, and cardiovascular disease.

Weight Gain (Especially around the Middle) or Difficulty Losing Weight

Weight gain is very common when women have elevated male hormones. High testosterone and DHEA lead to insulin resistance and weight gain in the condition, if you have CAH, it could be genetically transmitted to your children. Genetic testing is readily available for the most common form of CAH and is recommended for women and their partners who are planning families. Treatment of CAH in pregnancy may be necessary, especially if the baby is a girl, to prevent masculinization.

Hypothyroidism

Hypothyroidism causes symptoms similar to PCOS, such as menstrual cycle abnormalities, weight gain, and insulin resistance. Women with PCOS are at increased risk for having hypothyroidism. See chapter 7 for more on hypothyroidism.

Pituitary Gland Problems

A prolactinoma is a pituitary tumor that can cause androgen excess and is often misdiagnosed as PCOS. Increased production of the hormone prolactin can cause a woman to produce breast milk even if she is not breast-feeding. Acromegaly is a condition caused by a pituitary gland tumor that produces excess growth hormone and can cause symptoms of androgen excess. Acromegaly is also associated with other pituitary hormone deficiencies, insulin resistance, and diabetes, like PCOS. For more information on acromegaly, see chapter 12. Cushing's syndrome, most commonly caused by a pituitary gland tumor, can cause androgen excess along with excess cortisol. For more information on Cushing's syndrome, see chapter 11.

Premature Menopause

Premature menopause can cause symptoms similar to PCOS and should always be tested for.

midsection. My patients with androgen excess struggle with their weight despite valiant attempts at improving their diets and lifestyles. Improving insulin resistance lowers androgen levels and can make weight loss easier.

Testing for Androgen Excess

The purpose of testing for androgen excess is to look for all the imitators of PCOS, especially cancer. If you have symptoms and all your tests are perfectly normal, then you have the effects of androgen excess known as hyperandrogenism. In fact, many women with PCOS have completely normal labs. Why? Because tests are not perfect, and when measuring androgens, science still has a long way to go. Laboratories are particularly inaccurate at measuring androgen levels. Even though we're testing for androgen excess, high female androgen levels are still only one-tenth those of men. The lower the androgen level, the more difficult it is to measure accurately. The other problem is that the normal range is not clearly defined. Most experts believe that the upper part of the normal range is probably not normal, but high. Many women that I see with symptoms of androgen excess have "normal" levels that are in the upper end of the normal range. If someone has symptoms of hyperandrogenism, I consider these levels high.

Experts agree that if you have features of hyperandrogenism such as menstrual cycle problems, facial hair growth, or adult acne and yet have normal lab tests, then you probably have hyperandrogenism despite the normal results on the blood test. When diagnosing hyperandrogenism, symptoms are more important than lab tests. Also critical is a careful physical exam, looking for signs of androgen excess. We grade hirsutism using a scale known as the Ferriman-Gallwey scale. Do not be shocked if your physician requires a pelvic exam or asks to inspect your vulva and clitoris. Tell your doctor if you have a family history of obesity, diabetes, high cholesterol, or high blood pressure.

Androstenedione

Androstenedione is a lesser-known and weaker androgen made primarily by the ovary. Androstenedione can be converted by the body into testosterone or into estrogen. Androstenedione testing is not always required in the evaluation of hyperandrogenism, but it can be helpful, especially if the ovary is the source of hyperandrogenism.

Cholesterol Profile

High LDL (bad) cholesterol, low HDL (good) cholesterol, and high triglyceride levels are associated with hyperandrogenism. All women with hyperandrogenism should have a fasting lipid profile. For more information on cholesterol testing, see chapter 6.

Dehydroepiandrosterone Sulfate

Dehydroepiandrosterone is an androgen hormone made by the adrenal gland. The DHEA test is not very accurate, and dehydroepiandrosterone sulfate (DHEA-S) is considered a better test. DHEA-S is commonly elevated with

PCOS, but very high DHEA-S levels are a tipoff to an adrenal gland problem such as congenital adrenal hyperplasia, Cushing's syndrome, or adrenal gland cancer. A study from Taiwan found that elevated DHEA-S levels are associated with insulin resistance and an increased risk for diabetes. The same study found that women with high DHEA-S levels have less abdominal obesity but worse acne.

Endometrial Biopsy

Androgen excess can cause a buildup of the lining of the uterus, known as *endometrial hyperplasia,* which is a risk for cancer of the uterus. An endometrial biopsy should be done to screen for uterine cancer (known as *endometrial carcinoma*) in women who go more than three months without a menstrual cycle.

Estrogen

Estrogen levels are a helpful test, especially if there are symptoms of premature ovarian failure, such as irregular menstrual cycles, hot flashes, or vaginal dryness. Estradiol is the best test, but estrone or estriol can also be measured.

Glucose Testing

Blood sugar problems, insulin resistance, and hyperandrogenism are closely linked. Thirty to 40 percent of women with PCOS have blood sugar problems, and 10 percent have full-blown diabetes. All women with hyperandrogenism should have glucose testing to check for prediabetes or diabetes. The most basic test is a fasting glucose level. Other tests, including the hemoglobin A_{1c} and oral glucose tolerance test (OGTT), should also be done. If you have PCOS, I recommend that you have an oral glucose tolerance test every couple of years. For more on glucose testing, see chapter 6.

Hemoglobin and Hematocrit

Heavy menstrual cycles can result in low red blood cell counts, known as anemia. Red blood cell counts are measured by hemoglobin and hematocrit tests.

Insulin-Like Growth Factor-1

Excess growth hormone produced by a tumor of the pituitary gland is a cause of excess androgen levels. Insulin-like growth factor-1 (IGF-1) is a hormone produced by the liver that is used as an indicator of growth hormone levels. If the IGF-1 level is high, a growth hormone suppression test should be done to further evaluate growth hormone levels. For more information on growth hormone, see chapter 12.

Insulin Testing

Insulin testing is helpful for lean women with symptoms of hyperandrogenism to assess for insulin resistance. Insulin testing is not necessary if you are overweight or obese, because your weight on the scale is a better indicator of insulin resistance. In fact, many women with insulin resistance have low insulin levels. For more on insulin testing, see chapter 6.

Liver Function Tests

Because liver disease can be associated with female hormone problems, liver function tests should be checked periodically. Alanine transaminase (ALT), aspartate aminotransferase (AST), gamma-glutamyl transpeptidase (GGT), alkaline phosphatase, bilirubin, albumin, and prothrombin time are all tests of liver function.

Lutenizing Hormone and Follicle Stimulating Hormone

The pituitary hormones, lutenizing hormone (LH) and follicle stimulating hormone (FSH), also known as gonadotropins, give doctors information about the pituitary gland and hypothalamus and their regulation of testosterone and estrogen and are key for maintaining female hormone balance. Women with hyperandrogenism usually have gonadotropin levels in the normal range, but they can still be out of balance. Typically, the LH level is at least double that of the FSH level. This is called an elevated LH/FSH ratio. If the LH/FSH ratio is more than 2:1, it is highly suggestive of hyperandrogenism; however, one-third of patients with hyperandrogenism do not have elevated LH/FSH ratios.

Pelvic Ultrasound

A pelvic ultrasound is useful to check for cancer of the ovary. It also can detect cysts in the ovary. Thirty percent of women with cysts in their ovaries do not have androgen problems, and not all women with androgen problems have detectable ovarian cysts.

Progesterone

Progesterone testing is helpful to determine whether you are ovulating. Progesterone levels should be measured on days eighteen through twenty-one of the cycle. A progesterone level of less than 2 nanograms/milliliter (ng/mL) suggests that you are not ovulating. A progesterone level of 10–15 ng/mL is ideal. You can also take progesterone measurements during other times of the cycle to determine what phase of the cycle you are in.

Prolactin

Elevations of prolactin may indicate a pituitary tumor, a common cause of hyperandrogenism. Mild prolactin elevations without a pituitary tumor can also occur in women with PCOS. All women with features of hyperandrogenism should have prolactin levels measured.

17-Hydroxyprogesterone

A 17-hydroxyprogesterone test is done to check for congenital adrenal hyperplasia, a cause of hyperandrogenism. This test is frequently overlooked, but it is important because the treatment of congenital adrenal hyperplasia is different from other treatments for hyperandrogenism.

Sex Hormone Binding Globulin

Sex hormone binding globulin (SHBG) is a blood protein that binds both testosterone and estrogen. Hyperandrogenism, birth control pills, and insulin resistance can cause low SHBG levels. SHBG measurement is important, because it helps put the total testosterone test into perspective and allows calculation of free testosterone levels. Women with insulin resistance and PCOS commonly have low SHBG levels.

Testosterone

Measuring testosterone levels in women can be complicated. For a number of reasons, testosterone levels may be inaccurate or misleading. Test quality and variability, hormonal fluxes, and blood proteins all affect testosterone measurements. The techniques for testosterone measurements in women are the same as for men. For more information on laboratory evaluation of testosterone, see chapter 10.

Total testosterone measures all of the testosterone in the blood—both free and bound to proteins. Testosterone that is bound to proteins is not readily available to the tissues and is said to be inactive. Women with hyperandrogenism frequently have a normal total testosterone level but a high *free testosterone*. Very high total testosterone levels (above 200–300 nanograms/deciliter (ng/dL)) are suggestive of cancer of the ovary or adrenal gland.

Thyroid Testing

Women with androgen excess are at increased risk for having an underactive thyroid. Many of my patients with PCOS also have Hashimoto's hypothyroidism. Each condition can intensify the symptoms of the other. For more information on thyroid testing, see chapter 7.

Urinary Lutenizing Hormone and Fertility Monitors

Urinary LH levels are a good way of testing for the LH spike, which is indicative of ovulation. Ovulation problems are a common feature of androgen excess. LH testing kits for home use are available without a prescription. A fertility monitor is an electronic device that tracks the monthly cycle with urinary LH levels and notifies you when it detects the LH spike. Fertility monitors are a more accurate and reliable way of knowing when you are ovulating than measuring daily basal body temperature.

Treatments for Androgen Excess

Androgen excess can be treated using several approaches. Androgens can be lowered directly by using androgen blockers known as antiandrogen medications. Androgens can also be lowered by treating insulin resistance. Insulin resistance causes the ovaries and the adrenal gland to produce excess androgen hormones. Improving insulin resistance lowers androgen production. Experts believe that treating insulin resistance is the best way to treat androgen excess, especially if you have PCOS, because it also reduces the risk for complications of PCOS such as diabetes and heart disease. If you are overweight, the most important first step to improving insulin resistance is weight loss. The treatments for androgen excess and insulin resistance work best when combined with a healthy diet and regular physical activity.

Metformin

Although metformin is approved by the FDA for the treatment of type 2 diabetes, it is the most prescribed medication to treat PCOS. Metformin helps PCOS by lowering blood sugar and improving insulin resistance. Metformin can improve menstrual cycle problems and skin problems, and can help control sugar cravings and therefore help with weight loss. For more information on metformin, see chapter 6.

Birth Control Pills for PCOS	
Apri, Desogen, Reclipsen, Solia, Otho-Cept (desogestrel 0.15 mg and ethinyl estradiol 30 mg)	Ortho Tri-Cyclen, TriNessa, Tri-Previfem, Tri-Spritec (norgestimate 0.18–0.25 mg and ethinyl estradiol 35 mg)
Mircette, Kariva, Azurette (desogestrel 0.15 mg and ethinyl estradiol 20 mg)	Ortho Tri-Cyclen Lo, Tri Lo Sprintec (norgestimate .18–0.25 mg and ethinyl estradiol 25 mg)
Natazia (dienogest 2–3 mg and estradiol valerate 1–3 mg)	Yasmin, Ocella (drospirenone 3mg, and ethinyl estradiol 30 mg)
Ortho-Cyclin-28, MonoNessa, Previfem, Sprintec (norgestimate 0.25 mg and ethinyl estradiol 35 mg)	Yaz, Beyaz, Gianvi (drospirenone 3mg and ethinyl estradiol 20 mg)

Nutrition and Physical Activity

Even though there are medications for PCOS, they are never a substitute for nutrition and physical activity. The Hormonal Health Diet is the ideal diet for PCOS. Weight loss improves insulin resistance, which leads to lower androgen levels and improved symptoms. Physical activity helps with weight loss and improves insulin resistance.

Birth Control Pills

Birth control pills are a tried-and-true way of treating androgen excess. Birth control pills decrease androgen levels because they shut down androgen production in the ovaries and they increase production of blood proteins. Blood proteins bind to androgens, making them inactive.

Birth control pills contain synthetic progesterone, called *progestin*. Progestin is not exactly like real progesterone, because it acts like both progesterone and an androgen. Progestins have more androgenic activity than natural progesterone. Because women with PCOS already have high androgens, I recommend using birth control pills that have the least androgenic progestins,

Drospirenone

Yasmin, Yaz, Ocella, and BeYaz are products that contain a unique progestin, drospirenone, that blocks some of the effects of androgens. Drospirenone is similar to spironolactone (see page 228), which blocks testosterone action. Drospirenone is a mild diuretic, which means less fluid retention and bloating compared to other progestins. A side effect can be potassium levels that are too high, so regular blood tests are necessary. Because Yasmin and spironolactone have similar actions and both can raise potassium levels, it is not recommended to take both of these medications at the same time.

A study published in the *British Medical Journal* found that women who use birth control pills that contain drospirenone are three times more likely to develop blood clots than women who take other oral contraceptives. As a result, drospirenone has been the source of a great deal of Internet buzz and lawsuits. Drospirenone is also thought to increase the risk for depression. Many of my patients have had side effects with drospirenone, but others have done very well with this progestin.

---

drospirenone, desogestrel, or norgestimate. Avoid the progestins levonorgestrel, norgestrel, and norethindrone, which have the most androgenic activity.

Side effects of all birth control pills include acne, headaches, breast tenderness, nausea, PMS, and depression. Birth control pills with androgenic progestins can increase insulin resistance, raise blood sugar, and cause weight gain. Life-threatening blood clots, heart attacks, and strokes are a real risk with birth control pills. The risk is highest if you smoke cigarettes. If you smoke, you should not use birth control pills.

Progesterone

Progesterone and progestins (synthetic progesterone) are used in the treatment of androgen problems such as PCOS, primarily to induce a menstrual cycle. Not having a cycle for three months or more is a risk factor for cancer of the uterus. Progesterone in the form of synthetic medroxyprogesterone (Provera) or natural progesterone capsules (Prometrium) is usually taken for ten days every three

---

Variable Weight Effects of Birth Control Pills

Researchers have conducted countless studies on birth control pills and body weight. Ten million U.S. women take the pill, and despite fifty years of hand wringing and warnings from anti-birth control forces, "the pill" has become an accepted part of the American scene. The main synthetic estrogen used in birth control pills is ethinyl estradiol. All estrogen—synthetic or natural—raises the risk of blood clots, stroke, or heart attack in women over thirty-five, especially those who smoke.

Most studies show that birth control pills don't have much effect on weight. In my experience, some women do gain weight when they take the pill. Studies that carefully measure body composition have found that when women gain weight from taking birth control pills, the weight is mainly fat, not fluid or muscle.

Birth control pills come with synthetic estrogen in varying amounts: low, medium, and high. When your weight is a concern, the medium-dose estrogen is the best (30–40 mcg ethinyl estradiol). High-dose birth control pills that contain 50 mcg of ethinyl estradiol (Ovcon-50, Ogestrel 0.5/50-28, and Zovia 1/50) frequently cause weight gain. Most doctors know about this side effect, and the 50 mcg dose is rarely used anymore. Some studies have shown that lower-dose birth control pills can help boost metabolism and cause weight loss.

---

months to induce a menstrual cycle. Progesterone gel (Crinone, Prochieve) is a vaginal gel made of natural micronized progesterone (also derived from yams). A premeasured applicator ensures that you get the right amount into the vagina. The progesterone is absorbed through the lining of the uterus and works quite well at protecting the lining of the uterus. Only about 4 percent of the medication is absorbed into general circulation, so there is fluid retention and weight gain, compared to progesterone taken by mouth. Progesterone-containing intrauterine devices (IUD) (Progestasert and Mirena) release small amounts of progesterone into the lining of the uterus. Little progesterone is transferred to the rest of the body. Other than stimulating a menstrual cycle and lowering the risk of uterine cancer, progesterone does not do much to help the underlying cause of PCOS.

Natural Estrogen Birth Control

Natazia is the first birth control pill to contain natural estradiol instead of synthetic estrogen. The thought is that the natural estrogen will have fewer side effects, but no definite proof exists. Natazia also has a new progestin known as dienogest. Dienogest has an androgen-blocking effect similar to drospirenone but claims to have fewer side effects.

Spironolactone (Aldactone)

Spironolactone is a diuretic medication that also blocks the effects of androgens and can help reduce acne, hair loss, and facial hair growth. The main effect is mild, and it works best when combined with a birth control pill. In my experience, women need to take a minimum of 100 mg twice daily for at least one year to see any benefit. Blood tests are required to monitor potassium levels and check for liver problems, a rare side effect. Spironolactone can cause birth defects and should not used unless a woman is using some form of birth control.

Clomiphene Citrate (Clomid)

A medication usually used as a fertility drug, clomiphene citrate, is an effective treatment for PCOS in women who want to get pregnant.

Finasteride (Proscar, Propecia) and Dutasteride (Avodart)

Although approved for use in men, these medications are sometimes used to treat androgen excess in women. Finasteride and dutasteride work by blocking the enzyme 5-alpha reductase, which converts testosterone into the more active form, dihydrotestosterone (DHT). Although effective, these medications cause birth defects and should be used only under careful supervision.

Don't Consume Too Much Lime Juice

A 2010 study published in the journal *Endocrine Practice* showed that 100 percent of female rats who were given lime juice had irregular menstrual cycles. Lime juice appears to block ovulation and likely decreases fertility.

Getting Rid of Excess Hair

Hirsutism is cosmetically disfiguring as well as detrimental to women's emotional and social lives. All of the treatments mentioned may slow the progression of hirsutism but may not make the hair go away entirely. The best and most effective ways of eliminating hair are mechanical.

Bleaching and depilating creams are helpful but can also cause inflammation of the skin.

Eflornithine hydrochloride (Vaniqa) is a cream approved for the treatment of unwanted facial hair. The medication works by inhibiting the biosynthesis of hair proteins. The cream must be applied twice a day for at least two months to have any effect. Unfortunately, if the cream is stopped, the hair grows back.

Electrolysis claims to permanently remove the hair, but it can be painful, and multiple treatments are usually necessary.

Laser hair removal has still not been perfected. It's expensive, and the hair tends to grow back with time. In the future, better laser techniques may make this the hair removal therapy of choice.

Plucking and waxing can lead to inflammation and infection in the skin and are not as good as shaving.

Shaving is one of the best ways to remove excess facial hair. Incidentally, it is a myth that the hair will grow back thicker.

Self-Confidence

Many women with PCOS have problems with poor body image. The fear of social rejection can make a woman become socially isolated. Poor self-esteem and self-image can even lead to depression. Women with PCOS may need to work on developing better social skills and more self-confidence. It is helpful to understand PCOS as a medical/hormone problem. It is not your fault that you have PCOS. Many mental health professionals specialize in treating body image problems related to PCOS.

Progesterone Causes Insulin Resistance and Androgen Excess

Progesterone refers to the hormone produced in the ovary. Progesterone medications are those produced from a natural plant source (typically yams) but still chemically identical (bioidentical) to human progesterone. In contrast, *progestin* refers to a hormone that is synthetically produced and differs in many ways from natural progesterone. When classifying medications, the term *progestogen* refers to either natural progesterone or synthetic progestins. Progestins were originally developed because natural progesterone is not easily absorbed in pill form. Progestin pills are absorbed into the blood without trouble. Today, several natural progesterone products have been developed to overcome absorption problems. Despite this fact, use of synthetic progestins remains commonplace. Nearly all birth control pills and combination hormone replacement products still contain synthetic progestins.

Progestins do not always act as progesterone would in the tissues. While synthetic progestins may imitate some of progesterone's actions, they can cross-react with receptors for other hormones or cause other unwanted effects. The three main problems caused by synthetic progestins are insulin resistance, effects of androgen excess, and disruption of prolactin balance. Each progestin is slightly different in its ability to cause hormonal imbalance. Too much natural progesterone or unwanted effects from synthetic progestins can disrupt hormonal balance and start a cascade of other hormone problems that have a negative impact on health and body weight.

For reasons that still not completely understood, synthetic progestins, and to a lesser extent natural progesterone, increase insulin resistance and raise blood sugar levels. Synthetic progestins have a more potent effect on insulin sensitivity and have been known to cause diabetes in many cases. Most women who take progestins for long periods of time experience weight gain in the belly. Increased belly fat worsens insulin resistance, raises blood sugars, and increases the risk for developing diabetes. Many common side effects of progestins are thought, in part, to be complications of insulin resistance. Side effects include blood clots in the legs and lungs, cholesterol problems, gall bladder problems, liver problems, menstrual cycle problems, fluid retention, insomnia, fatigue, depression, and anxiety.

Progestins can make you hungry, especially in high doses. One medication, megestrol (Megace) is used as an appetite stimulant in patients with cancer or AIDS. Progestin medications are known to lower HDL (good) cholesterol and raise

LDL (bad) cholesterol. Progestins cause fluid retention responsible for bloating and cyclical edema. Progestins can cause depression, irritability, and mood swings. It's thought that the effects of progestins on brain chemicals such as serotonin and norepinephrine compound with insulin resistance to influence mood. Depo-Provera, an injectable progestin, is notorious for causing severe depression in some women.

Progestins have the ability to stimulate the receptor for male hormones—the androgen receptor—resulting in excess androgens, facial hair, and acne. The androgenic potential varies among progestins, but in general the ones that have the most androgenic effects also have the most detrimental effects on insulin resistance, blood sugar, and cholesterol. Progestins disrupt the balance of another important female hormone, prolactin. Breast tenderness and breast milk production are side effects in some women who take progestins.

Medroxyprogesterone acetate (Provera) is a highly androgenic progestin that causes side effects such as weight gain, bloating, depression, and hot flashes. Research from the University of Texas has shown that women who used medroxyprogesterone had an increase in both glucose and insulin levels. Medroxypro-gesterone has also been associated with bone loss because it decreases estrogen production, but the effect may be reversible after stopping the drug. If you take Depo-Provera, it is important to get adequate calcium, vitamin D, and exercise to protect your bones.

Birth control pills containing the progestins levonorgestrel, norgestrel, and norethindrone are the worst for the effects of excess androgen, insulin resistance, and weight gain. Pills with the progestins desogestrel, norgestimate, and drospirenone are less androgenic.

Progesterone creams, extracted from Mexican yams, are a natural alternative reported to be effective in relieving the hot flashes of menopause. Local pharmacies compound these creams, so there is tremendous variability among different preparations. Some creams can be exceptionally potent, ten to twenty times more potent than pills. I have seen many women gain weight from using progesterone creams, so be sure to use a reliable compounding pharmacist.

If progesterone therapy is necessary, try micronized progesterone (Prometrium) or compounded natural progesterone. It causes less weight gain but also makes you sleepy. Take it before you go to bed.

Birth Control Pills in Obese Women

There has been some debate about the safety and effectiveness of birth control pills in women who are obese, because they have been reported to have 3 percent failure rate, compared to a 2 percent failure rate in women with normal body weight. Obese women who take birth control pills also have an increased risk of blood clots. Experts recommend using the lower dose pills with 20–35 micrograms (mcg) of estrogen. There is no proof that the 35 mcg dose is more effective or that the 20 mcg is safer.

Hormone Imbalance: Hypothalamic and Pituitary Gland Disorders

Studies show that as many as 15 percent of women with androgen excess have an undiagnosed noncancerous tumor in their pituitary gland. Most pituitary gland tumors are small and don't cause any problems. Most women aren't even aware of the tumors, because most of the time the tumors don't do any harm. Problems arise, however, if the tumor is a prolactinoma, or prolactin-secreting tumor. High prolactin levels shut down production of estrogen and progesterone, causing a woman to have symptoms of menopause. Tumors that cause high prolactin levels are associated with breast milk production and cessation of periods.

Tumors can also cause problems if they grow too large. A large tumor will compress the rest of the pituitary gland, which can result in multiple hormone deficiencies. Sometimes pituitary tumors make hormones that cause other problems in association with female hormone problems, such as Cushing's syndrome (see chapter 11), acromegaly, or growth-hormone deficiency (see chapter 12).

Hormone Imbalance: Premature Menopause

Premature menopause is on the rise. Women as early as their teens or twenties may experience early menopause symptoms, such as hot flashes and night sweats, because their bodies stop producing female hormones. Symptoms of early menopause can be subtle and may present as irregular periods or depression. One study found that 67 percent of women with early menopause feel depressed.

Menopause is considered normal anytime after the age of forty-five, but the average age of menopause is fifty-two. Most women will have menopause at the

Symptoms of a Possible Pituitary Gland Tumor		
Anger	Fatigue	Menstrual cycle problems
Breast milk production	Headaches	Mood swings
Depression	High blood pressure	Sexual dysfunction
Diabetes	Infertility	Vision problems
Facial hair growth	Insomnia	Weight gain
	Memory loss	

same age as their mothers. Early menopause (also called POF, for premature ovarian failure or primary ovarian insufficiency) can be caused by an overactive immune system that destroys the ovaries. POF can increase your risk of having other autoimmune conditions, such as Hashimoto's hypothyroidism (chapter 7) and Addison's disease (chapter 11). Smoking causes damage to the ovaries as well.

Testing for Early Menopause

Follicle Stimulating Hormone

Follicle stimulating hormone is a hormone made by the pituitary gland. As the ovary makes less and less estrogen, the brain responds by increasing FSH levels. Although both LH and FSH are made by the pituitary gland to control the ovaries, FSH is the first hormone to rise in menopause. The elevation of FSH with a normal LH level is a common situation in early menopause. If you are still menstruating, the best time to measure an FSH level is on the second day of the

Symptoms of Early Menopause	
Symptoms before age forty-five	Irregular or absent menstrual cycles
Depression or mood swings	Loss of libido
Fatigue	Poor sleep
Hot flashes	Vaginal dryness or discharge

Hypothalamic Amenorrhea: Another Cause of Early Menopause

Hypothalamic amenorrhea means loss of the menstrual cycle caused by problems with the hypothalamic region of the brain. Problems with female hormones are commonly seen with problems that affect the brain, which includes brain tumors and head trauma. Starvation and excessive exercise can also cause the brain to shut down female hormone production. When a woman's body fat drops too low, the brain shuts the ovaries down as a form of self-protection. It's the reason why many women with anorexia nervosa as well as female athletes stop having periods. Blood tests can determine whether early menopause is caused by either hypothalamic amenorrhea or by premature ovarian failure.

---

menses. If the FSH level is more than 10 mIU/mL, the ovaries are beginning to fail. FSH levels above 4 mIU/ml suggests menopause but should be confirmed by a second test. FSH levels fluctuate wildly, so repeat testing often gives very different results. A low FSH level can indicate a hypothalamic amenorrhea or pituitary gland tumor such as a prolactinoma.

Estrogen Levels

The best test to directly measure estrogen is estradiol, but estrone and estriol levels can also be measured. Estradiol is an indicator of healthy estrogen levels. Estradiol levels drop in menopause, but estrone (the estrogen made from fat) may go up. If you are still menstruating, estradiol should be checked on day two or three of your menstrual cycle (follicular phase). An estradiol level less than 80 picograms/milliliter (pg/ml) is suggestive of estrogen deficiency, and levels below 50 pg/ml are highly suggestive of estrogen deficiency. Levels up to 200 pg/ml are considered normal. Estradiol levels can fluctuate wildly during perimenopause.

Lutenizing Hormone

LH is also made by the pituitary gland. During the normal transition to menopause, LH will rise, but not as quickly as FSH. A low LH level can indicate a problem with the hypothalamus or pituitary gland.

Your Action Plan for Early Menopause

Get checked for related medical disorders. Early menopause is associated with an increased risk for osteopenia or osteoporosis, hypothyroidism, pernicious anemia, and other autoimmune disorders (see chapter 7).

Exercise. Daily moderate intensity physical activity eases symptoms, boosts mood, and gets metabolic rate back on track.

Stop smoking. Smoking is a known toxin to the ovary, inducing early menopause. Women who smoke go through menopause one to two years earlier than women who do not smoke.

Avoid endocrine disruptors. A 2011 study published in the *Journal of Clinical Endocrinology and Metabolism* found that chemicals in plastics are linked to early menopause. Human-made chemicals known as perfluorocarbons are found in many household products, including clothing and food storage containers, and act as endocrine disruptors. These chemicals are also known to cause cardiovascular disease and impair the immune system. See "Practical Strategies for Intelligent Weight Loss," beginning on page 327, for more on endocrine disruptors.

Take a hormone replacement. Although taking hormones is still controversial for women with normal menopause, most experts recommend taking hormones until the age of natural menopause (forty-five or fifty). Hormone replacement therapy or birth control pills are recommended for women who have had premature ovarian failure, at least until the age of forty-five. For more on hormone replacement, see chapter 9.

Early Menopause and Your Blood Type

According to a study presented at the American Society for Reproductive Medicine, women with blood type O have decreased ovarian reserves, leading to lower estrogen levels when compared to women with other blood types.

Thyroid Testing

Thyroid problems frequently occur in association with premature menopause, both of which can be autoimmune disorders. Ask your doctor to check thyroid stimulating hormone (TSH), free T3, and free T4 (see chapter 7).

Chapter Review

In addition to familiar female hormones such as progesterone, women also need a balanced supply of male hormones so that normal monthly cycles occur on schedule.

The chapter discussed in detail a class of male hormones known as androgens that are essential for female health throughout life. Elevated levels of any one of the three male hormones can set in motion a cascade of health problems, some potentially life threatening.

The chapter discussed typical situations in which female hormone imbalances occur; the first as a result of early puberty. The chapter noted that 25 percent of girls today show early signs of puberty by age seven with the associated consequence that many of these girls tend to be overweight.

Premenstrual syndrome is another common hormone-related condition and is connected to food cravings, food binges, weight gain, depression, anxiety, and other health consequences. PMS also causes insulin resistance, and it raises blood sugar levels, which in turn causes weight gain.

The chapter offered a number of ways to treat PMS, including dietary changes, exercise, reducing stress, and increasing the intake of calcium and B, C, and E vitamin supplements. The impact of androgen excess, known as hyperandrogenism, was also discussed.

Excess androgen is linked to high blood pressure, diabetes, and increased cancer risk, among other health consequences. Typical symptoms range from weight gain and the appearance of facial hair or excess body hair to irregular periods and decreased libido.

The most common hormonal disorder in women is a genetic condition known as polycystic ovary syndrome. While most of these women are obese, about 25 percent of this group is of normal weight.

The chapter discussed a variety of ways to test and treat both PCOS and androgen excess. The tests are not perfect and sometimes offer inconclusive results that force answers to be sought through a process of elimination by a physician. Accurate testing is also affected by variations in a woman's normal monthly cycle and the hormone levels produced by or perhaps associated with another disease.

Excess androgen levels may be treated through the use of androgen blockers known as anti-androgen medications or by beginning treatment protocols for insulin resistance. Female hormone imbalances may be addressed through changes in nutritional intake and increased physical activity, the taking of certain drugs such as birth control pills, or by the introduction of synthetic progesterone.

The next chapter expands on the discussion in this chapter and discusses in detail the hormones associated with menopause.

CHAPTER

9

Women's Hormones II
Survive Perimenopause and Menopause

Many people associate menopause and perimenopause with weight gain. Menopause is frequently associated with weight gain—on average, several pounds—but not all women gain weight, and others gain quite a lot. Obviously other factors come into play: heredity, weight distribution, and diet.

Perimenopause is the time of transition just before a woman enters menopause, and it's not always a gentle time. For a time—years, in some women—a woman may have alternating periods of low estrogen mixed with surges of very high estrogen levels. Symptoms wax and wane, causing even more problems. It's commonly misdiagnosed as a thyroid problem or manic depression. Perimenopause is also a time when many women gain weight, especially in the belly. Women who have always carried their weight on their hips and buttocks may experience a shift in the distribution of body fat to the middle section.

When estrogen levels become low, women frequently experience vasomotor symptoms. The most common is the *hot*

Low Libido, Low Androgens

Although androgen excess receives more attention, low androgen levels can be problematic for some women with low libido. Androgens help maintain muscle mass and determine body fat distribution in men and women. Androgens are responsible for the appearance of body hair; they make the skin oilier; as in men, they contribute to sex drive. Just as in men, women's androgen levels decline with age. Androgen decline at menopause is considered part of the natural aging process. (They actually start declining when a woman reaches her thirties.)

Estrogen medications suppress testosterone production by the ovaries, so women on estrogen replacement therapy or birth control pills usually have low androgen levels. Symptoms of androgen decline include loss of sexual desire, weight gain (or sometimes, weight loss), increased fat in the belly, loss of muscle, tiredness, lack of energy, decreased sense of well-being, depression, loss of shine in the hair, dry skin, lack of mental clarity, anemia, urinary incontinence (from loss of muscle tone in the pelvis and the bladder), and osteoporosis.

Most endocrinologists consider androgen therapy for women controversial. Testosterone is sometimes prescribed for low libido, but this treatment remains controversial and is not approved by the U.S. Food and Drug Administration. Androgen therapy can have many side effects. Among the most concerning are the risk of birth defects, negative effects on the cholesterol profile, and a possible risk of heart disease. Other side effects include acne, hair growth in male areas (face, chest, nipples, and back), voice deepening, overactive sex drive, irregular bleeding, hair loss, and enlargement of the clitoris.

flash or *hot flush,* the latter term the one preferred by endocrinologists. Sleep disturbance is one of the most common symptoms of perimenopause. Sleep problems then cause multiple hormone disruptions that lead to weight gain, including low growth hormone, insulin resistance, and leptin resistance.

Symptoms of Menopause

Anger	Irritability	Pain with intercourse
Anxiety	Loss of libido	Urinary tract infections
Depression	Memory loss	Vaginal dryness
Disrupted sleep	Migraine headaches	Weight gain, especially around the belly
Fatigue	Mood swings	
Hot flashes or flushes	Osteopenia or osteoporosis	

During perimenopause, menstrual cycles may become irregular. Estrogen surges at times, causing episodes of very heavy bleeding. The estrogen surges can also contribute to the growth of benign uterine tumors known as fibroid tumors, simply called fibroids or fireballs. They almost never cause cancer, but they are one of the most common reasons for needing a hysterectomy. Some fibroids can become quite large. One patient of mine gained 40 pounds when she was in her early forties. All the weight was up front, leading her (and many of her friends) to believe she had become pregnant. The truth turned out to be far less joyous: she had a 40-pound fibroid uterine tumor. She underwent a successful operation, and her weight is now back to normal. Since then, another patient read about this case in a previous edition of *Hormonal Balance* and came to me with similar symptoms. Sure enough, she had a huge noncancerous ovarian tumor that was successfully removed.

During perimenopause, along with the estrogen surges—which cause increased appetite and bleeding—come periods of low estrogen levels. At this time, women begin to lose the protective effect of estrogen. The risk of heart disease increases, bad cholesterol goes up while good cholesterol tumbles, osteoporosis sets in, and fat distribution changes. Usually estrogen (especially estradiol) causes fat to go to hips, buttocks, and under the skin, but as estradiol levels drop in the early stages of menopause and estrone takes on increasing importance, fat moves to the belly. Visceral fat or abdominal adiposity is the bad fat I discussed in chapter 2. Many women note their breasts and hips get smaller but they gain weight in their bellies during this time. When menopause is complete, this effect

Endocrinology of Estrogen

Estrogen is a steroid hormone, chemically almost identical to other steroid hormones such as testosterone, dehydroepiandrosterone (DHEA), androstenedione, or cortisol. The term steroid refers to the chemical structure of the hormone, which is derived from cholesterol. Calling a hormone a steroid says nothing about what the hormone does. Small changes in the structure of steroid hormones turn them into other hormones with completely different activities.

Your brain controls the production of all steroid hormones through the pituitary gland and the hypothalamus. The gonadotropin-releasing hormone (GnRH) is produced by the hypothalamus in tiny pulses to stimulate the pituitary gland to make follicle stimulating hormone (FSH) and luteinizing hormone (LH). These hormones act on the ovary, stimulating it to produce estrogen, progesterone, and

testosterone. The small bursts of this potent hormone stimulate the pituitary gland to make its two hormones, FSH and LH. These hormones work collectively to control the production of hormones from the ovary. DHEA, which is made by the adrenal gland, is regulated by the pituitary gland hormone adrenocortitrophic hormone (ACTH), which I discuss in chapter 11. Each of these hormones feeds back to the brain in a check-and-balance type system. There are three major types of estrogen.

Estrone is the main type of estrogen made by fat. Yes, fat makes hormones just like any other gland does. (See chapter 2 for more on fat as an endocrine organ.) Unlike other hormones, fat makes estrogen by converting androgens. The estrone that fat produces promotes storage of more fat in the belly and around the organs.

on weight distribution is even more pronounced. Menopause is a stressful time. Stress causes hormonal changes, including insulin resistance, low thyroid hormone activity, high cortisol, and low growth hormone, that slow your metabolism and promote weight gain.

Menstrual cycles become irregular; hot flashes, sleep disturbances, vaginal dryness, weight gain in the belly, and shrinkage of breasts may occur. The fluctuations in hormones cause emotional instability. Perimenopausal women

As discussed in chapter 3, this type of fat causes insulin resistance, which is why many doctors refer to estrone as a "bad estrogen." Young women have low levels of estrone, because the ovaries can easily convert estrone into estradiol. After menopause, the ovary loses this ability. Menopause is associated with a decline in healthy estradiol and a rise in unhealthy estrone.

Estradiol is produced by the ovary and is the predominant estrogen in young women. Estradiol promotes storage of "healthy" fat around the hips and buttocks. This fat distribution improves insulin resistance and blood sugar levels. Estradiol is responsible for the majority of the positive benefits attributed to estrogen and is known as a "good estrogen." Estradiol is responsible for the female body appearance. The fat in the hips and buttocks is "safe fat" compared to fat in the belly. When estradiol is low, fat accumulates in the belly. Some women have problems with birth control pills or hormone replacement therapy because they take estrogens that disrupt the normal healthy balance of estradiol and estrone.

Estriol is produced by the placenta during pregnancy. This weaker form of estrogen has a neutral effect on metabolism. Estriol is a component of many bioidentical hormone medications.

Each type of estrogen prompts slightly different actions, and each one can be converted into the other, which is why they are generally thought of as simply estrogens, but all estrogens are not the same. This misconception has led to some of the misunderstandings about estrogen.

should carefully consider the risks and benefits of hormone replacement therapy, because estrogen deficiency causes changes in the body. In particular, perimenopause is a time when there is rapid bone loss, leading to osteopenia and osteoporosis. The average woman goes through menopause at age fifty-one and dies at age eighty, giving her thirty years of postmenopausal life. On average, women gain about 10 pounds in the first few years after menopause that often goes to the belly. Why this weight gain? Is it the fault of menopause?

Fat Makes Estrogen

Although most people associate the hormone estrogen as coming from the ovary, fat tissue is responsible for producing a significant amount of estrogen in the body. This is even true for men, as I discuss in chapter 10.

Your body contains more than 30 billion fat cells. The fat cell contains an enzyme known as aromatase, which converts androgens to estrogens—primarily estrone. Estrone is the estrogen that gains dominance after menopause, when the ovaries shut down; before that, estradiol is the primary form of estrogen in the body. Given that fat cells convert androgens to estrogen, and that estrogen is primarily estrone, people who are overweight also have a lot more estrone than average; remember, estrone is the "bad estrogen" that causes insulin resistance.

In terms of weight gain, women are not alike. Young women tend to gain weight where they already have fat—the buttocks and hips. Older women (and men) tend to gain weight in the belly. The classic pear shape is thought of as *gynoid;* the apple shape is called *android.* When estradiol production declines and estrone levels rise during and after menopause, fat in women tends to follow the same pattern as fat in men—going to the belly. This shape, the apple shape, is associated with a greater risk of insulin resistance, metabolic syndrome, hypertension, diabetes, and cardiovascular disease.

Estrogen + Leptin + Insulin = Cancer

Breast cancer is the second leading cause of cancer death in women, killing 500,000 women every year. Obese women who get breast cancer have worse outcomes and are more likely to die than normal weight women who get the disease. It is well known that excess estrogen increases the risk of female cancers, most notably breast cancer. Obesity increases the risk for breast cancer by 40 percent, in part because fat makes extra estrogen. Taking estrogen medications, especially hormone replacement therapy (HRT) in menopause, also increases breast cancer risk. The Women's Health Initiative was a landmark government-sponsored study that discovered the health risks of hormone use in menopause. This study stunned doctors when researchers reported in 2002 that the risk of hormone replacement therapy outweighed any benefits. Since that time, hormone use has sharply declined, but questions remain about this study. In a follow-up study, researchers found that the risk of breast cancer, in addition to that for strokes and blood clots, seems to disappear about ten years after stopping hormone replacement therapy.

Breast tumors can have receptors to estrogen, progesterone, or a protein called HER2. Being overweight not only increases the risk for estrogen-dependent

---

Estrogen Dominance

Estrogen dominance is a term that alternative medicine providers use, and it also appears on the Internet. Dr. John Lee, author of *What Your Doctor May Not Tell You about Menopause,* claims to have coined the term. The term is not used by traditional medicine providers, however. There are no articles with the term *estrogen dominance* in the title on PubMed.gov, the U.S. National Library of Medicine, National Institutes of Health website, which summarizes most of the scientific publications in the past twenty-five to thirty years.

Whether or not estrogen dominance is a real medical term, the fact is that being overweight means that your body is producing too much estrogen. Getting your body weight back to normal is the best way to overcome estrogen dominance.

---

tumors but also increases the risk of non-estrogen-dependent cancers. Obese women have an increased risk of developing a deadly form of breast cancer known as triple-negative breast cancer. This type of breast cancer occurs in 10–20 percent of cases and is not fueled by estrogen. These tumors are called triple-negative because they lack receptors for estrogen, progesterone, or HER2, the receptors that are the targets for breast cancer drugs. Tumors that are missing the receptors make treatment (and survival) difficult.

Increasing evidence shows that obesity plays a role in the development of breast cancer and other cancers through fat cell hormones such as leptin and adiponectin (see chapter 5). Leptin levels are elevated in obese women, and excess body weight has been shown to increase breast cancer risk, so it makes sense that leptin plays a role in the development of breast cancer. Leptin stimulates expression of aromatase, a fat cell enzyme that increases estrogen levels through the chemical modification of androgens. Adiponectin is a fat cell hormone that is thought to have a protective effect against cancer. Adiponectin levels are highest in lean, healthy people. The levels decline as a person gains weight and develops insulin resistance. Insulin resistance also results in high insulin levels, which can stimulate growth hormone pathways known to increase the risk for getting cancer (see chapter 12).

The risk for breast cancer and other obesity-related cancers, therefore, comes from more than just estrogen. Leptin, adiponectin, insulin, and many other variables also play important roles in making people with excess fat at increased risk for cancer.

Menopause: What Tests Do You Need?

Most hormone tests aren't the be-all and end-all for diagnoses. Many variables come into play, so many mistakes can be made. You should always make sure that your doctor is very familiar with your diet and lifestyle and that he or she is aware of how to properly interpret test results before you allow the diagnosis to stand.

During menopause, and especially perimenopause, there are additional variables. Levels of female hormones undergo tremendous fluctuations over the course of a day, a week, and a month, something that is simply part of the female cycle. Symptoms of menopause—such as vaginal dryness, hot flashes, and loss of sex drive—in combination with cessation of menstrual periods are about as good an indicator as any blood test. Most women do not need, and have never needed, a blood test to tell them they are menopausal. If problems are suspected, LH, FSH and the hormones discussed in the section on early menopause should be tested.

Health Maintenance During Menopause

The transition to menopause should be a reminder to make sure you are up to date with regular health maintenance, such as having a physical examination with your primary care physician. Your examination should include cholesterol and blood sugar testing, a mammogram, bone density testing, a colonoscopy, and an EKG or cardiovascular stress test.

A Healthy Lifestyle Prevents Breast Cancer

In 1997, an important study showed the relationship among physical activity, weight, diet, and the risk for breast cancer. Since then, more than sixty studies have reinforced the benefits of exercise in lowering the risk of breast cancer. The Women's Health Initiative Dietary Modification trial showed a beneficial effect of a low-fat diet on prevention of breast cancer. Alcohol use, on the other hand, has been found to increase the risk for breast cancer.

Balance Your Hormones: The Decision to Take Hormones in Menopause

Hormone replacement therapy and bio-identical hormone replacement therapy (bHRT) remains controversial among endocrinologists. Taking hormones is a smart move for some women, while other women are better off not taking hormones.

Hormone Replacement Therapy

The biggest concerns about HRT include cardiovascular disease (heart attacks and strokes), cancer, blood clots, gall bladder problems, and the unknown, all of which have scared women off HRT at one time or another. In fact, most women do not take hormone replacement therapy. It is estimated that only 10–15 percent of women who *could* take hormones are given the opportunity to by their physicians, and among those who are prescribed HRT, half stop taking the hormones within the first year.

Estrogen has both positive and negative effects. For the cardiovascular system, the effect is controversial. Early studies indicated that estrogen was good for the heart, but the Women's Health Initiative and other studies have demonstrated that HRT increases the risk for cardiovascular disease. There is a growing opinion, however, that for younger women who start HRT shortly after menopause, cardiovascular risk is low, but older women may have increased cardiovascular risk.

The average age of menopause is fifty-two. This average hasn't changed since records about this life change were first kept, about 600 AD. In the perimenopausal years, estrogen production declines. In menopause, the aging ovary shuts down and stops making estrogen entirely. One of the most concerning features of estrogen deficiency is bone loss. Osteoporosis, or the milder version, osteopenia, is a painless, silent disease. Unless tested for it, most people have no idea they even have it, unless they break a bone, and once a bone is broken, the chances of acquiring another condition—such as pneumonia or a blood clot—are greatly increased. Fractures of the spine, known as compression fractures, make women shorter as they age and give them that all-too-familiar humped back known as kyphosis. Indeed, many women die within a year of their first broken bone from osteoporosis.

Some people claim that estrogen can improve vitality and insulin resistance, two key factors in battling the bulge. Estrogen replacement therapy usually will not do much for your weight, though. It may redistribute fat to the chest and hips, where it was in more youthful days, instead of the stomach, where it tends to go during and after menopause. Twenty-five percent of women who take estrogen gain weight, even if only a couple pounds of fluid retention.

Studies confirm that women who take estrogen have more muscle and less fat than those who do not, so while estrogen medications do not cause significant weight gain, you may notice an increase in lean tissue (muscle and bone) and a decrease in fat, which may lead to a small increase in weight (but a smaller body).

The liver is an important organ in the insulin resistance game; it's through the liver that estrogen improves insulin sensitivity. As a result, each formulation of HRT has its advantages and disadvantages. Estrogen pills are absorbed through the intestines to the bloodstream and then transported to the liver, where they are metabolized. This process is known as the "first-pass effect." For the most part, estrogen pills improve insulin resistance. The estrogen patch avoids the liver, though, and therefore has less effect on insulin. Estrogen in patches is absorbed through the skin and then transported directly into general circulation, so the effects on the liver are greatly diminished, though not eliminated. Estrogen pills decrease LDL (bad) cholesterol and increase HDL (good) cholesterol, but the patch's impact is, again, diminished. Estrogen pills, ironically, can increase triglycerides, but the patch can lower them. The patch causes fewer blood clots and possibly fewer migraine headaches and gall bladder problems than the pill.

HRT has remained controversial over the past ten years. The standard advice given by many of the professional organizations is that HRT should be used only to treat the symptoms of menopause, primarily hot flashes. It is also recommended that the lowest possible dose of HRT be taken for the shortest possible amount of time, usually two years. Nausea and breast tenderness are the most common side effects of estrogen. It usually helps to start at a very low dose and increase gradually. Also weight gain, vaginal discharge, acne, and headaches may accompany HRT.

Studies like the Women's Health Initiative have brought estrogen's safety into question. Nevertheless, many women do benefit from HRT. Each woman needs to discuss all the risks and benefits with her physician to determine whether HRT is right for her. The risks of HRT include an increased risk for cardiovascular disease, blood clots, breast cancer, gall bladder disease, liver disease, elevated triglyceride levels, high blood pressure, and headaches.

Estrogen benefits include increasing "safe" fat. Without estrogen, bad fat increases, making insulin resistance worse. HRT pills raise good cholesterol (HDL cholesterol) and lower bad cholesterol (LDL cholesterol), more so than the patch. Estrogen prevents menopausal bone loss, but that's not the best reason for taking HRT, since other medications are available to prevent bone loss. Estrogen's affect on bones also helps women prevent the loss of teeth. Estrogen helps skin retain collagen and prevents early wrinkling. Although controversial, estrogen is thought to protect against ovarian cancer and may also protect you from colon cancer. Many women who take HRT report feeling younger and more vibrant.

A women's decision to go on hormone replacement therapy is a personal one. You must look at all the advantages and disadvantages yourself; everyone is different. For example, if you have a strong family history of breast cancer or heart disease, you may be less inclined to take estrogen than if the opposite situation exists. If you are at particular risk for osteoporosis or have side effects from osteoporosis medications, you may take the slight risk of breast cancer or cardiovascular disease for the positive effects on bones. The bottom line is that each woman has to weigh her own risks and benefits and come to a decision with her physician.

Most estrogens come from natural sources, but natural does not always mean better. Premarin, which is considered a natural hormone, is extracted from the urine of pregnant horses and contains estrogens that are foreign to humans. There is no "cookbook" dose of estrogen. In my experience, women usually have to try two or three (sometimes more) different doses or brands of estrogen until they find the one that suits them. If you've had problems with estrogen in the past, don't give up—it's likely you'll find a regime that works for you. I usually start with a low dose of estradiol and increase the dose over the next six to twelve months. If this doesn't do the trick, I switch to a different form of estrogen. As always, a healthy lifestyle is an important aspect of female hormonal balance. Even if you don't take HRT, you can still do many things to help balance your female hormones. Regular physical activity and the Hormonal Health Diet are as important as medications and enhance the effects of HRT.

Compounded bHRT

In recent years, there has been a lot of controversy about bHRT regarding its safety and efficacy. Some physicians do not advise using bHRT, while others wholeheartedly endorse it. Preparations of bioidentical hormones made by a qualified compounding pharmacist include estriol, which is a form of estrogen that, although regarded as being safe, has not been approved by the FDA. Although unapproved, estriol products are legal if prescribed by a physician and compounded by a qualified pharmacist. One hundred percent estriol tablets or cream can be used, or estriol can be combined as Biest (20 percent estradiol, 80 percent estriol) or Triest (10 percent estrone, 10 percent estradiol, 80 percent estriol). Progesterone and testosterone are sometimes added as a component of bHRT.

Bioidentical Hormone Replacement Therapy

Bioidentical hormones are also called "natural" hormones, because they are chemically identical to the hormones made naturally by the body. They are available as prescription products approved by the FDA and as custom-made products made by compounding pharmacies. If you need a compounded product, I recommend using a quality compounding pharmacy with a pharmacist who keeps up to date with the latest techniques and quality control.

Bioidentical hormones can be taken as pills, creams, gels, or patches. As with all hormone products, prescription products are preferred over compounded products, because the quality control is much better. Having too much estrogen in the blood, whether natural or synthetic, can cause problems. If you take bHRT, it is important to see your doctor regularly.

Estradiol

Estradiol is the most commonly prescribed bHRT. Pure estradiol in the form of 17-beta estradiol is natural estrogen extracted from plants. Many women do well with one mg of estradiol taken once daily as a bioidentical natural hormone that is available as a generic prescription at a standard pharmacy. Prescription estradiol pills are made using a special manufacturing process called micronization that produces a pill that dissolves into tiny pieces, which allows the estradiol to be easily absorbed into the system. Estradiol the most abundant in the body during the reproductive years and is responsible for many of the positive benefits attributed to estrogen.

Estradiol patches have advantages and disadvantages. The patch has less benefit for insulin resistance and improving cholesterol. However, the patch is associated with fewer blood clots, less triglyceride elevation, and less cardiovascular disease. The blood clot issue makes the patch a better alternative for smokers, too.

The patch provides the steadiest levels of estrogen. Estrogen levels spike, then fall after taking the pill, but remain constant on the patch. But there are problems to be aware of: the patch can fall off or irritate the skin. Dosing is inflexible—if you need something in between the available patch doses, you are out of luck.

Micronized estradiol cream (Estrace cream) is excellent for vaginal and urinary symptoms (known as atrophic vaginitis). Only small amounts of estrogen enter the general circulation, so the effect stays localized to the vagina. Estring is a flexible, time-release source of estrogen that is inserted into the vagina like a diaphragm. It can be left in place for up to three months. Like the cream, not much of the estrogen from the ring is absorbed into the bloodstream and is best for vaginal dryness and urinary problems.

Conjugated Estrogens

Conjugated equine estrogens (CEE) such as Premarin are one of the most common types of estrogen used for HRT. Many think Premarin is a synthetic estrogen, but as I mentioned, Premarin is a natural form of estrogen, just not natural to humans. CEE is a collection of estrogens extracted from the urine of pregnant mares, thus *pre-mar-in*. The exact components of Premarin have never been completely characterized, but the substance contains at least ten different estrogens. The most abundant of these is estrone. Estrone is the type of estrogen that is associated with insulin resistance and weight gain. Another concern with CEE is that besides estrone, CEE contains other forms of estrogen not natural for humans; these are estrogens for horses known as equilenin and equilin. Conjugated estrogen cream (Premarin cream) is also available to treat vaginal symptoms. Conjugated synthetic estrogen (Cenestin) is a synthetic estrogen product that contains high levels of estrone.

Esterified Estrogens

Estratab and Menest, known as esterified estrogens, contain several types of estrogens derived from plants. Estrone is the primary ingredient.

Estropipate

Ogen and Ortho-Est are brands of estropipate, which is considered a natural estrogen. This estrogen is very similar in chemical structure to estrone. Estrone is a "bad estrogen" and can contribute to insulin resistance and weight gain, but there is no proof, in the proper doses, that estropipate does the same thing. It's another natural estrogen and worth a try if other estrogens have not worked for you. Estropipate cream (Ogen cream) is also available for vaginal symptoms.

Estrogen Progesterone Combination Therapy

If you have a uterus, you will need to take progesterone in combination with estrogen. Progesterone or synthetic progestins are added to hormone replacement therapy for only one reason: to prevent uterine cancer. If you have had a hysterectomy, there is no reason to add progesterone to your HRT.

There are several ways to take progesterone. With cyclic dosing, a larger dose of progesterone is added to the daily estrogen for five to fourteen days a month. You will continue to have monthly cycles. The natural hormonal cycles are mimicked in this regime, but it is far from being exactly like the natural hormonal ebb and flow. Expect to have a short and light menstrual period six hours or so after the last dose of the month. The periods will be very regular. This form of HRT can also result in PMS, something most women would like to avoid.

With continuous dosing, a smaller dose of progesterone, in combination with estrogen, is taken every day. You may have irregular and unpredictable spotting for up to six months, but then there should have no further bleeding. Most women prefer this to the cyclic dosing. Continuous dosing protects from uterine cancer better than cyclic dosing. Twenty percent of women taking cyclic

---

Raloxifene (Evista)

One alternative to estrogen is a SERM (selective estrogen receptor modulator), also known as a designer estrogen. SERMs have some of the positive effects of estrogen with less of the negative effects and may be an alternative if you cannot take estrogen. They have selective agonist and antagonist properties—remember the lock and key of chapter 2—and thus stimulate the estrogen receptors in some tissues while blocking the receptor in others. Doctors call this "tissue specific" or "mixed agonist/antagonist."

There are some disadvantages to SERMs. They're not quite as good as estrogen for bones, although they remain a great choice. They do not help the symptoms of menopause, such as hot flashes, and they may even make the symptoms worse, but the biggest problem is lack of knowledge. The drugs are too new to have had any long-term research or patient experience to draw from. The other problem is that there is no "perfect SERM." The perfect SERM would act like estrogen at the level of the bones, the heart, and the blood vessels but block estrogen at the level of the breast and uterus. It would lower breast cancer and uterine cancer risk, prevent osteoporosis, and help the heart and blood vessels. Raloxifene is a good SERM, but better SERMs and more specialized SERMs are in development. Maybe one day a special SERM for women who want to lose weight will even be developed.

---

dosing will stop having periods after a while. This is okay: the lining of the uterus has simply become inactive. A new regime for HRT is known as pulsed progestin HRT. Here the progesterone is given for three days on, three days off. This method may have fewer side effects and better protection against uterine cancer than traditional continuous dosing, without the withdrawal bleeding that occurs with cyclic dosing.

Balance Your Hormones!
Nonhormonal Treatments for Symptomatic Menopause

Clonidine (Catapres)

Clonidine is a widely used high blood pressure medication available in both pill and patch forms. It's another potent regulator of body temperature. Clonidine is commonly used to treat the symptoms of menopause. The main limitation of clonidine is that it makes many women very sleepy.

Gabapentin

Studies have shown that the antiseizure medication Gabapentin (Neurontin) can reduce the severity of menopausal hot flashes. The usual dose is 100–200 mg at bedtime.

SSRI Medications

A study supported by the National Institute of Aging showed that the selective serotonin reuptake inhibitor (SSRI) escitalopram quickly and effectively decreases the severity and the frequency of menopausal hot flashes. A dose of 10–20 mg has been shown to be almost as effective as estrogen, and it starts working within one week. Researchers aren't sure exactly why antidepressant medications reduce hot flashes. It is thought that serotonin, and perhaps other brain hormones, play a role in causing hot flashes.

Vitamin D

Menopause is a time when women have bone problems, and although bone loss has been partially attributed to estrogen deficiency, vitamin D deficiency is a major cause of bone problems in the United States. Vitamin D is a steroid hormone, one that allows your gut to absorb calcium. Without it, most of the calcium you eat passes right out into your stool. Most people do not get enough vitamin D from sunlight and dairy products. Vitamin D deficiency can cause bone pain and fatigue. I recommend 2000–4000 IU of Vitamin D every day.

Calcium

Calcium, a key mineral, becomes even more important to women as they age. If a person suffers from a lack of calcium, the body will take the difference out of the skeleton, leading to bone loss. Studies have shown that consuming calcium, particularly in the form of low-fat dairy products, can also accelerate weight loss. It's thought that somehow calcium speeds up fat-burning enzymes in the body. Before a woman enters menopause, physicians recommend a minimum of 1000 mg of calcium in food and/or supplements. During and after menopause, at least 1500 mg of calcium is recommended. Keep in mind that the average American consumes less than 800 mg a day.

Consume calcium over the course of the day, not all at once, and always with plenty of water. All humans should drink plenty of water anyway—not only does it help with absorption, as in the case of calcium, but it also flushes the system.

Unfortunately, high-fiber diets interfere with the absorption of calcium, so you should take this fact into consideration when taking calcium supplements. Better to get your calcium as part of such a diet, not in addition to it. Calcium itself interferes with the absorption of iron, so iron supplements and calcium supplements should not be taken at the same time.

All calcium preparations contain elemental calcium for a simple reason: calcium is an element, number 20 on the periodic table, but it cannot exist alone and must be bound to another atom or molecule to be stable. For this reason, not all calcium supplements are created equal. Calcium carbonate, for example, has about 40 percent calcium, so the typical 1250 mg tablet has about 600 mg of elemental calcium. Calcium citrate, however, contains only 21 percent calcium, so an equivalent tablet has almost 300 mg less elemental calcium. It's an old saw, but true: Always read those labels!

Calcium carbonate is the most common calcium preparation available. It's got the highest percentage of calcium and is readily available in sources ranging from oyster shells to antacid tablets. The most common side effect of calcium carbonate is gas or upset stomach. Calcium citrate is a good alternative for people who experience side effects from calcium carbonate. Calcium itself is a mineral in milk, cheese, yogurt, collard greens, kale, broccoli, and sardines.

Acupuncture

Studies have shown that acupuncture can decrease the symptoms of menopause.

Physical Activity

Weight-bearing exercises such as walking and lifting weights are ideal for menopausal women because they prevent bone loss. Physical activity helps add lean body mass, aids with fat loss, and improves insulin resistance.

(Continues)

Balance Your Hormones!
(*continued*)

Natural Menopause Supplements

Many of the natural menopause products available in grocery stores, drug stores, and health food stores contain soy isoflavones. Isoflavones are chemicals extracted from plants (such as soy beans) that are similar to, but not exactly the same as estrogen. I hesitate to recommend these products, because concentrations of isoflavones vary tremendously from brand to brand and pill to pill. In addition, because isoflavones are not identical to estrogen, the effects are not identical to estrogen. Recent studies have shown that natural menopause supplements don't do very much and may even increase the frequency of hot flashes.

Estrogen and Progesterone in Foods

Natural estrogens and estrogen-like substances found in nature are known as phytoestrogens (plant estrogens). More than three hundred different plants—including soybeans, wholegrain wheat, lentils, whole grain cereals, dried seaweed, rice, dates, flaxseed oil, bean sprouts, pomegranates, cherries, and coffee—have been found to contain estrogen-like substances. A number of herbs contain estrogen, too, including parsley, garlic, licorice, red clover, thyme, turmeric, hops, and verbena. Black cohosh *(Cimicifuga racemosa)* and red clover *(Trifolium pratense)* are the best-known herbal sources of estrogens and estrogen-like substances. Red clover contains a phytoestrogen called coumestrol, which is also found in bean sprouts.

At least twenty naturally occurring estrogen-like compounds with names such as lignans and isoflavonic phytoestrogens have been identified. All have slightly different actions in how they stimulate or block the two estrogen receptors. In general, they're weaker than estrogen, and they don't build up in tissues the way estrogen does, but they seem to have a positive effect against several types of cancer, including breast cancer, uterine cancer, and prostate cancer.

Their usage dates back centuries, even to the time of Hippocrates. Despite their long history of use, phytoestrogens haven't been studied much, so their effect on weight and various organs remains unknown.

Another common nutrient that has a positive, estrogen-like effect on women is soy. Soy products may reduce risk of breast cancer, lower cholesterol, and prevent heart disease. (Asian women, who typically consume more soy than Westerners, have traditionally had an easier time with menopause than Western women.) Several soy phytoestrogens, known as flavonoids and isoflavonoids, have been identified. Among the best known are diadzen, genistein, glycitein, and coumestrol.

Just like phytoestrogens, there are phytoprogesterones. Mexican yams and yam root in general are the most common source of progesterone and are contained in the medications discussed previously. The chemical substance disogenin is the progesterone-like component of the yam. Other herbs with progesterone properties include oregano, verbena, turmeric, thyme, red clover, and damiana.

Chapter Review

This chapter focused on six hormones associated with female hormone balance and discussed how these hormones work together to maintain good health. The chapter also covered in detail a host of health complications that typically occur in menopausal women and what can be done to control or mediate associated health problems due to hormonal imbalance.

The three key female hormones discussed—estrogen (responsible for female shape), progesterone (typically associated with water retention, PMS, and menstrual regulation), and prolactin (key for breast health and milk production)—all work in concert to promote basic, normal female functions. Male hormones—testosterone, androstenedione, and dehydroepiandrosterone (DHEA)—are important for normal female hormonal balance as well as promoting the building of muscle and lean body mass.

The three major types of estrogen were discussed, including estradiol (responsible for healthy fat around hips and buttocks of young women) and estrone (associated with pre- and post-menopausal weight and fat gain). Most overweight women tend to have more of this type of fat than any other. A third type, estriol, is produced by the placenta during pregnancy and plays only a minor role in the balancing act.

The many consequences of an imbalance in these hormones in pre- and postmenopausal women was discussed, including typical issues such as weight gain, irregular menstrual cycles, hot flashes, problems sleeping, many others.

Finally, testing and treatment for the hormonal impact of menopause were discussed. It was noted that most women do not need a test to know they have entered their menopausal phase. Tests are available, but the results are hard to interpret.

Treatment, although controversial, is available using hormone replacement therapy and bio-identical hormone replacement therapy.

Nonhormonal therapies include the use of drugs used for other conditions (such as high blood pressure medications), vitamin supplements, increased physical activity, and changes to diet. Specific dietary changes include the introduction of foods containing natural estrogen or estrogen-like substances (soybeans, whole grain wheat, bean sprouts, coffee soy products and common herbs such as oregano and thyme).

The next chapter covers important, specific details about the essential role male hormones play in the hormonal balance of men.

10

Men's Hormones
Enhance and Restore Testosterone

The term *androgen* comes from the Greek *andros*, meaning "man," and *gennan*, meaning "to produce." Androgen hormones are best known for male sexual characteristics and include testosterone, androstenedione, and dehydroepiandrosterone (DHEA). Androgens have potent effects on body weight and body composition. In fact, one of their primary functions is to increase muscle and decrease fat. Androgens have a powerful effect on the brain, influencing mood, sexual desire, desire to exercise, and energy level.

Testosterone is the most important and most potent androgen. Testosterone is made in special cells in the testicles called leydig cells. The weaker androgens, androstenedione and DHEA, are made in the outer portion of the adrenal gland called the adrenal cortex.

Men's Hormones Are Steroid Hormones

A steroid hormone is any hormone that has a chemical structure derived from cholesterol. Yes, cholesterol, what you thought was bad, is also beneficial. All steroids have a common structure that contains four rings made of carbon, the backbone of the cholesterol molecule (see Figure 10.1). In a

In This Chapter

- ▶ How Androgens Affect Male Hormonal Balance
- ▶ Normal Levels of Testosterone
- ▶ Causes of Low Testosterone
- ▶ Diagnosing and Treating Low Testosterone in Men

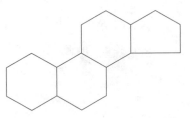

Figure 10.1   The Four-Ring Structure of Steroid Hormones

All steroid hormones are derived from cholesterol. The four-carbon-ring backbone is common to all steroid hormones.

series of steps, specific enzymes modify cholesterol to become each of the various steroid hormones. The enzymes in each gland determine the final hormone produced. Steroid hormones include testosterone, androstenedione, estrogen, aldosterone, DHEA, pregnenolone, progesterone, cortisol, and even vitamin D. The term *steroid* simply describes the chemical structure, not the action of the hormone.

Androgen hormones are known as anabolic steroids. The term anabolic means a metabolic process that promotes tissue growth. Anabolic steroids specifically promote the growth of muscle tissue. All steroid hormones exert their action by controlling your genes. Anabolic steroids turn on genes that make muscles grow.

Anabolic steroid medications were originally developed as a treatment for cancer patients and victims of starvation. The positive effects of anabolic steroids have made them attractive to people who do not have medical conditions that warrant their use, which is known as anabolic steroid abuse. Because of anabolic steroids' muscle- and strength-building qualities, athletes and body builders take them in an attempt to gain a competitive edge. The International Olympic Committee, Major League Baseball, and most American team sports have banned anabolic steroids, but secretive use is widespread. Illicit "designer" androgens help athletes gain an unfair competitive edge while avoiding detection. Anabolic steroid abuse is a problem not only among elite athletes. The epidemic of abuse has spread to local fitness centers as well as to college and high school athletes. Even young boys have been caught using anabolic steroids, which is a shame, because of steroids' negative side effects, from testicular shrinkage to breast development and permanent sterility.

Testosterone and Your Brain

Androgens affect the brain by controlling the "maleness" in our personalities. The most notable actions of testosterone are to increase sex drive and aggression. Even women's personalities are affected by androgens, a subject I discuss in chapter 8.

Testosterone is essential for hormonal balance, and men with low testosterone invariably feel depressed, anxious, or just plain tired. They report a decrease in zest for life and don't feel like being social. Testosterone replacement therapy improves many of the psychological symptoms of hypogonadism.

Ironically, however, not only do androgens affect the brain, but the brain also affects androgens by regulating the levels of these substances in our bodies. The production of testosterone is dependent on the pituitary gland and the hypothalamus, a region in the brain that also regulates appetite and body weight. The pituitary gland makes two hormones—luteinizing hormone (LH) and follicle stimulating hormone (FSH)—that turn on androgen production as well as sperm production in the testicles. If the pituitary gland can't make enough LH or FSH, the testicles will not make testosterone.

In stressful situations, the brain can prompt more testosterone production by boosting LH and FSH production. If it senses that the body needs more—such as before a sporting event or if the testicles are failing—the brain signals the testicles to produce more testosterone. The opposite is also true: if the brain, by way of the pituitary, senses an abundance of testosterone, it will decrease LH and FSH production.

This information brings us back to bodybuilders, athletes, and other people who use anabolic steroids. Invariably, they all have small testicles. With all that extra testosterone floating around, the brain tells the testes that there is no need to produce more testosterone. LH and FSH levels plummet, and the testicles turn soft and shrivel. In endocrine circles it's called L-M-N-O-P syndrome: lots of meat, and no potatoes!

Steroid Hormones Easily Convert to One Another

All steroid hormones can be converted to one another, and testosterone is no exception (see Figure 10.2). A blood enzyme known as 5-alpha reductase can

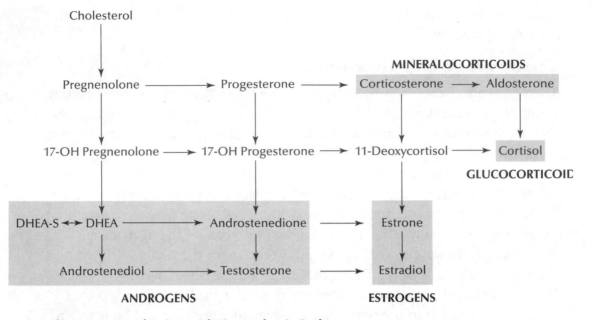

Figure 10.2   The Steroid Biosynthesis Pathway

All steroid hormones are synthesized from a common precursor, cholesterol. The enzymes present in each gland determine the final hormone produced. Steroid hormones can be converted to one another.

convert testosterone into a form called dihydrotestosterone, or DHT. DHT is responsible for two distinctly male characteristics: male-pattern balding and benign growth of the prostate. Alternatively, androgens can be converted to estrogens from an enzyme called aromatase. Androstenedione is converted into estrone, and testosterone is converted into estradiol, by the aromatase enzyme. Estrogens are important in men because they are responsible for bone health, but too much estrogen can make testosterone go low.

Finasteride (Proscar) and dutasteride (Avodart) are used to shrink an enlarged prostate gland by blocking the 5-alpha reductase enzyme. Propecia—yes, the hair growth medicine—is also finasteride. It helps men with male-pattern baldness grow some of their hair back by blocking the actions of DHT in the scalp. Testosterone may make men more virile, but it's also the reason men lose their hair. (No wonder women are attracted to bald men!)

A class of drugs known as aromatase inhibitors blocks the conversion of testosterone to estrogen. Anastrozole (Arimidex), exemestane (Aromasin), and

Testosterone Resistance

Testosterone works like other hormones. To exert its actions, a hormone must bind with a receptor. Think of the "lock-and-key" concept I discussed in chapter 2. Steroids, like other hormones, have very special and specific receptors. The receptor is either on the actual DNA, or it binds to the steroid and the steroid-receptor unit then binds to DNA. Either way, the steroid hormone works by turning genes on and off in our cells directly and controlling certain genes that are known as steroid-responsive genes. Different receptors may have different activity levels or amounts in different people.

The way that testosterone interacts with a receptor varies from person to person. Here's an extreme example of receptor viability: there's a condition called androgen insensitivity syndrome, in which the androgen receptors don't work at all. The DNA of an individual with this syndrome does not detect androgen even though the levels are sky high. Meanwhile, the body keeps making more and more keys—the androgen itself—but the lock—the androgen receptors—is broken. If this happens during fetal development, a baby will develop as a female because of the lack of androgen, but it will be a male genetically, with a Y sex chromosome.

A person with androgen insensitivity syndrome has testicles hidden in the abdomen and a blind vaginal pouch—there's no uterus or ovaries. Because to all appearances, this genetic male is a female, the condition often doesn't make itself known until puberty, when there will be no onset of menstruation. Some of these children grow into adults without realizing they have this condition until they try to get pregnant. Overall, most live their lives as normal women, but they can't have children. In time, they should see a doctor to have their testicular tissue removed, because it can become cancerous if it remains in its original condition.

I bring up this extreme example because more subtle examples also exist. There are situations in which testosterone levels may be normal or even high, but the testosterone cannot function properly because the receptor is defective. This testosterone resistance is similar to other types of hormone resistance, such as insulin resistance (see chapter 6) and thyroid hormone resistance (see chapter 7). Medications such as spironolactone (Aldactone) and others can block the androgen receptor and cause symptoms of hypogonadism.

Age-Related Testosterone Decline

Age-related testosterone decline, which still has not been precisely defined, goes by many names: male menopause, mild testicular failure, andropause, viropause, male climacteric, male gonadopause, late onset hypogonadism, ADAM (androgen deficiency of the aging male) syndrome or PADAM (partial androgen deficiency in the aging male) syndrome. These names all suggest a phenomenon that parallels female menopause, which may be the wrong message to be giving men with age-related testosterone decline.

Fewer than 15 percent of older men with low testosterone take testosterone replacement therapy. Androgen therapy is not well accepted to treat normal aging. But some doctors worry about even treating men with medically significant hypogonadism. Critics note that long-term safety studies on TRT have not been done. The concern parallels the controversies that continue for treating menopausal women with estrogen. Estrogen replacement therapy, once considered the standard of care for menopausal women, has become increasingly controversial, because of the results of long-term safety studies that showed increased risks for blood clots, cardiovascular disease, and breast cancer. Despite this information, many women still take estrogen. Although the television airwaves have been filled with ads about "low T," there is some controversy about men over the age of sixty taking testosterone. Some research has suggested that testosterone could increase the risk having a heart attack in older men.

Although many men experience lower testosterone levels as they age, it is not inevitable. Studies have shown that decreased testosterone is more likely a consequence of illnesses men acquire as they get older, such as excess body fat, high blood pressure, and high cholesterol. Staying healthy is the best way to keep your testosterone levels normal.

letrozole (Femara) have become blockbuster medications in the fight against breast cancer.

In men, aromatase activity increases with age and with the level of obesity, which means that older or obese men have lower levels of testosterone and higher levels of estrogen. Aromatase inhibitors are sometimes given to men who take testosterone replacement therapy (TRT) to boost testosterone levels and prevent conversion into estrogen. I don't recommend this process because it can lead to bone loss.

Low T

Low T or low testosterone production, known as hypogonadism, is estimated to affect 4–5 million men in the United States. Hypogonadism, or inadequate functioning of the testicles (also known as *gonads*), can affect men at any age. Hypogonadism can be genetic, or it can be caused by a variety of medical problems.

The risk of hypogonadism increases with age. All men experience a gradual decline in androgen levels as they get older, beginning as early as twenty-five years of age. By the age of seventy, more that 80 percent of men have testosterone levels below the normal range. Studies have shown that very healthy men have less of an age-related decline in testosterone levels.

Being overweight or having other medical problems like high blood pressure, diabetes, high cholesterol, rheumatoid arthritis, liver disease, kidney disease, or HIV, or even being in chronic pain increase the risk of hypogonadism. Low testosterone levels are associated with decreased muscle size and strength, increased body fat, sexual dysfunction, bone loss, depression, fatigue, diminished sense of well-being, and increased risk for heart disease. Declining androgen levels can occur slowly or abruptly, and the rate varies from person to person. If the symptoms come on abruptly, you may have a more serious form. At whatever rate it occurs, however, overly low testosterone levels are a concern.

Symptoms of Hypogonadism

Anemia

Anemia means decreased red blood cell counts. Testosterone is one of the factors responsible for red blood cell production. Men with hypogonadism typically have mild anemia that gets better with testosterone replacement therapy.

Bone Loss

Thinning of the bones, known as *osteoporosis* or *osteopenia,* is traditionally thought of as a disease that women get after menopause, but bone problems are commonly seen in men with hypogonadism. Bone loss is one of the most serious

> ## Androgen Deficiency in Aging Males (ADAM) Questionnaire
>
> 1. Do you have a decrease in libido (sex drive)?
> 2. Do you have a lack of energy?
> 3. Do you have a decrease in strength and/or endurance?
> 4. Have you lost height?
> 5. Have you noticed a decreased enjoyment of life?
> 6. Are you sad and/or grumpy?
> 7. Are your erections less strong?
> 8. Have you noticed a recent deterioration in your ability to play sports?
> 9. Are you falling asleep after dinner?
> 10. Has there been a recent deterioration in your work performance?
>
> If the answer is "Yes" to question 1 or 7 or at least three of the other questions, low testosterone may be present.

complications of male hypogonadism. Testosterone is required for proper bone health. Mild bone loss, osteopenia, can progress to the more severe form, osteoporosis. Bone loss puts men at increased risk of fracturing a bone. The most common bones to be fractured are the hip, wrist, or spine. A fracture of the spine, called a spinal compression fracture, can result in loss of height and a humping of the back.

Breast Growth

Low testosterone can result in growth of male breast tissue (gynecomastia). Gynecomastia is typically more pronounced in obese men, but lean men can also get it. Testosterone replacement therapy can improve gynecomastia, but gynecomastia can also be a side effect of testosterone replacement therapy. Some men have permanent breast enlargement even after the hypogonadism is treated. Breast reduction surgery is a treatment for men who have bothersome gynecomastia.

Decrease in Frequency of Shaving

Testosterone is responsible for facial hair growth. Some men with hypogonadism report a decrease in their need to shave.

Decreased Sex Drive (Libido)

Testosterone exerts its effect on the brain by regulating sex drive. Many men with hypogonadism have decreased libido; however, some men do not. A normal libido does not exclude the possibility of having hypogonadism.

Depression or Anxiety

Men with hypogonadism report changes in mood, such as nervousness, irritability, anger, negative thinking, a diminished sense of well-being, or an increase in depressed moods. Clinical depression is common in men with hypogonadism; men with untreated hypogonadism typically have a poor response to antidepressant medications. Many men with hypogonadism just feel terrible. They have completely lost their interest in life. Testosterone replacement therapy reverses these symptoms, but sometimes antidepressants or anti-anxiety medications are also required for complete relief of symptoms.

Diminished Quality of Life or Lowered Sense of Well-Being

A lowered sense of well-being or the feeling that life has lost its quality is one of the most overlooked symptoms of hypogonadism. Men treated with testosterone replacement therapy report dramatic improvements in their quality of life and sense of well-being.

Erectile Dysfunction or Decreased Sexual Performance

Sexual problems are the most well-known symptom of hypogonadism. Adequate testosterone levels are required for proper sexual functioning; however, most people with hypogonadism still get erections from time to time. Men with hypogonadism complain about the quality of their erections; they are not as strong or as frequent as they used to be, or they can't be maintained for as long as they used to be. Men with a poor response to the medications Viagra, Levitra, or Cialis are at risk for having hypogonadism. Some men with hypogonadism have completely normal sexual function, so the absence of this symptom does not exclude the diagnosis of hypogonadism.

Fatigue

Low energy is one of the most common complaints in men with hypogonadism. Men frequently report falling asleep after dinner or being too tired to exercise. Decreased muscle strength, poor sleep, depression, and anemia are all contributing factors to the fatigue.

Hot Flashes or Excessive Sweating

Sensations of warmth, flushing, or excessive sweating can occur, especially at night, which is a symptom similar to what women experience when they are going through menopause.

Insomnia

Insomnia, which can contribute to fatigue, is sometimes a symptom of hypogonadism.

Loss of Body Hair, Chest Hair, Pubic Hair, or Armpit Hair

Along with facial hair, hair follicles on other parts of the body require testosterone for proper growth. Testosterone deficiency can result in loss of body, chest, pubic, and armpit hair.

Low Sperm Count

Testosterone and pituitary gland hormones known as gonadotropins (LH and FSH) are required for normal sperm production. Men with hypogonadism may have a low volume of ejaculate and poor sperm quality or low sperm counts. Testosterone replacement therapy generally does not improve sperm quality or sperm counts. Some men with hypogonadism can improve sperm counts using hCG or clomiphene citrate (Clomid).

Muscle Weakness, Loss of Endurance, or Decreased Muscle Mass

The normal effect of testosterone is to build muscle, so it's logical that hypogonadism is associated with muscle weakness, decreased endurance, or loss of muscle mass. Some men report deterioration in their ability to play sports.

Poor Memory and Lack of Concentration

It is normal to experience an age-related decline in mental capacity, but the declines seen with hypogonadism are more severe than those seen with normal aging. Many men report deterioration in their work performance.

Premature Aging

Hypogonadism speeds up the normal aging process. Men with hypogonadism look older and feel older. Testosterone replacement therapy makes a man look younger and feel younger.

Shrinking or Softening of the Testicles

Hypogonadism may result in either shrinking or softening of the testicles.

Softening of the Voice

Low testosterone has effects on the vocal cords that can result in a softer voice.

Weight Gain (Especially around the Middle)

Hypogonadism is a common cause of weight gain. Typically there is muscle loss and increased fat, which cause decreased metabolism. Men with hypogonadism have less desire to exercise, which also contributes to weight gain.

Causes of Hypogonadism

Determining the cause of hypogonadism is very important. Low testosterone can be a result of many different conditions that require additional treatments beyond traditional testosterone replacement therapy. Hypogonadism can be a sign of a more serious medical condition. Anyone with hypogonadism should have a full evaluation to determine the cause. There are two main categories of hypogonadism: central hypogonadism and testicular failure.

Testicular Failure	Central Hypogonadism
Testicular failure occurs when the testicles become injured or diseased and are unable to produce testosterone.	Disorders of the pituitary gland and other parts of the brain can cause hypogonadism through decreased production of LH and FSH. It's called central hypogonadism because the problem lies in the central nervous system.

Causes of Central Hypogonadism

Obesity or Excess Body Fat

Excess body fat is a common cause of low testosterone. Forty percent of obese men have low testosterone levels. Obesity itself can lower androgen levels for many reasons. Being overweight worsens the age-related decline of androgens. Other hormone signals, such as leptin, estrogen and cortisol, can lower androgen levels to a significant extent, and these two hormones' levels increase as you gain weight. Fat cells produce hormones called inflammatory cytokines or adipokines that lower testosterone by slowing signals from the hypothalamus and pituitary gland, increasing the risk of hypogonadism in overweight men. Overweight men have increased levels of aromatase, the enzyme that converts androgens into estrogens. Low testosterone results in higher estrogen levels and lower growth hormone levels (see chapter 12) leading to further decreases in muscle mass and increases in body fat. It's a vicious cycle: being overweight (or having a high percentage of body fat) disrupts androgen balance and overall hormonal balance, making you lose muscle and gain fat.

Diabetes, Prediabetes, or Insulin Resistance

Men with insulin resistance, type 2 diabetes, prediabetes, and metabolic syndrome are at very high risk for hypogonadism. The link between diabetes and low testosterone has been confirmed in several studies and occurs in as many as 50 percent of these men. Studies have found that men with both diabetes and low testosterone have more symptoms, especially erectile dysfunction and fatigue. The Endocrine Society recommends that all men with type 2 diabetes have their testosterone levels checked regularly.

It's thought that insulin resistance, increased estrogen production from fat cells, high blood sugar, and chronic illness combined with excess fat (especially in the upper body) and age-related androgen decline all play a role. These factors synergize to cause medically significant hypogonadism. Men who have diabetes and untreated hypogonadism gain fat and lose muscle and have difficulty getting their blood sugar under control. Improving insulin resistance can improve testosterone levels, but they usually don't go all the way back to the normal range. Although low testosterone is common in men with insulin resistance and diabetes, there aren't many studies to show that replacing testosterone improves insulin resistance. (For more on insulin resistance, see chapter 6.)

Pituitary Tumors

A tumor of the pituitary gland, known as a pituitary adenoma, commonly causes hypogonadism. One variant of a pituitary tumor, known as a prolactinoma, almost always results in hypogonadism. This tumor produces excessive amounts of the hormone prolactin, which is responsible for milk production in women. Prolactinomas can cause male breast growth, and in rare cases, they have been known to cause breast milk production in men.

Chronic Pain

Men with chronic pain, especially those on prescription pain medication, are at very high risk for hypogonadism. Narcotic medications are well known to cause hypogonadism by exerting a toxic effect on the testicles as well as the hypothalamus and pituitary gland. Chronic pain also results in insulin resistance (see chapter 6) and increased cortisol production (see chapter 11), which lower testosterone levels.

Head Injury

Head injuries are a common cause of pituitary gland dysfunction. Men with head injuries, even from many years earlier, may develop low testosterone alone or along with other pituitary gland hormone deficiencies. It is very common to see growth hormone deficiency in conjunction with a head injury, and many of the symptoms of growth hormone deficiency overlap with those of hypogonadism (see chapter 12).

Hereditary Hemochromatosis

Hereditary hemochromatosis is a genetic disease in which the body absorbs too much iron and deposits it in organs, causing tissue damage. Hereditary hemochromatosis frequently causes endocrine dysfunction because of iron deposits in the glands, especially the pancreas and the pituitary gland. Pancreatic dysfunction results in insulin deficiency and a form of type 1 diabetes. Iron deposits in the skin give it a bronze color, so it's sometimes called bronze diabetes. The most common pituitary gland dysfunction is hypogonadism.

Hereditary hemochromatosis is more common than most doctors realize; 1 out of every 500 people have hereditary hemochromatosis. It's one of the most common genetic diseases in Caucasians, yet it's hard to diagnose early because the symptoms are so subtle. On average, it takes ten years from the first symptom to diagnosis. The most common early symptoms are fatigue, joint aches, and a decreased sex drive. Other symptoms include abdominal pain, tanning of the skin (without being out in the sun; the skin will eventually become more and more bronzed), and depression. Tests for blood counts, iron metabolism, and the hereditary hemochromatosis gene can diagnose the condition. Because of the high risk of cirrhosis of the liver, most doctors recommend that patients with hemochromatosis have a liver biopsy.

If left untreated, hemochromatosis can lead to insulin resistance, diabetes, arthritis, hepatitis, hypogonadism, heart failure, cirrhosis of the liver, and liver cancer. Treatment for hemochromatosis is a periodic phlebotomy, removing of the blood. If you have symptoms of hemochromatosis or have a family history of hereditary hemochromatosis, you should discuss it with your physician.

Sarcoidosis

Sarcoidosis is a disorder of unknown cause that is characterized by the formation of substances known as granulomas. Granulomas can occur anywhere in the body and are most common in the lungs. When sarcoidosis affects the brain, it is known as neurosarcoidosis. Neurosarcoidosis can cause central hypogonadism when it damages the hypothalamus and pituitary gland. Typically, neurosarcoidosis causes multiple deficiencies of pituitary gland hormones. Sarcoidosis is more common in young adults and in African Americans, and it tends to run in families. If you have sarcoidosis and symptoms of hypogonadism, you should discuss it with your physician. A magnetic resonance imagining (MRI) scan of the pituitary gland can be helpful to diagnose neurosarcoidosis.

Excess Cortisol

Whether from corticosteroid medications or produced abnormally by the adrenal gland, excess cortisol can lower testosterone levels in men. For more information on cortisol, see chapter 11.

Exposure to Female Hormones

Unintended exposure to female hormones, from a spouse's estrogen cream, for example, can cause male hypogonadism. Environmental estrogens such as Bisphenol A (BPA) and phthalates can lower male hormone levels (for more information, see chapter 7). Rare cases of testicular tumors can produce high amounts of estrogen as well. The pituitary gland responds to estrogen just as it does to testosterone. Excess estrogen decreases LH and FSH levels, resulting in decreased testosterone production.

Causes of Testicular Failure

Autoimmune Disease

Immune system destruction of testosterone-producing cells in the testicles known as Leydig cells can lead to hypogonadism. Along the same lines as type 1 diabetes and autoimmune thyroid disease, the body makes antibodies that attack and destroy a gland. Any gland can be a target for attack, and the testicles are no exception.

Trauma or Injury to the Testicles

I have seen many patients with previously untreated hypogonadism who have a remote history of injury to their testicles. I have also seen many patients with hypogonadism who have had one testicle removed years before and never realized it put them at risk for hypogonadism.

Infection

An infection of the testicles, known as orchitis, can result in hypogonadism. Mumps is infamous for causing testicular failure. Male hypogonadism is the most common cause of hormone deficiency in men infected with the HIV virus. In fact, HIV patients are one of the largest groups of men taking testosterone medications.

Alcohol, Drugs, and Tobacco

Believe it or not, one of the most pernicious toxins to the testicles is alcohol. Drinking too much can permanently damage the testicles and inhibit testosterone production. Tobacco smoke, marijuana, cocaine, heroin, and other drugs have a similar effect. Narcotic medications are well known to cause hypogonadism by exerting a toxic effect on the testicles as well as the hypothalamus and pituitary gland.

Fluid Retention

Liver problems, kidney problems, and congestive heart failure can cause fluid retention in the body and sometimes in the scrotum or testicles, which can cut off the blood supply to androgen-producing cells, decreasing production of testosterone.

Urologic Problems

Urologic conditions such varicocele, hydrocele, spermatocele, and even testicular cancer can cause swelling in the testicles, which can cut off the blood supply to testosterone-producing cells. Not everyone with these conditions gets hypogonadism, but having any of these conditions does increase your risk. A complete examination of the testicles and scrotum followed by a testicular ultrasound is a good way to check for these conditions.

Vasectomy

Although controversial, it is thought that having a vasectomy can increase your risk for hypogonadism. The surgery may disrupt the blood supply to the testicles, causing a decline in function. Unfortunately for some men, the problem is less subtle. Infections and bleeding are complications of a vasectomy or vasectomy reversal surgery that can lead to more severe cases of hypogonadism.

Testing for Hypogonadism

Despite problems with testing, establishing a diagnosis of hypogonadism requires laboratory confirmation of low testosterone levels. Several types of testosterone measurements may be necessary to fully evaluate someone's testosterone status. Because there is no perfect test, the diagnosis of hypogonadism can be a judgment call on the part of the physician.

Total Testosterone

Total testosterone is the test most commonly used to diagnose hypogonadism, but this test is not always the most accurate measurement. Different laboratories employ differing testing methods, so there can be a tremendous variation in test results. The total testosterone test measures the total amount of testosterone in the blood—both free and bound to proteins, primarily sex hormone binding globulin (SHBG) and albumin, but since up to 60–80 percent of total testosterone is bound to SHBG, this test is highly dependent on SHBG levels.

Testosterone that is bound to SHBG is not readily available to the tissues and is said to be inactive. If SHBG levels are normal, the total testosterone level is usually accurate, but abnormal SHBG levels will throw the test off. Higher SHBG levels will make the total testosterone level appear normal when it is actually low.

Although the "normal range" is still debated, most laboratories report a reference range for total testosterone of around 260–1000 nanograms/deciliter (ng/dL). But many endocrinologists agree that a total testosterone level below 300 ng/dL may be medically significant. Testosterone levels between 300 and 500 ng/dL represent a gray zone and require further testing.

The traditional method for measuring total testosterone is immuno-histochemical luminescence, or radioimmunoassay. A new laboratory technique called liquid chromatography tandem mass spectrometry is even more

---

Diagnosing Hypogonadism

Measure testosterone, LH, and FSH before 10:00 A.M.

Confirm abnormal tests with a second test.

Make a diagnosis:

    Central hypogonadism: Low testosterone, low or normal LH and FSH

    Testicular failure: Low testosterone, high LH and FSH

Determine the cause.

---

accurate and more reliable than traditional methods of measuring testosterone. The total testosterone is used to determine free testosterone levels, so if the measurement is inaccurate to start with, the free testosterone level will also be inaccurate.

Measured Free Testosterone

Free testosterone represents testosterone that is not bound to proteins. This test measures the most active component of testosterone and is not affected by SHBG levels. The preferred methods for measuring free testosterone are equilibrium dialysis or tandem mass spectrometry. The problem with free testosterone measurements is that most laboratories use testing methodology that is unreliable. Make sure that the free testosterone measurement isn't being done using an inferior technique called the analog method. The analog method is cheap and easy to perform but is not reliable.

Calculated Free Testosterone

In most situations, the calculated free testosterone can be more accurate than either the total testosterone or the measured free testosterone. A sophisticated mathematical equation gives a value for the free testosterone based on total testosterone, albumin, and SHBG level. The formula for this calculation can be found on the website of the International Society for the Study of the Aging Male at www.issam.ch/freetesto.htm.

The Challenges of Measuring Androgens

Androgen measurements remain one of the great challenges in endocrine laboratory testing. Even with all the advances in the field, diagnosing hypogonadism can be difficult. Tests for androgen levels can be variable and inaccurate for many reasons.

Test reliability. Testosterone is one of the most difficult hormones to measure. Many tests are available, but so far there is no perfect test. Most tests are fairly good at measuring normal or high testosterone levels. The challenge is measuring low levels of testosterone. In today's managed care environment, a particular test may be done because it is cheaper, and not because it is better.

Lab imperfection. Doctors are not perfect and neither are labs. Androgen testing is notorious for a high degree of variability. I have sometimes taken a blood sample from a patient, divided it in half, and sent the blood to two different labs for the same test. The results can be very different. Doctors call this disparity "assay variability." Endocrinologists will try to minimize this problem by sending all of their hormone tests to a single lab. Even so, there can be problems with quality control and variability, and each lab has its own reference range—that is, its own definition of normal—so the normal range also varies from lab to lab.

Hormone fluxes. Testosterone is secreted in cyclic patterns; diurnal rhythms, diet, activity level, and even sun exposure will affect testosterone production. Testosterone usually peaks first thing in the morning,

---

Bioavailable Testosterone

Bioavailable testosterone represents all the testosterone that is readily available to the tissues and includes free testosterone and weakly bound testosterone. Free testosterone makes up about 2 percent of the total circulating testosterone. Another 20–40 percent of total testosterone is loosely bound to the blood protein albumin. This albumin-bound testosterone can be easily extracted and is said to be a bioavailable component. Knowing how much testosterone is tightly bound and how much is bioavailable to the tissues is very important. The bioavailable testosterone test is calculated based on a variety of measurements, including total and free testosterone levels as well as albumin and SHBG.

which is why men often wake up with an erection. This fact is also why I recommend measuring testosterone levels before 10:00 A.M. To control for minute-to-minute hormone fluxes, endocrinologists will sometimes draw three separate blood samples twenty minutes apart, combine the blood, and send the combined samples to the lab for a single test. The complete sample, known as a pooled sample, provides a more integrated measure of hormone secretion.

Blood proteins. Ninety-eight percent of testosterone is attached to proteins in the blood. Sex hormone binding globulin holds 60–80 percent of the testosterone. Testosterone bound to SHBG is not biologically active. Twenty to 40 percent of testosterone is bound to another protein, albumin. Albumin-bound testosterone can come free and is biologically active, unlike SHBG-bound testosterone. The total testosterone measures SHBG-bound, albumin-bound, and free testosterone in aggregate. Variations in SHBG or albumin will cause the total testosterone measurement to be unreliable.

Normal? Testosterone experts still debate what is truly a normal testosterone level. Many doctors now agree that the normal range is not accurate and should be reevaluated. Some laboratories are now reporting normal values according to how old the patient is. Currently, efforts are being made to set a more precise normal value with a standardization of the testosterone assay.

Luteinizing Hormone and Follicle Stimulating Hormone

Gonadotropin hormones—luteinizing hormone and follicle stimulating hormone—give doctors information about the pituitary gland and hypothalamus and their regulation of testosterone. Testosterone follows a traditional endocrine feedback loop with LH and FSH. If the production of testosterone from the testicle is diminished, LH and FSH levels increase in an attempt to stimulate the testicle to produce more testosterone. In other words, testicular failure results in low testosterone and high LH and FSH levels. If the problem comes from the brain or pituitary gland, testosterone will be low and LH and FSH will also be low. Sometimes the testosterone level is low but the LH and FSH levels are normal. In this situation, the LH and FSH are said to be "inappropriately normal," because if the pituitary gland were working properly, levels would be higher.

Sex Hormone Binding Globulin

SHBG is the main protein that carries testosterone in the bloodstream. Sixty to 80 percent of testosterone is bound to SHBG. SHBG binds testosterone very tightly and makes it inactive. SHBG is important because most of the testosterone that is measured in a total testosterone test is bound to SHBG, yet this form of testosterone is not active in the body. When SHBG levels are normal, total testosterone is a fairly reliable test, but when SHBG is either too high or too low, the total testosterone does not accurately represent the body's testosterone status. It's important to know SHBG levels to determine the reliability of testosterone levels, but abnormal SHBG levels don't necessarily mean a medical problem. SHBG levels increase with aging. Obesity and diabetes also cause higher SHBG levels. Low SHBG is a risk factor for insulin resistance. Liver problems, kidney problems, genetics, and many medications can affect SHBG levels.

Prolactin

Elevations of prolactin may indicate a pituitary tumor, a common cause of hypogonadism. All men with low testosterone, and especially those with low or normal LH and FSH levels, should have prolactin levels measured.

Albumin

Twenty to 40 percent of testosterone in the body is bound to the blood protein albumin. The testosterone bound to albumin is weakly bound and can be easily extracted for use in the tissues. Albumin-bound testosterone is said to be bioavailable. Abnormal albumin levels are not as common as abnormal SHBG levels, and in the grand scheme of things, albumin is less important than SHBG in testosterone measurement. Obesity, malnutrition, and liver disease can affect albumin levels. Albumin levels are generally part of a standard blood test called a complete metabolic panel.

Dihydrotestosterone

Dihydrotestosterone is made from testosterone by the enzyme 5-alpha reductase. DHT levels are sometimes helpful in diagnosing hypogonadism or monitoring therapy. DHT is primarily responsible for negative effects of testosterone, such as prostate enlargement and hair loss.

Estrogen

Elevated estrogen levels can be a cause of hypogonadism. The most common test performed is for estradiol, but estrone and estriol levels can also be measured. Liver problems, obesity, and accidental exposure to estrogen are all causes of high estrogen levels. Testosterone replacement therapy can also result in elevated estrogen levels, so estrogen levels may be measured to monitor for this complication.

Liver Function Tests

Because liver disease is frequently associated with hypogonadism, liver function tests should be made periodically. Alanine transaminase (ALT), aspartate aminotransferase (AST), gamma-glutamyl transpeptidase (GGT), alkaline phosphatase, bilirubin, albumin, and prothrombin time are all tests of liver function.

Hemoglobin and Hematocrit

Hypogonadism causes low red blood cell counts (anemia). Red blood cells are measured by hemoglobin and hematocrit tests. Testosterone replacement therapy increases red blood cell counts but can cause too much blood, a side effect known as polycythemia. Hemoglobin and hematocrit should be monitored at least every six months during testosterone replacement therapy.

Prostate-Specific Antigen

Testosterone has effects on the prostate gland, and monitoring prostate health is an important part of testosterone replacement therapy. Prostate-specific antigen (PSA) should be measured before starting testosterone replacement therapy, and if elevated, should be fully evaluated by a urologist before determining if testosterone replacement therapy is appropriate. PSA is monitored every three months for the first year on testosterone replacement therapy and every six months thereafter.

Bone Density Testing

Because low testosterone is an important causal factor in thinning of the bones, any man with hypogonadism should have bone density testing or bone mineral density (BMD) testing performed. Dual-energy X-ray absorptiometry (DEXA) is the most accurate and advanced test available for measuring bone density. The test is quick and painless and gives very important information about the density of bones.

Other Tests

Men with hypogonadism are at increased risk for a variety of medical problems. Blood sugar, cholesterol, and thyroid testing should be done in all men with hypogonadism. Other androgen levels, including androstenedione and DHEA-S, can be tested. Sometimes it's useful to measure multiple androgen levels; but testosterone is usually the most informative.

Testosterone Replacement Therapy

The goal of treating testosterone deficiency is to alleviate the symptoms of hypogonadism and bring testosterone levels into the normal range. Testosterone-replacement therapy comes in a variety of formulations. Testosterone pills should not be used in men, because this form of TRT causes liver toxicity.

Testosterone Injections

Testosterone enanthate and testosterone cypionate are the two most common types of injectable testosterone. These are long-acting testosterone medications and are given as a deep muscular injection. The testosterone is dissolved in oil, and the injections are given anywhere from once a week to every four weeks.

There are two problems with testosterone injections. First, the shot is difficult to take. Because testosterone is dissolved in sesame oil (enanthate) or cottonseed oil (cypionate), a large needle must be used, and the injection is given very deep into the muscle. The testosterone forms a reservoir that is slowly released into the bloodstream. The second problem is that testosterone levels do not remain steady. Hormone levels peak about twenty-four to seventy-two hours after an injection and decline over the next several days to weeks, leading to fluctuations in mood, appetite, sex drive, and energy level. To minimize these problems, I recommend taking a lower dose injection (100–150 mg) once a week. This method gives more stable blood levels and decreases the volume of the injection, allowing a smaller needle that doesn't have to go as deep into the muscle.

Testosterone Gel (Androgel, Testim, Fortesta, Axiron)

Testosterone gels are convenient and easy to use, and they provide fairly constant blood levels of testosterone, which eliminates the highs and lows seen with testosterone injections. I have found that some men require the maximum dose of testosterone gel to get their testosterone levels into the normal range. Sometimes even the maximum dose of testosterone gel is not adequate. In these cases, there is usually a problem with the gel's penetration of the skin, a good reason to change over to a different type of testosterone replacement, such as shots, pellets, or higher-concentration compounded testosterone gel. If you use testosterone gel, you must be careful that you do not let wet gel touch the skin of anyone, especially not children or your partner.

Androgel has become the number one most prescribed type of TRT. It is an alcohol-based gel that contains either 1 percent or 1.62 percent testosterone. The gel is applied to the upper arms and shoulders every morning. Androgel comes in single-use packets or a pump.

Testim is a formulation of 1 percent testosterone gel that uses a compound known as pentadecalactone as the base for the gel. Pentadecalactone is very good at penetrating the skin, getting more testosterone into the bloodstream. Testim comes in 5 gram tubes that have a screw top. The main problem with Testim is that it has a peculiar odor (the manufacturers call it a scent). Some people say it smells like musk oil; others say it smells like fishy perfume. Endocrinologists joke about the smell; they know someone is on Testim from the instant they meet him just by the smell. The gel is sticky or tacky and can feel uncomfortable on the skin. Despite these inconveniences, Testim is the TRT of choice for many men. If there are problems with the gel feeling sticky or if the smell is bothersome, I recommend the following: rub the gel in for at least two minutes, which allows the gel to penetrate the skin, and the stickiness goes away. Apply the gel to the thighs, lower back, and calves. The farther away from the nose, the less you will smell it. Apply talcum powder or baking soda after rubbing in the gel. When following these steps, most men do very well with Testim.

Fortesta and Axiron are newer brands of 2 percent testosterone gel that seem to work just as well as the other products.

Compounded Testosterone Gel

I have found that custom-compounded formulations of testosterone gel, which can be created by an experienced compounding pharmacist, can be extremely helpful for men with hypogonadism. As with all pharmaceuticals made by compounding pharmacies, the quality of the products can be poor. I have seen a tremendous amount of variability in the testosterone levels in patients who use compounded testosterone gels. Custom-compounded testosterone gel can be made as strong as 5 percent, which is more than twice as potent as other testosterone gels. As with all compounded products, it is important to use a reliable compounding pharmacist.

Striant

Striant is a testosterone tablet that is not swallowed but is placed between the cheek and gum. It's called a mucoadhesive sustained-release buccal tablet. The tablet is placed on the upper gums, where it gradually softens into a waxy glob that conforms to the shape of the gum. The usual dose is one 30 mg tablet twice a day, and patients are instructed to wipe the residual portion out of their mouths before applying a new tablet. I have found that some patients can do well with using the tablet once a day and not wiping out the residual portion. Many men find Striant difficult to get used to, but when used properly, it helps most men achieve normal testosterone levels. Striant is a great choice for obese men who frequently have problems with gel penetrating the skin. Striant is also reported to cause lower DHT levels, the testosterone byproduct that contributes to prostate enlargement and hair loss. The main complaint I hear about Striant is that it is inconvenient and that it can cause mouth sores.

Testosterone Patches (Androderm and Testoderm)

Testosterone skin patches, or transdermal testosterone patches, come in two varieties. Testoderm is applied to the scrotum. Androderm is applied to the upper arms, back, or abdomen. Skin patches are effective, but they are not a popular form of TRT. Up to 30 percent of men experience rashes or skin irritation, and up to 12 percent have blister formation. The patches can be inconvenient and can fall off during exercise.

Testosterone Pellets (Testopel)

Testosterone pellets can be implanted under the skin to provide testosterone for three to six months. Some men prefer this therapy because they don't have to bother with rubbing in gel every day.

Anastrozole (Arimidex), Exemestane (Aromasin), and Letrozole (Femara)

This class of drugs, known as aromatase inhibitors, works by blocking the conversion of testosterone into estrogen. The drugs are approved for use in women for the treatment of breast cancer and are increasingly being used as an adjunctive therapy to TRT. Most experts consider the use of aromatase inhibitors in men to be very risky, because aromatase inhibitors cause bone loss.

Oxandrolone (Oxandrin)

Oxandrolone is a synthetic androgen available in pill form. It's very expensive and not commonly used for male hypogonadism.

Clomiphene Citrate (Clomid)

Approved as a fertility drug in women, clomiphene is also effective for raising testosterone levels and sperm counts in men. The usual dose is 25–50 milligrams (mg) daily.

Human Chorionic Gonadotropin

Injections of human chorionic gonadotropin (hCG) can be used in men with central hypogonadism to increase testosterone levels, increase testicular size, and increase sperm counts. Treatment with hCG can be complex and may require injections of LH and FSH as well. This treatment is primarily reserved for men who want to increase their sperm count and improve fertility.

Future Therapies

New delivery systems for testosterone are always in the works. A nasal spray formulation looks promising. Research is also being done on injecting microcapsules and a long-acting version of testosterone, testosterone undecenoate, which lasts three months instead of a few weeks. Synthetic versions of testosterone-like hormones are being developed that may have advantages to traditional TRT.

Side Effects of Testosterone Replacement Therapy

Once the correct dose is determined, most men do not have side effects from testosterone replacement therapy. The biggest complaint about testosterone replacement therapy is the method of delivery, since a simple pill is not available. I have heard patients complain about every type of treatment. Some people hate rubbing gel into the skin every day; others can't stand the thought of a shot. Testosterone can have serious side effects that can be seen with any of the delivery devices. There can be an increase in the level of anger or aggression. Some men get a huge increase in their sex drive, which can be too much for their wives or partners to handle. There can be breast growth or tenderness, acne, liver problems, high blood pressure, fluid retention, headaches, prostate enlargement, decreased sperm counts, and increased blood counts. Sometimes, therapeutic phlebotomy is required to draw excess blood caused by Testosterone replacement therapy (TRT). TRT has been reported to cause a worsening in sleep apnea, but I have never seen a patient experience this complication. Testosterone decreases sperm counts and causes testicular shrinkage.

There is always the potential for anabolic steroid abuse among men. Some men have a psychological condition called body dysmorphic disorder, in which they're convinced that their bodies are horribly unattractive. Their concerns can be focused on many parts of the body, from their hair to their legs, but for many, it's the physique that's disappointing. They work out, and to help their workouts along they abuse testosterone. Anabolic steroid abuse is associated with permanent sterility, erectile dysfunction, breast tissue growth, psychological problems, cholesterol problems, and premature cardiovascular disease.

To date, there is no evidence that testosterone replacement therapy causes prostate cancer, but it is known that TRT causes existing prostate cancer to grow. Therefore, any man planning to start TRT should be evaluated for prostate cancer with a PSA test and a digital rectal examination. PSA should be monitored every three months for the first year and every six months thereafter. TRT can make male breast cancer worse, so this condition is a contraindication to the use of testosterone. There is also the risk of the unknown. Large long-term prospective trials of TRT have not been performed, so the clinical benefits and long-term safety are unknown.

Androgen Supplements

Thanks to professional athletes and the birth of anti-aging medicine, interest in androgen supplements is high, but do they really work?

Androstenedione

This hormone, almost identical to testosterone, is available as a dietary supplement without a prescription. Andro, one of the major brands, had more than

$100 million in sales in 1999, thanks in no small part to baseball slugger Mark McGwire's revealing that he took the supplement during his record-setting 1998 season.

It is thought that androstenedione supplements are converted to testosterone and have effects on increasing muscle mass and reducing fat mass. Several studies have failed to show that androstenedione can live up to its claims, however. In fact, it appears that androstenedione tends to raise testosterone and estrogen levels, the latter putting you at risk for breast growth. Androstenedione also lowers HDL (good) cholesterol. In 2004, the U.S. Food and Drug Administration issued a warning on products containing androstenedione because they pose the same risks as long-term anabolic steroid abuse. The consensus among endocrinologists is the same. Other versions of androstenedione, such as androstenediol, 19-norandrostenedione, and 19-norandrosterone, are available as dietary supplements but have not proven to be any safer.

Dehydroepiandrosterone

DHEA is considered a "weak" androgen. DHEA can be converted to androstenedione and testosterone. Unfortunately, DHEA can also be converted to other hormones, such as estrogen. What happens in your body when you take DHEA? No one really knows.

DHEA is naturally made by the adrenal gland. DHEA has been called the "youth hormone" because levels peak when people are in their twenties and then decline dramatically with advancing age. The decline has been given the name adrenopause. Among the claims for DHEA: it increases lean body mass; it improves insulin resistance; it boosts energy levels and libido; it improves mood. All these claims remain unproven.

There are some troubling side effects. The most notable is a theoretical risk of prostate cancer. Doctors who do recommend DHEA disagree on dosage levels, ranging from 10 mg on up to as high as 1600 mg per day. I typically do not recommend DHEA supplements, but sometimes I prescribe very low doses of DHEA for hypogonadal men who also have adrenal gland deficiencies.

Muscle-Boosting Tips

Although taking testosterone isn't for everyone, there are still some things you can do to build your muscle mass. Even if you do take testosterone, these tips may help your hormones work more effectively.

Check Your Growth Hormone

Growth hormone is another hormone that has a major effect on muscles. Growth hormone deficiency has many of the same symptoms as hypogonadism. For more information, see chapter 12.

Exercise

Physical activity of any kind boosts testosterone levels. Exercise makes muscles physically stronger and metabolically stronger. Exercise is an important step in achieving hormonal balance.

Do Resistance Training

To significantly improve your body composition, you must do resistance training. There are many ways to do resistance training. You can lift free weights, use weight machines or bands, or do isometric exercises. If you have never lifted weights before, start with very low weights and slowly work your way up to higher weights. You may also want to consider two or three sessions with a personal trainer to perfect your technique. Many lifters debate which is better, free weights or machines. My answer: both are great. Just remember, if you use free weights, you need to use a spotter. Many weightlifting injuries can be prevented by the use of a spotter. You should plan to do resistance training at least twice a week. Consistency is key. A twenty-minute weight training session twice a week will have a significant effect on your body composition in as little as four weeks.

Address Your Stress

Stress lowers androgen levels by reducing hormonal signals from the brain. Stress has a negative effect on many hormones, creating a hormonal imbalance that slows metabolism. Stress, either psychological or physical, will reduce muscle mass and increase fat mass.

Get Plenty of Sleep

Your hormones are ruled by circadian rhythms. Androgens and growth hormone are both secreted while you sleep. When you don't get enough sleep, these hormones are not made in sufficient quantities. A study published in the *Journal of the American Medical Association* found that testosterone levels fall as much as 15 percent after one week of sleep restriction of five hours a night.

Take Protein Supplements

Protein provides the building blocks for healthy muscles. Make sure you get your minimum protein requirements (see chapter 2). Egg whites, low-fat dairy products, fish, and lean cuts of meat are excellent sources of protein.

Lose Weight

Stay away from fad, muscle-building diets. It is important to get the right number of calories and have a healthy balance of carbohydrates, protein, and fat.

Avoid Creatine Supplements

Studies on creatine are mixed. Some show no benefit at all. Other studies show only a short-term benefit.

Chapter Review

Androgens profoundly affect men's body weight and muscle composition and have a powerful effect on the brain, overall mood, sexual desire, and energy levels.

Anabolic steroids promote muscle tissue growth and control typical male characteristics including sex drive and aggression. Testosterone is essential for male hormonal balance.

The chapter pointed out that low testosterone ("low T") makes men feel anxious, depressed, and tired. Most obese men have lower levels of testosterone and higher levels of estrogen. Low T production affects about 4–5 million men in the United States.

A low testosterone level normally occurs as men get older, but being overweight, conditions such as diabetes, high cholesterol, or liver and kidney disease exacerbate the problem.

While the root causes of low testosterone (insulin resistance, pituitary tumors or gland malfunction, testicular failure due to injury or disease) may be hard to determine, a whole host of identifiable consequences are possible, including erectile dysfunction and decreased sexual performance, low libido, weight gain, fatigue, depression, anxiety, insomnia, breast growth, premature aging, loss of body hair, and others.

The chapter pointed out various ways to test for low T in men, including specific protocols for interpreting blood tests, but noted that sometimes diagnosing is a physician's judgment call.

Treatment options are somewhat limited and include testosterone replacement therapy in the form of injections, gels, tables, patches, and drugs. All treatment methods come with their own sets of benefits and risks. If these treatments are not possible, exercise, stress reduction, increased sleep, and weight loss show some benefit.

The next chapter discusses why maintaining a normal cortisol hormone level is important for your health.

CHAPTER

11

Calm Your Adrenal Gland to Lower Cortisol

Although cortisol is thought of as a stress hormone, you need it to live. Too much cortisol, however, increases your appetite and cravings and leads to weight gain. Excess cortisol causes fat accumulation in the midsection, similar to the belly fat of insulin resistance. A condition known as Cushing's syndrome results in extremely high cortisol levels and can be caused by tumors in the pituitary gland or the adrenal gland. Even if you don't have Cushing's syndrome, cortisol can be produced in excess by an adrenal gland that's under too much stress.

Weight Gain from Stress

Many of my patients gain weight because of stress. Early on, they may not notice the effects of excess stress—putting on a few extra pounds, catching a cold more easily, lowered sex drive, less energy, and poor memory. They may blame just "getting older," but the real problem may be stress on the adrenal gland. For the most part, the adrenal gland can handle demands from stress. Some stress is normal, and our bodies can deal with it as long as it is at a manageable level. If there's too much stress, though, the adrenal gland makes excess stress hormones, most notably, cortisol. Elevated cortisol combined with an

> **In This Chapter**
>
> ▶ Elevated Cortisol Levels Linked to Weight Gain
>
> ▶ Health Effects of Excess Cortisol
>
> ▶ Treating and Controlling Excess Cortisol

unhealthy diet accelerates and amplifies weight gain in the abdomen and upper body. At the same time, cortisol causes large muscles in the shoulders, upper arms, and thighs to deteriorate, which leads to lowered metabolism, fatigue, and more weight gain.

Today nearly everyone is susceptible to stress. A recent study found that more than half of all adults report being under too much stress. It's that out-of-control stress that makes us sick, tired, and fat. People under chronic stress have shorter lives. As the *Journal of the American Medical Association* noted in 1999, "Chronic stress ... that evokes prolonged distress can influence cardiovascular, immune, and endocrine function, and these alterations are sufficient to enhance a variety of health threats."

Stress at work, too many activities, or financial stress will cause cortisol levels to climb. The result is usually weight gain. Family stress of any type is one of the most potent types of stress that frequently causes people to gain weight. Researchers from Ohio State University found that after a divorce, men tend to gain weight but women usually lose weight. The study did not determine why this occurs. The weight loss among women is common enough to have received the nickname the "divorce diet." Divorce attorney Randall M. Kessler, Esq., says, "A lot of my female clients lose weight in the beginning because they feel a sense of worry. Once they become engaged in the divorce process, they gain hope and they eat healthier to help with the healing process."

Excess weight, environmental endocrine disruptors, chronic illness, and excessive alcohol consumption also cause stress on the adrenal gland and kick it into overdrive. Dieting itself is stressful. Yo-yo dieting, in particular, can increase levels of cortisol. Studies in mice found that repeated dieting and regaining weight may reprogram the brain, affecting how future stress and emotions drive feeding behaviors and promoting binge eating, which is thought to be one of the main reasons why diets eventually fail.

Stress increases the risk for gaining weight; that's a common fact. But we tend to overlook the hormonal reasons: high stress leads to high cortisol. High cortisol leads to insulin resistance. Cortisol and insulin resistance boost appetite and cause uncontrollable carbohydrate cravings. Leptin, neuropeptide Y, and other hunger hormones follow suit, magnifying the effect of stress, increasing appetite, and slowing metabolism even further. Eventually the body's hormones become entrained in a mode best suited to adapt to stress but not ideal for your weight. The good news is that by following the plan in this chapter, you can learn to calm your adrenal gland and reduce the impact of stress on your appetite, metabolism, and weight.

Effects of Excess Cortisol

Excess cortisol boosts appetite and causes carbohydrate cravings, resulting in weight gain in the belly. Muscle loss in the arms and legs leads to a slower metabolism and profound fatigue. Cortisol excess lowers the levels of hormones that build muscle: androgens and growth hormone. Cortisol excess also inhibits thyroid function, further slowing metabolism. Cortisol excess causes the breakdown of vital tissues, such muscle, bone, tendons, ligaments, and skin. This tissue destruction causes muscle weakness, thinning of the bones, and easy bruising. Studies have linked elevated cortisol to high blood pressure, elevated cholesterol and triglycerides, acid reflux, ulcers, and memory loss. High cortisol is tied to mood disorders such as depression, anxiety, and mood swings. Cortisol lowers the immune system and can make you more susceptible to infections, colds, and the flu.

Cortisol affects the brain and can cause depression or anxiety. Cortisol excess can cause severe mood swings and even euphoria. In some cases cortisol excess has even been known to cause psychosis with wild hallucinations. Cortisol influences the release of brain chemicals such as serotonin and dopamine, and cortisol excess disrupts the delicate balance between the pituitary gland and the adrenal gland. Cortisol elevations cause mood problems, but these problems can also result in higher cortisol levels. In fact almost any psychiatric illness, even a mild one, may result in cortisol excess.

Cortisol excess can have many negative effects, including the following:

Acne	Decreased well-being
Anxiety	Depression
Binge eating	Facial hair (women)
Bone loss (osteoporosis and osteopenia)	Facial redness
Bruising	Facial rounding
Carbohydrate cravings	Fatigue
Decreased muscle mass	Fractures
Decreased sex drive	Frequent infections
	Frequent colds or flu

Gastroesophageal reflux disease

High cholesterol

High triglycerides

Increased appetite

Increased blood pressure

Increased blood sugar

Increased body fat, especially in
the belly

Insomnia

Kidney stones

Menstrual cycle problems

Mood swings

Muscle wasting

Overeating

Poor concentration

Poor memory

Poor sleep

Poor wound healing

Slow metabolism

Stretch marks

Stomach ulcers

Thin arms and legs

Thin skin

Upset stomach

Weakness

Weight gain

Some of these symptoms deserve particular attention, so let's discuss them.

Weight Gain

Cortisol increases the amount of fat in your body and in a particular distribution. Excess cortisol leads to fat buildup in the belly, chest, and face, creating a body with an apple shape, the worst type of fat. This fat buildup can cause many of of the symptoms of insulin resistance and leptin resistance.

Increased Appetite and Carbohydrate Cravings

Anyone who has ever taken a steroid medication can tell you they can never get enough to eat while taking steroids. Cortisol stimulates hunger centers in the brain and in particular increases cravings for high-carbohydrate foods.

Tissue Breakdown

Cortisol causes muscle breakdown, leading to muscle weakness, slowed metabolism, and insulin resistance. For this reason, cortisol is known as a catabolic hormone because it breaks down muscle tissue. Muscle wasting means less muscle, and with less muscle, your metabolism slows. You feel weak and tired. You don't want to exercise, even though it would be good for you (and would probably reduce some of that stress naturally). Cortisol also causes the breakdown of other tissues, such as bone and skin. Bone loss leads to osteoporosis,

Adrenal Fatigue

Many of my patients have been told that they are gaining weight because their adrenal glands are burned out or they have a condition called adrenal fatigue. You may have heard the terms *adrenal fatigue, adrenal burnout,* or *adrenal exhaustion.* Proponents of this condition claim that the condition is caused by the effects of chronic mental, emotional, or physical stress on the adrenal gland.

The Endocrine Society, the professional organization for endocrinologists, notes that "adrenal fatigue is not a real medical condition." Proponents recommend saliva testing for cortisol to diagnose adrenal fatigue; however, the Endocrine Society states, "There are no tests that can detect adrenal fatigue."

Supporters of adrenal fatigue recommend improving lifestyle by quitting smoking and ceasing to drink alcohol, getting more sleep, exercising regularly, and eating healthy foods. These important health behaviors will make you feel better no matter what the diagnosis. Websites about adrenal fatigue have permeated the Internet and promote a variety of unproven herbal supplements, animal glandular extracts, and even cortisol medications to treat the condition. According to the Endocrine Society, though, "Supplements and vitamins made to treat adrenal fatigue may not be safe. Taking these supplements when you do not need them can cause your adrenal glands to stop working and may put your life in danger."

Whatever you want to call it—adrenal fatigue, exhaustion, or burnout—it is not a real hormonal condition. Adrenal fatigue is a fake diagnosis that has no scientific basis. If you have been told you have adrenal fatigue, get a second opinion from a board-certified endocrinologist.

Unlike adrenal fatigue, Addison's disease is a real medical condition that occurs when the adrenal glands cannot make enough cortisol. People with deficiencies of cortisol lose weight and feel tired all the time. As cortisol levels continue to drop, the body shuts down and goes into shock. The condition is often misdiagnosed as shock from a severe infection. It can sometimes come on very suddenly, especially when a person is exposed to stress. As President John F. Kennedy did, patients with Addison's disease must take cortisol medications in order to live. Without treatment the condition is fatal.

and skin breakdown leads to easy bruising, stretch marks, or thin skin with a ruddy appearance.

Immune Suppression

Cortisol keeps the immune system in check. It has potent anti-inflammatory properties but also interacts with white blood cells to suppress your immune system, which is why people under a lot of stress tend to get sick: the immune system has been weakened by stress with cortisol. Regardless, doctors prescribe cortisol-like medications, such as cortisone or prednisone, to treat medical disorders and severe allergies caused by immune overactivity. It's a difficult balance.

Cortisol Is Necessary for Life

Cortisol is not all bad. Your body needs cortisol to function properly. In fact, cortisol helps the body cope with the stress of daily life. Cortisol is regulated by the pituitary gland and the hypothalamus. This link is known as the hypothalamic-pituitary-adrenal (HPA) axis. The HPA axis senses our level of stress and directs the adrenal gland to pump out hormones accordingly. Normally the body produces cortisol according to a circadian rhythm or regular twenty-four-hour cycle. Cortisol peaks around 8:00 A.M. (to get us going in the morning) and gradually falls throughout the day to hit its lowest levels around 3:00 A.M. Even during times of extreme stress, cortisol still tends to maintain this circadian rhythm. Cortisol-containing medications or tumors of the adrenal gland or pituitary gland can disrupt this rhythm, though, which is why timing is critical when a blood or saliva test is done.

The brain sends signals to the pituitary gland by way of the hypothalamus, which is also the most important part of the brain for regulating appetite and body weight. The hypothalamus produces a hormone called corticotrophin-releasing hormone, or CRH for short. CRH stimulates the pituitary gland to release its hormone, adrenocortitrophic hormone (ACTH), which in turn tells the adrenal gland to make glucocorticoids. Normally, when cortisol levels go up, a signal is sent to the brain to ease up on CRH or ACTH production. This careful balance ensures that you have the right amount of cortisol.

The adrenal glands are triangular-shaped glands on top of each kidney, and—as with the kidney and many other organs—there are two of them. Also like the kidney, you need only one to survive. Cortisol is just one of many hormones made by the adrenal glands. Each adrenal gland is really two organs

Adrenaline Rush

The most immediate hormonal stress response of the adrenal gland is the fight-or-flight response caused by the hormone adrenaline (also known as epinephrine). Some people refer to this as the "adrenaline rush." Adrenaline makes your heart beat faster and revs up your body. Adrenaline levels rise and fall from minute to minute and respond at a moment's notice to the situation at hand. Adrenaline is used as an emergency medication to boost blood pressure and restart the heart when someone is in shock

rolled into one. The outer portion of the adrenal gland, known as the adrenal cortex, is responsible for making steroid hormones, most notably cortisol. The middle part of the adrenal gland is called the adrenal medulla. It's like a separate gland and produces adrenaline, which is also a stress hormone.

Cortisol is known as a steroid hormone. The term *steroid* is a generic term for any hormone with the classic four-ring structure derived from cholesterol. Steroids include androgens, estrogens, progesterone, and many others. Cortisol belongs to a specific class of steroid hormones known as glucocorticoids or corticosteroids. These hormones raise blood sugar levels, in part by breaking down muscle tissue (glucose = glucocorticoid). This class of steroid hormones has a major role in the control of glucose and other nutrients. Corticosteroids are not to be confused with anabolic steroids, discussed in chapter 10. Anabolic steroids build muscle tissue and promote fat loss. Corticosteroids have the opposite effects—they promote fat accumulation and muscle loss.

Like all steroid hormones, cortisol interacts directly with your genes. Glucocorticoids bind to a glucocorticoid receptor inside the cell, and this entire complex binds to DNA, turning genes on and off. As I described in chapter 2, cortisol and the receptor work in the classic lock-and-key design for hormone-receptor interactions.

Cushing's Syndrome

Cushing's syndrome was named after a famous Boston neurosurgeon, Harvey Cushing, who first described the condition. Cushing discovered the most common cause of the syndrome was a small tumor in the pituitary gland. Other

Presidential Adrenal Glands

Presidents Dwight D. Eisenhower and John F. Kennedy both had very famous adrenal glands. Although adrenal gland problems are rare, they can cause severe symptoms or even death. Thanks to modern medicine, diagnosis and treatments are much better now than they were in the 1950s and 1960s.

President Eisenhower was known to have erratic blood pressure as early as the 1930s. He suffered a massive heart attack during his first term as president in September 1955. Eisenhower died from complications of this heart attack fourteen years later. An autopsy confirmed that the late president had a small pheochromocytoma in his left adrenal gland. A pheochromocytoma is an adrenal gland tumor that produces surges of adrenaline, resulting in episodes of sweating, flushing, rapid heartbeat, and anxiety. People who have this rare condition usually have very high and labile blood pressure, which can lead to a heart attack or stroke. Special medications are needed to treat the high blood pressure, and ultimately surgical removal is required. Ten percent of pheochromocytoma tumors are cancerous. Gene tests for pheochromocytoma are available and are recommended if you have a family history of pheochromocytoma. If you have symptoms of a pheochromocytoma, see your doctor right away.

President Kennedy was a famous sufferer of another adrenal gland condition called Addison's disease. Addison's disease, or adrenal insufficiency, is most frequently caused by autoimmune destruction of the adrenal gland. Addison's disease can be

cortisol-excess conditions are syndromes; only the pituitary cause is the *disease*. The condition is fairly rare; fewer than 1 in 1,000 people who have symptoms actually have it, but not everyone has been diagnosed. Women are four times as likely to develop Cushing's as men, and some overweight people have Cushing's but don't know it. Cortisol-like medications can also cause symptoms as severe as those of a tumor. Although the severity of Cushing's syndrome can be highly variable at presentation, most people have much more severe manifestations than those with cortisol excess from chronic stress.

Some people with Cushing's syndrome gain huge amounts of weight in a short period of time. Even with slower weight gain, body fat distribution can be slow and smoldering, with symptoms of tiredness, abdominal pain, weight loss, and tanning of the skin. Kennedy had to take cortisol medications that replaced his deficient hormone. A simple blood test for cortisol may not be reliable enough to diagnose mild adrenal insufficiency. The best test for Addison's disease is called a cosyntropin stimulation test. A blood sample is taken to test for cortisol, and then an injection of the medication cosyntropin is given. Cosyntropin is a synthetic version of the pituitary gland hormone that stimulates the adrenal glands. Thirty to sixty minutes after the injection is given, a second cortisol blood test is taken. Sometimes doctors will take three or more blood samples over time. Normally, the cosyntropin injection will cause the cortisol level to rise. If it does not go up high enough, the diagnosis of Addison's disease is made. When adrenal insufficiency is caused by autoimmune destruction of the adrenal glands, it is frequently associated with other autoimmune diseases. Adrenal insufficiency increases the risk of other autoimmune syndromes, such as Hashimoto's thyroiditis and type 1 diabetes. Patients with adrenal insufficiency should be monitored for autoimmune conditions (see chapter 7). Sometimes an infection of the adrenal gland can cause a more sudden and more complete loss of cortisol, which is a bad situation. It's unusual to see such a severe situation, known as acute adrenal insufficiency, but it illustrates the fact that cortisol is necessary for life.

an indicator of cortisol excess. Along with fat that accumulates in the abdominal region, fat may also build up in the hollow space over the collar bones (known as supraclavicular fat pads), the back of the neck between the shoulder blades (known as dosocervical fat pad or buffalo hump), and in the face (known as moon face). Doctors refer to this appearance as Cushingoid body habitus. Although not all people who have Cushingoid body habitus have Cushing's syndrome, this appearance should trigger your doctor to measure your cortisol levels.

Patients with Cushing's syndrome usually have muscle weakness and wasting. While the midsection grows, the arms and legs become very thin. The muscles may become quite weak, to the point that it is difficult to rise from a chair.

The thigh and shoulder muscles are particularly affected, which is known as proximal muscle weakness, because the muscles close to the torso are affected more than distal muscles, such as the calf and forearm. Stretch marks (known as striae) are common in many people with cortisol excess, but the striae of Cushing's syndrome may take on a peculiar appearance. The striae may develop quite rapidly and may develop on the belly, armpits, forearms, groin, or other parts of the body. The striae of Cushing's syndrome are usually wide (more than a half-inch) and may be red or purple. Pink or flesh-colored striae are less suggestive of Cushing's syndrome.

Skin problems are also common with cortisol excess. If you are young, thinning of the skin can be a warning sign for Cushing's syndrome. (Thinning of the skin is a normal part of the aging process and often appears in older folks.) The skin of the face can become thin, resulting in a red or ruddy complexion. Other skin problems, such as acne, easy bruising, and poor wound healing, can also occur but are not as specific for Cushing's syndrome.

High blood pressure that is difficult to control can be a warning sign of Cushing's syndrome. High blood pressure is a common condition and can be linked to a variety of hormone problems, including insulin resistance, thyroid problems, growth hormone excess, and others. High blood pressure caused by Cushing's syndrome may go up and down or may be difficult to control on multiple medications (more than three types of blood pressure medications).

Psychological problems are extremely common in Cushing's syndrome. Depression and anxiety are common in all types of cortisol excess; however, in the setting of other features of Cushing's syndrome, problems with mood may be a warning sign. Patients with Cushing's syndrome have reported all degrees of psychological problems, including poor sex drive, poor memory, poor sleep, high anxiety, inability to concentrate, severe depression, and even psychosis.

Infections can occur in patients with Cushing's syndrome because of the immune system-lowering effects of cortisol. Common infections include colds, sinus infections, yeast infections, and bladder infections. Patients with Cushing's syndrome may also come down with exotic infections typically seen in AIDS patients.

It is very unusual to have Cushing's syndrome and not have menstrual cycle problems; therefore, women with normal menstrual cycles almost never have Cushing's syndrome. Sometimes adrenal gland overactivity leads to excessive production of male hormones. Female facial hair growth can be severe and may be associated with balding (in a pattern similar to a man), deepening of the

Warning Signs for Cushing's Syndrome

Cushingoid body habitus	Menstrual cycle problems
Depression or anxiety	Muscle weakness
Elevated blood sugar	Rapid or excessive weight gain
Facial hair growth (in women)	Severe cystic acne
Frequent infections	Stretch marks that are red, purple, or wider than half an inch
High blood pressure	
Low potassium levels	Thinning of the skin (under the age of forty-five)
Male-pattern balding (in women)	

voice, and growth of the clitoris into what may resemble a small penis. While male hormones cause hormone problems other than Cushing's syndrome, these extreme effects are always a cause for concern. For more information on male hormone problems in women, see chapter 8.

Adrenal gland cancer is a potential cause of Cushing's syndrome, but most of the time Cushing's syndrome isn't cancer at all, but a benign, hormone-producing tumor in the pituitary gland that can be removed surgically. The main causes of Cushing's syndrome are

- Pituitary gland tumors (also known as Cushing's disease)

- Adrenal gland tumors

- Rare cancers that produce ACTH (known as ectopic ACTH-producing tumors)

- Exposure to steroid medications (iatrogenic Cushing's syndrome)

Glucocorticoid Medications

Glucocorticoid medications, sometimes referred to as steroids or corticosteroids, are cortisol-like medications that come in all forms: pills, creams, eye drops, nasal sprays, gels, enemas, lung inhalers, and injections, and with names such as prednisone, prednisolone, dexamethasone, triamcinolone, cortisone, or hydrocortisone. You've probably heard of the most common, prednisone and cortisone, and the terms people use when they're taking them: "on cortisone" or "on steroids." These medications treat medical conditions caused by an overactive immune system—conditions such as inflammatory bowel disease, lupus, sarcoidosis, arthritis, kidney disease, and liver disease. Because of the immune suppression ability of these medications, they are used frequently in organ transplant patients. Even some types of cancer may be treated in part with glucocorticoids.

Although very effective in treating many conditions, glucocorticoid medications have horrible side effects. They flood the body with extra corticosteroids and induce what doctors call a "disease state," in which diseases like Cushing's syndrome can suddenly take root. Incidentally, many pets are given steroids to help with allergies, yet they can get all the same problems as humans.

Because these medications are so frequently prescribed, patients, and even physicians, forget about the serious side effects. Let me remind you, the side effects of these medications can be as serious as having Cushing's syndrome. If you take any of these medications, especially the pills, daily, you should be closely monitored by your physician. Work with your physician to take the lowest possible dose of steroids and create a plan to taper the steroids even further. In my career, I have had very few patients who could not eventually stop taking steroid medications. Many doctors think it is too dangerous to stop the steroids, but I believe it is more dangerous to continue taking them.

If you have been taking steroids for more than thirty days, your body is dependent on them; some would say addicted. If you stop taking them abruptly, you face serious medical consequences, because your adrenal gland has turned off its steroid production. Your steroid dose must be slowly tapered. Most endocrinologists will tell you that you need to take about as many days to taper the steroids as you have been taking them. For example, if you have been taking corticosteroids for a year, you should slowly decrease your dose over the course of one year before completely discontinuing the medication. I do not recommend that you taper off the medication by yourself; it requires careful monitoring by an endocrinologist.

Testing for Cushing's Syndrome

Testing for Cushing's syndrome can be tricky and should be done through a qualified physician. Many general practice physicians are able to run screening tests for Cushing's syndrome, but all abnormal screening tests should be referred to an endocrinologist. There are a several types of tests, and experts still disagree about which test is best. Testing is not perfect, and often a series of tests is required to confirm the diagnosis of Cushing's syndrome. Although there are many causes of Cushing's syndrome, the initial testing is the same for all forms. The first set of testing is to determine whether you have an overproduction of cortisol. If so, your endocrinologist will give you additional tests to determine which type of Cushing's you may have.

Twenty-Four-Hour Urine Free Cortisol

The twenty-four-hour test Urine Free Cortisol (UFC) remains the current standard screening test for Cushing's syndrome. Yes, you have to collect all your urine into a container over a twenty-four-hour period. This test can determine that you do not have Cushing's syndrome; however, a positive UFC does not guarantee Cushing's syndrome. The higher the level, the more likely Cushing's syndrome; levels more than four times the upper limits of normal are almost always Cushing's syndrome. Obesity, depression, pregnancy, excessive exercise, and excessive alcohol use have been shown to cause mild elevations of the UFC.

The term *pseudo-Cushing's syndrome* has been given to the condition that has many of the symptoms and physical features of Cushing's syndrome and excess cortisol but without the physical presence of a tumor. Urine cortisol levels are usually mildly elevated, but further testing rules out Cushing's syndrome. Chronic stress, as well as obesity, depression, excessive exercise, diabetes, pregnancy, and excessive alcohol use can all elevate cortisol levels and cause pseudo-Cushing's syndrome. The remedy for pseudo Cushing's syndrome calls for treating the underlying illness and removing the stress.

Serum Cortisol Level

The serum cortisol level is one of the best tests for Cushing's syndrome, but timing is everything. To assess for excess cortisol production, a blood test for cortisol is reliable only if it is done at midnight. Although the midnight serum cortisol level test is accurate, it is very inconvenient. Serum cortisol levels from other times of the day are not useful for diagnosing Cushing's syndrome.

Salivary Cortisol Level

Although most saliva tests are considered unreliable, salivary cortisol testing is an exception. The midnight salivary cortisol test is a very accurate and reliable way to measure cortisol. The test is valid only for diagnosing cortisol excess. It is not reliable for diagnosing cortisol deficiency.

A sample of saliva is collected into a small cotton cylinder and sent to a laboratory for analysis. The key to this test is that you should not eat, drink, or exercise for at least two hours prior to taking the sample. Sometimes I ask my patients to obtain two or more samples throughout the day in addition to the midnight sample. Most laboratories will report the normal range according to the time of the day. Normally, cortisol is high in the morning and low late at night. Loss of this diurnal rhythm can be a sign of cortisol excess.

Suppression Testing

A test known as the overnight dexamethasone suppression test is a reliable test for Cushing's syndrome. Like the UFC, this test can be falsely positive, especially if you have the conditions that lead to pseudo-Cushing's syndrome. You must take a 1 milligram (mg) tablet of dexamethasone at midnight, the night before your test. At 8:00 A.M. the next day, blood is collected and cortisol is measured. Under normal circumstances, dexamethasone, a synthetic glucocorticoid, will suppress the adrenal glands' natural cortisol production. If the cortisol level is above 3.5 micrograms/deciliter (mcg/dL), Cushing's syndrome is suspected.

Confirmatory Testing

Most of the time, additional testing is required to confirm a diagnosis of Cushing's syndrome. Testing protocols vary among endocrinologists and can be cumbersome and lengthy. Confirmatory tests include more sophisticated versions of the dexamethasone suppression test, a dexamethasone-suppressed CRH stimulation test, other stimulation and suppression tests, magnetic resonance imaging (MRI) and computed tomography (CT) scans, and even directly measuring blood hormone levels from the pituitary gland.

How to Lower Your Cortisol Levels

By following the suggestions listed, you can lower your cortisol levels. Your appetite will stop surging, and you will be able to use your calories to give you increased energy instead of having those calories turn into fat.

> ## Cautions about Testing for Cushing's Syndrome
>
> - Testing for Cushing's syndrome is one of the most controversial subjects in the field of endocrinology. Experts have heated arguments about testing protocols.
>
> - Testing is still crude. Tests that are easy to perform usually give unreliable results. The more reliable tests usually require you to take medication (sometimes for days) or even receive injections of very expensive medications prior to blood testing. These "stimulation" and "suppression" tests must be performed by an up-to-date endocrinologist, because protocols frequently change.
>
> - Many people are inappropriately tested for Cushing's with a simple blood cortisol test. Because cortisol levels in your blood will fluctuate, a simple blood test alone is rarely helpful. Unless the doctor draws your blood at a specific time, serum cortisol is useless.
>
> - Many people with symptoms suggestive of Cushing's are not tested by their doctors. If you think you have it, ask your doctor to test you.
>
> - An elevated test does not mean you definitely have Cushing's. Confirmatory tests are almost always needed. If your levels are high, do not get overly concerned that you have adrenal gland cancer or some other horrific problem. Your levels are most likely elevated because of excess stress or excess weight.
>
> - On the other hand, a normal test does not always mean you are okay. Sometimes cortisol is produced episodically and can be missed on initial testing. If you have symptoms that are very suggestive of Cushing's but have a normal test, ask your doctor to repeat the test. I have had patients who had negative testing the first two tries, but on the third were positive and subsequently the patients were found to have tumors.

Eat Right

The Hormonal Health Diet is a plan that allows you to lose weight permanently without feeling stressed out about it. The balance of carbohydrates, protein, and fat, as well as the small, frequent meals, are ideal for lowering cortisol levels,

I Have a Positive Test for Cushing's . . . What Do I Do?

Don't panic! Most people with positive tests do not have Cushing's. Merely being overweight can cause you to produce excess cortisol in levels high enough to make your test abnormal. Stress, either emotional or physical, or heavy drinking can also raise cortisol levels. If you have a positive test, your endocrinologist must perform further tests to determine whether you have true Cushing's or pseudo-Cushing's syndrome. The term pseudo-Cushing's has been given to the situation when someone has a false positive UFC or dexamethasone suppression test and has many of the symptoms of Cushing's syndrome without the physical presence of a tumor. Many people with pseudo-Cushing's syndrome are overweight with central obesity, a moon-shaped face, diabetes, and high blood pressure.

If confirmatory tests show that you have Cushing's, treatment includes surgical removal of the offending tumor. If possible, the surgery should be performed at a major medical center with an experienced endocrinologist and neurosurgeon working as a team.

controlling cravings, and reducing hunger. See chapter 4 for more information on the Hormonal Health Diet.

Improve Insulin Resistance

Elevated cortisol causes insulin resistance, which leads to hunger and carbohydrate cravings. The action plan for overcoming insulin resistance is outlined in chapter 6, and it includes eating slow carbohydrate foods, eating on a schedule, getting enough sleep, and exercising regularly, all of which reduce insulin resistance as well as lower cortisol levels.

Keep Sodium Consumption Below 2700 mg Daily

Because of the side effects of high sodium intake—bloating and high blood pressure—a low-salt diet will help you. Salt makes you retain water. Salt also deprives bones of calcium. Keep sodium consumption below 2700 mg daily and check your blood pressure regularly.

Cut Down on Alcohol

Heavy alcohol use makes the adrenal gland overreact and may induce pseudo-Cushing's syndrome. Drinking in moderation (one drink a day) is okay, but don't overdo it.

Drink Caffeine in Moderation

Drinking more than two or three cups of coffee a day can raise cortisol levels. Does coffee make you gain weight? No. Caffeine in fact raises your metabolism, decreases the risk for diabetes, and improves lung function and exercise performance. Coffee and other caffeinated beverages do not need to be avoided, but limit consumption to no more than three cups a day.

Avoid Steroid Medications

Doctors prescribe steroid medications for many conditions. In my experience, steroid medications are rarely necessary and often do more harm than good. I've seen steroid medications overprescribed to treat sinus infections and bronchitis. I've also seen a lot of patients who get steroid injections in the back, knee, or other joints. Alternative nonsteroid treatments are often available, but your physician may not prescribe them unless you specifically ask.

Address Your Stress

Lowering your stress may be the hardest thing you can do. Many people use food as a way of coping with stress. Food is enjoyable; food is comfortable. When we are in a stressful situation, whether it be emotional or physical, it's natural to want food. It may not make the stress go away, but it seems to ease the mind, if only for a few minutes, and most stress is in the mind.

Here comes that vicious circle again: you get stressed, you eat, you gain weight, you feel more stressed, you eat again. You have to break the cycle. Find new stress reduction techniques. When you relieve stress, you take a double step closer toward balancing your hormones. Not only do your cortisol levels drop, but also your insulin doesn't spike, which eliminates a major spark to those cycles.

Here are a few ways you can lower cortisol by reducing stress:

■ **Increase physical activity.** Physical activity helps your body better handle stress by improving cardiovascular and musculoskeletal systems. Exercise improves insulin resistance. If your body is healthier, it will be better able to withstand the physical drain of stress. Note: The best type of exercise for lowering cortisol is slow and steady. Extreme exercise, such as marathon running, can raise your cortisol. Do you have no time to exercise, or are you too tired to exercise? These excuses for not exercising are the most common. The vast majority of people who are "too tired to exercise" report having increased energy and less fatigue after exercising. Exercise is critical for optimal cortisol levels and hormonal balance. Exercise helps the body handle stress by improving cardiovascular and musculoskeletal systems. Exercise dramatically reduces insulin resistance. A healthy body is better able to withstand the physical drain of stress. The best type of exercise for lowering cortisol is slow or moderate, and the key is consistency. Make physical activity part of your daily routine by making it a priority. Many people enjoy waking up an hour earlier and performing some physical activity before they begin their day, an effective strategy I have used myself. After a while, you will not feel as good if you miss a morning of exercise. Exercise does not have to be done all at once. Small bouts of a variety activities (for example, shopping, gardening, walking, cleaning the house, marching in place) can be done for a few minutes at a time for a cumulative effect. If you have Cushing's syndrome, or are taking steroid medications, you should exercise with caution. Your muscles have become weakened from the excess steroids and are susceptible to breakdown. If even very light exercise exhausts you, it could be a sign of Cushing's syndrome or another serious medical condition, such as heart disease, lung disease, kidney failure, liver failure, muscular disorder, or a neurological disorder.

■ **Lower your intake of high-calorie foods.** Most people use food as "anti-stress medicine." Stress eating is a common reaction to nervous tension and contributes to weight gain. People tend to gravitate toward comfort foods during times of stress. What is comfort food? Food that makes you feel good. Comfort foods do help relieve stress. The problem is they also make you gain weight. For many people, comfort foods are home-cooked foods such spaghetti and meatballs, macaroni and cheese, or fried chicken and mashed potatoes. For others, comfort food is fast food or junk food. Comfort foods are usually high in fat, carbohydrates, and calories, but they don't have to be. Perhaps an apple will do just as well as a slice of apple pie, and the apple is much better for you.

- **Practice positive self-talk and improve your self-esteem.** Tell yourself, "I can do it." You talk to yourself every day. Think about what you are saying. Are you hard on yourself? Do you give up easily? You control how you talk to yourself. Tell yourself that you are in control. As you see results, it will be easier and easier to give yourself mental rewards. Don't worry about failure. Remind yourself that the road to better health is not an easy one, but you can take it.

- **Learn meditation, yoga, tai chi, or chi gong.** All are all excellent ways to lower stress. They combine strength, stretching, breathing, and meditation, and almost anyone can do them. Yoga has become a growing fitness craze and has expanded to specialty yoga classes such as power yoga, disco yoga, bikram (hot) yoga, and even doga (with your dog), invented by Suzi Teitelman. Meditation relaxes your mind. Yoga combines meditative techniques with stretching, one of the most overlooked parts of exercise. While performing all of these methods—in fact, during all forms of exercise and stress reduction, period—drink lots of water.

- **Get massages.** Massage works the muscles, loosening the knots and freeing the toxins that have collected during stressful times.

- **Make time for yourself.** Too busy all the time? Many people are stressed because they have too much to do. Organizing and simplifying your life can be a powerful way to lower stress levels, especially for type A personalities. I recommend *Organizing the Good Life: A Path to Joyful Simplicity—Home to Work and Back* by Celia Rocks, as well as the classic, *The Seven Habits of Highly Effective People* by Stephen Covey.

- **Spend time with friends and family.** Your friends and family members are your greatest support. Let them know what is going on with your life. If you are trying to lose a meaningful amount of weight, involve them in the process. You will receive support up front and also get ongoing congratulations every time they see that you have lost more weight.

Chapter Review

Maintaining a normal cortisol hormone level is important for your health. An elevated level of this "stress hormone" increases appetite and cravings, leading to weight gain that accumulates in the midsection and upper body. At the same time, excess cortisol deteriorates large muscles in the shoulders, upper arms, and thighs, which leads to lowered metabolism, fatigue, and more weight gain.

The chapter noted that high cortisol levels lead to insulin resistance, which is linked to uncontrollable carbohydrate cravings. Leptin, neuropeptide Y, and other hunger hormones further magnify the effect of stress, increasing appetite and slowing metabolism even further.

The effects of cortisol excess include nearly fifty conditions, including acne, binge eating, decreased sex drive, frequent colds, menstrual cycle problems, stretch marks, and weight gain.

Clearly cortisol at normal levels provides positive benefits; it helps us get moving in the morning and is linked to self-preservation fight-or-flight responses. However, insufficient levels are consequences of serious diseases such as Cushing's syndrome, a disease characterized by muscle weakness and wasting.

The chapter concluded with a discussion of how testing is done for Cushing's syndrome—specific blood tests, saliva tests, and others—and suggested ways to improve the condition, including eating the right foods slowly and on a schedule, getting proper sleep and exercise, and reducing stress as well as coffee and alcohol consumption.

CHAPTER

12

Get Pituitary Support with Growth Hormone

During childhood, growth hormone is important for making children grow. Children who are deficient in growth hormone are very short. Growth hormone, sometimes referred to as hGH (for human growth hormone), was originally prescribed only by pediatric endocrinologists. If your child was short for his or her age, these professionals would prescribe growth hormone to make the child grow taller. Although growth hormone is so named because it makes children grow taller, it does much more than that. Even after you stop growing, growth hormone remains an important hormone, regulating body composition, energy level, and mood. It's an anabolic hormone—a muscle builder, like testosterone. Growth hormone and testosterone have similar effects on body composition, decreasing fat and increasing muscle mass.

Growth hormone has a different structure than the four-ring chemical structure of a steroid, though (see chapter 10). It's known as a peptide hormone, and unlike steroids, which are made from cholesterol, growth hormone is composed of amino acids, the building blocks of protein.

Today we are seeing a growth hormone in a new light. Growth hormone is used for its muscle-building and fat-burning effects.

In This Chapter

- ▶ Weight Gain Caused by a Deficiency
- ▶ Disorders Triggered by Growth Hormone Deficiencies
- ▶ Tests to Detect a Deficiency
- ▶ Treatments for Growth Hormone Deficiency

It is also used illegally by athletes to improve performance. It has been promoted as a cure for just about every ailment, from chronic fatigue and fibromyalgia to muscle wasting and osteoporosis. Adult growth hormone deficiency is now recognized as a real adult disease. Disorders of the pituitary gland can result in growth hormone deficiency, but a minor head injury or just being overweight can also result in lower levels of growth hormone.

For people who are deficient, treatment with growth hormone has a number of benefits: it reduces the amount of fat in the body and increases muscle mass; it improves heart function and exercise performance; it improves mood and the sense of well-being; it strengthens bones; and it helps wounds heal faster. But a caution: growth hormone is not a cure-all. Studies have found that returning growth hormone to normal levels can have a number of hormonal consequences, including increasing insulin resistance and leptin resistance. Too much growth hormone can cause more serious ailments, including diabetes, high blood pressure, carpal tunnel syndrome, heart disease, arthritis, and even cancer. Recent studies have found that growth hormone accelerates aging, which is ironic, since it has been promoted as an anti-aging hormone.

Most people don't necessarily need to take growth hormone—in a pharmaceutical form—to improve their health. Your body makes growth hormone naturally, and by following the advice in this chapter, you can help your pituitary gland boost its own production of growth hormone.

Growth Hormone and Body Composition

Growth hormone, whether produced naturally or taken as medication, has favorable effects on body composition. It has potent muscle-building and fat-burning effects that are important for long-term weight control, because these things determine your body composition. If you suffer from growth hormone deficiency, you'll notice a gradual gain in body fat and a loss of muscle mass. The change may be subtle at first, and your weight may not change. With time, though, lean body mass decreases, fat mass increases, and metabolism slows down. Eventually weight gain will set in. People with long-standing growth hormone deficiency have a very slow metabolism because their muscles have wasted away and have become replaced by fat. Fatigue and muscle weakness are common complaints from folks with growth hormone deficiency. Growth hormone deficiency is associated with central obesity: fat around the belly, the type of fat that is associated with insulin resistance, type 2 diabetes, high cholesterol, and cardiovascular disease, as I discuss in chapter 6. The problem gets worse as you get older. Just as fat lowers your growth hormone levels, so does aging. Talk about vicious cycles!

Being overweight, especially having excess abdominal fat or a high body fat percentage in and of itself, can cause the pituitary gland to slow growth hormone production. In some cases, growth hormone levels can be as low as someone who has a pituitary tumor. The medical term for this condition is obesity-related hyposomatotropism, and it is another example of the vicious circles created when the body is out of hormonal balance.

Scientists understand that fat cells play a major role in the obesity–growth hormone connection. Excess body fat produces many inflammation chemicals (see chapter 5), which inhibit the function of the pituitary gland, rendering it incapable of producing adequate amounts of growth hormone. These are the same inflammation chemicals that are responsible for a host of hormonal imbalances, including insulin resistance (chapter 6), leptin resistance (chapter 5), and T3 conversion problems (chapter 7), but the problems are not caused by inflammation chemicals alone. Growth hormone deficiency causes leptin resistance and insulin resistance to a greater extent than would be expected from just having excess body fat. By decreasing body fat, you support your pituitary gland in making more growth hormone while alleviating all these maladies.

Enhancing growth hormone by reducing body fat eventually leads to a higher metabolism. Moreover, removing that extra fat around the middle also reduces insulin resistance and leptin resistance. How does growth hormone do it? Growth hormone helps you lose fat by making the fat burnable as fuel. The by-product of this change is more energy.

Growth hormone counters the effects of insulin. It's an interesting contradiction. Insulin promotes fat accumulation, but growth hormone promotes fat breakdown. But here's where growth hormone can be dangerous, because excess growth hormone can raise blood sugar levels. Because it counters the effects of insulin, too much growth hormone can cause insulin resistance and even diabetes. A study from the National Institutes of Health in Bethesda found that growth hormone increased insulin resistance in adults, especially in women. Another study published in the *Journal of Clinical Endocrinology and Metabolism* found that growth hormone treatment was linked to diabetes. Some studies, however, show that boosting growth hormone from a low level to a normal level reduces insulin resistance. The upshot is that, as with all your hormones, balance is critical. Too much or too little growth hormone can be harmful to your health.

Growth Hormone Is a Typical Pituitary Gland Hormone

As with other hormones produced by the pituitary gland, growth hormone is a hormone strongly influenced by feedback (see chapter 2). When the body reports the need for more growth hormone, the pituitary springs into action. Similarly, when the pituitary notices a rise or fall in the level of growth hormone, it takes steps to regulate its production.

Special cells, called somatotrophs, in the pituitary gland make growth hormone. Signals come from the brain by way of the hypothalamus, which produces a growth hormone–releasing hormone, a hormone that stimulates the pituitary gland to make growth hormone. A second hypothalamic hormone, somatostatin, inhibits pituitary gland production of growth hormone. Somatostatin is also produced by the pancreas, and medications that mimic somatostatin cause dramatic weight loss in some people (see chapter 5). Obviously, growth hormone does not act by itself, but rather in concert with many hormones.

Just like other pituitary gland hormones, growth hormone works by telling another gland to make a second hormone. In this case, the liver functions as that second gland. Growth hormone tells the liver to produce a second hormone known as insulin-like growth factor-1 or IGF-1, also known as somatomedin C, a hormone whose chemical structure is similar to insulin. IGF-1 is extremely important; in fact, most of what we consider the action of growth hormone is the action of IGF-1. Most blood tests for growth hormone are tests for IGF-1.

Anti-Aging Hormone or Aging Hormone?

Growth hormone levels naturally decline as you get older. (See Figure 12.1.) Serving in the role of making children grow taller, growth hormone levels peak during the growth spurt of puberty. After puberty, growth hormone levels slowly fall throughout the rest of your life. By the time we reach age thirty or forty, our levels are half of what they were when we were teenagers. It is normal for growth hormone levels to go down as you get older. High growth hormone levels later in life are a risk factor for ailments associated with aging, such as cancer, diabetes, and heart disease. In recent years, a great deal of research has come out about how growth hormone signals the cells of the body to age. Studies have shown that mice with low growth hormone or those with mutations in the receptor for growth hormone live much longer than mice with normal growth hormone and normal growth hormone receptors. Having an "endocrine defect" may be beneficial, slowing the aging process by protecting us from cancer and other ailments of aging. Boosting growth hormone to unnaturally high

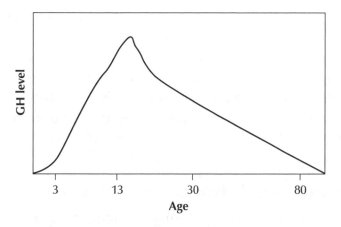

Figure 12.1 Growth Hormone Declines with Age

Growth hormone levels peak during puberty and then decline throughout life. By age thirty or forty, our levels are half of their pubertal peak.

levels (even if normal for a younger person) accelerates the effects of aging, even though someone may experience short-term benefits such as increased muscle mass and decreased body fat.

Ironically, a field of medicine called anti-aging medicine promotes the use of growth hormone as an anti-aging hormone. Proponents cite an article in the *New England Journal of Medicine* that states, "There is evidence that growth hormone deficiency in adults is deleterious, increasing the risk of death from

Growth Hormone and Cancer

High growth hormone levels have long been associated with an increased risk for cancer, notably colon cancer, lymphoma, breast cancer, and prostate cancer. Increased growth hormone levels have been linked to prostate cancer in men, and growth hormone has been shown to cause cancer in laboratory animals. Taking growth hormone or having a tumor that produces excess growth hormone will increase cancer risk, but even having naturally higher growth hormone level could also be of concern. For example, one study found that tall women had a higher cancer risk. "Cancer incidence increases with increasing adult height for most cancer sites," according to study author Dr. Jane Green of Oxford University.

cardiovascular disease." Many anti-aging physicians prescribe growth hormone medications or supplements for older individuals to help them feel younger. The goal is to restore growth hormone levels to the level of a thirty- to forty-year-old; however, most endocrinologists do not advocate the use of growth hormone as an anti-aging medication because of the known deleterious effects. The best way to mitigate the inevitable decline in growth hormone that comes with getting older is not by taking supplements but by getting healthier and naturally boosting growth hormone production.

Stress Causes Growth Hormone Problems

As we've seen many times, stress can disrupt hormonal balance in a manner that promotes weight gain. Stress can be physical or emotional, or it can come from diseases or conditions such as hypothyroidism, diabetes, liver disease, kidney disease, AIDS, or severe burns. The excess fat in our bodies can also cause physical and hormonal stress on the body. Stress causes a multitude of problems with growth hormone. Stress can lead to sleep problems, and since growth hormone is produced when you sleep, sleeping less means less growth hormone.

Even without sleep problems, stress can have a direct effect on your brain and pituitary gland, causing less growth hormone production. Stress also damages growth hormone receptors. When growth hormone receptors become damaged, the growth hormone does not function properly. The pituitary gland is already too pooped out to keep up with the demand. Stress can also lead to growth hormone resistance.

Growth Hormone Resistance

Resistance to any hormone can occur, and growth hormone is no exception. When the body resists the effects of growth hormone, it doesn't matter how much growth hormone you produce, it won't work. Because stress can cause growth hormone resistance, when you alleviate stress, you can naturally boost the effect of the growth hormone you have.

AIDS is a condition associated with high-level growth hormone resistance. As a result, doctors sometimes treat AIDS patients with megadoses of growth hormone, attempting to overcome this resistance. Growth hormone therapy improves muscle mass and muscle strength, but studies have not yet shown that it will prolong life. There is very limited information on long-term safety and proper dosing for growth hormone in AIDS patients.

Dwarves Hold Clues to Diabetes and Cancer

In small towns in Ecuador live groups of very short people with a rare type of genetic dwarfism known as Laron syndrome. People with Laron syndrome have severe growth hormone resistance because of a mutation of the growth hormone receptor. In these people, growth hormone levels are very high, but IGF-1 levels are low because the growth hormone can't tell the liver to produce IGF-1. The result is a human of very short stature who cannot be helped by treatment with growth hormone. Today a new medication is used to treat children with Laron syndrome. Mecasermin (Increlex) is a synthetic IGF-1 medication that bypasses the need for a functioning growth hormone receptor and allows children with Laron syndrome to grow taller.

People with Laron syndrome have an extremely low rate of diabetes and cancer. In fact, these diseases are practically unheard of; however, people with Laron syndrome don't have an extended life span. Scientists are studying their blood to see if they can find which factors are critical for protecting the cells from damage and helping with life extension. It is not known if taking mecasermin will negate the protective effect, but there is concern that it will.

Growth Hormone Deficiency

Even though there is still a lot of controversy about the benefits and risks of growth hormone, growth hormone deficiency is an accepted medical diagnosis in adults. The symptoms of adult growth hormone deficiency may be vague and often ignored. Symptoms may be mistaken for other hormonal imbalances.

The following are among the indicators of growth hormone deficiency:

Cholesterol problems

Decline in kidney function

Depression

Difficulties with sex life (loss of libido)

Difficulty relating to others

Emotional irritability

Heart disease

Increase in body fat

Insomnia

Lack of a sense of well-being

Fatigue, lack of energy

Loss of muscle mass

Poor general health

Poor memory

Premature aging

Reduced capacity for exercise

Social isolation, loss of zest for life

Thinning of the bones (osteoporosis or osteopenia)

Wrinkling skin, thin skin, or dry skin

Growth Hormone Deficiency and the Heart

Studies have shown that patients with severe growth hormone deficiency have twice the risk of dying from heart disease. A growth hormone imbalance of any type can cause heart problems. Growth hormone increases the thickness of the heart walls and affects their function. Growth hormone deficiency can cause a condition known as dilated cardiomyopathy, in which the heart gets big, floppy, and weak. The condition leads to heart failure.

Growth hormone deficiency is associated with premature atherosclerosis and with decreased HDL (good) cholesterol and increased LDL (bad) cholesterol. It's well known that high cholesterol is a cause of coronary artery disease and heart attacks. Restoring normal growth hormone levels can improve the cholesterol profile and the health of the heart.

Balance, again, is important. Growth hormone excess can cause heart problems as easily as growth hormone deficiency: the heart gets very big and thick and has trouble pumping (part of the phenomenon called acromegaly—see following). Heart disease is the number one cause of death in patients with growth hormone excess. A study from Amsterdam found that taking growth

Growth Hormone and Fibromyalgia

There has been some controversy about a link between low growth hormone levels and fibromyalgia. Studies have shown that patients with fibromyalgia have problems with growth hormone. Studies have identified both growth hormone deficiency and growth hormone resistance in patients with fibromyalgia. Some preliminary studies using growth hormone to treat fibromyalgia have been promising; however, most experts are hesitant to recommend using growth hormone for this purpose.

Congenital Growth Hormone Deficiency

The classic form of growth hormone deficiency is congenital, or childhood growth hormone deficiency. Children born with growth hormone deficiency do not grow, and pediatric endocrinologists use growth hormone to restore normal growth. If untreated, these children remain short. Most people with growth hormone deficiency, however, take on a pudgy appearance—keep in mind the effect growth hormone has on fat and muscle. In the past, patients stopped taking growth hormone when they achieved a normal height. Now most endocrinologists advocate lifelong treatment with growth hormone, though the dosages decrease after the patient achieves adult height.

---

hormone as a medication increases the likelihood of dying from a heart attack or stroke by 250 percent.

Causes of Growth Hormone Deficiency

There are many causes of growth hormone deficiency; the two main categories are congenital and acquired. Congenital means that you were born with it. Acquired means that tumor, disease, or trauma has injured the pituitary gland, resulting in a deficiency of growth hormone. As with all hormonal conditions, severe, moderate, and mild forms exist. The most severe cases of adult-onset growth hormone deficiency—90 percent, in fact—are usually caused by a tumor in the pituitary gland. Pituitary tumor patients can be deficient in many hormones, but growth hormone deficiency is the most common.

Pituitary Gland Tumors

Growth hormone deficiency is the most common hormonal abnormality caused by pituitary tumors or other brain tumors. Pituitary gland tumors may sound terrible, but most of them are tiny noncancerous growths. The main reason they cause problems is that they can decrease the pituitary gland's ability to make hormones. Even microscopic pituitary gland tumors can compress the normal cells of the gland, resulting in a hormone deficiency. Sometimes these tumors will also make too much of a particular hormone; for example, too much growth hormone causes acromegaly (see pages 323–324), while too much adrenocorti-trophic hormone (ACTH) causes Cushing's disease (see chapter 11). Sometimes pituitary tumor patients have multiple hormone deficiencies, including growth hormone, thyroid stimulating hormone (TSH), sex hormones, luteinizing hormone (LH), follicle stimulating hormone (FSH), and cortisol (ACTH). This condition is known as panhypopituitarism. Less frequently, the back of the pituitary is damaged. This part, known as the posterior pituitary gland, produces a hormone known as vasopressin, also known as an antidiuretic hormone, which prevents you from urinating too much. Without it, you may urinate up to five gallons (yes, five gallons) each day, a condition called diabetes insipidus, as opposed to the more common type of diabetes, which is called diabetes mellitus.

Obesity

When someone has growth hormone deficiency because of obesity alone, it's called obesity-related hyposomatotropism. Obesity can lower growth hormone levels for many reasons. Being overweight worsens the age-related decline of growth hormone. Other hormone signals, such as leptin and cortisol (see chapters 5 and 11), can lower growth hormone levels to a significant extent, and the levels of these two hormones increase as you gain weight. Fat cells produce hormones called inflammatory cytokines, or adipokines, that lower growth hormone by slowing signals from the hypothalamus and pituitary gland. It's a vicious cycle: being overweight (or having a high percentage of body fat) disrupts growth hormone balance and overall hormonal balance, making you lose muscle and gain fat. Growth hormone replacement therapy for obesity-related hyposomatotropism is not recommended.

Overeating

According to a 2011 study from the University of Michigan, growth hormone levels can be rapidly suppressed by overeating and lack of physical activity. In the study, subjects were encouraged to overeat for a two-week period, consuming about 4,000 calories a day. They were also told not to exercise. Growth hormone levels dropped dramatically after just a few days.

Head Injuries

Head injuries, even less traumatic ones, are a commonly overlooked cause of growth hormone deficiency. Severe head injuries can cause dysfunction of any or all of the pituitary gland hormones and is associated with a condition known as postconcussion syndrome. Growth hormone is one of the most susceptible to head injuries. Even minor head injuries that occurred several years prior have been known to cause growth hormone deficiency. If you have symptoms of growth hormone deficiency and a history of head trauma, discuss them with your physician.

Hereditary Hemochromatosis

In hereditary hemochromatosis, a genetic disease, the body absorbs too much iron, which is deposited in organs and causes tissue damage. Hereditary hemochromatosis frequently causes endocrine dysfunction because of iron deposits in the glands, especially the pancreas and the pituitary gland. Growth hormone deficiency is a common feature of hereditary hemochromatosis. Low testosterone, diabetes, increased amount of blood (known as polycythemia), and liver problems are also common with this condition.

Empty Sella Syndrome

Empty sella syndrome is caused by a small anatomical defect above the pituitary gland that increases pressure in a portion of the skull known as the sella turica. The pituitary gland flattens out along the walls of the sella turica. Empty sella syndrome is more common in overweight people and those with high blood pressure. Empty sella syndrome sometimes results in growth hormone deficiency or other pituitary hormone deficiencies.

Sarcoidosis

Sarcoidosis is a disorder of unknown cause that is characterized by the formation of substances known as granulomas, small masses of grainy tissue. Granulomas can occur anywhere in the body and are most common in the lungs. When sarcoidosis affects the brain, it is known as neurosarcoidosis. Neurosarcoidosis can cause growth hormone deficiency when it damages the hypothalamus and pituitary gland. Typically, neurosarcoidosis causes multiple deficiencies of pituitary gland hormones, but growth hormone may be the first to go.

Radiation

Anyone with a history of radiation exposure to the head or neck is at risk for growth hormone deficiency.

Testing for Growth Hormone Deficiency

Testing for growth hormone deficiency is usually more complicated than a simple blood test. Most of the time, a growth hormone stimulation test is required to make the diagnosis of growth hormone deficiency. Patients with multiple pituitary gland hormone deficiencies, known as panhypopituitarism, are virtually guaranteed of having growth hormone deficiency and do not need to be tested because the diagnosis is so certain.

Growth Hormone Levels

A simple growth hormone measurement is not a reliable test for diagnosing growth hormone deficiency. Growth hormone is secreted from the pituitary gland in pulses, so hormone levels fluctuate greatly. Even a level of zero could be normal.

IGF-1 Levels

A low IGF-1 level is very suggestive of growth hormone deficiency. Low normal IGF-1 levels are also consistent with mild growth hormone deficiency. IGF-1 levels have a normal range that is based on age.

Binding Proteins

There has been a lot of interest in measuring one of these proteins, insulin-like growth factor binding protein-3 (IGFBP-3) as a way of diagnosing growth hormone deficiency. At this time, however, this test is mostly used in research settings.

Stimulation Tests

The growth hormone stimulation test is the best and most accurate way of testing for growth hormone deficiency. The classic stimulation test is known as the insulin tolerance test. In it, a patient is given a large dose of insulin. The blood sugar drops to dangerous levels, which provokes growth hormone to be released. This test is good, but dangerous.

Medications that stimulate growth hormone secretion from the pituitary gland, such as arginine, clonidine, or glucagon, can be administered in a doctor's office as a safe and reliable stimulation test. Typically a baseline sample of blood is obtained, and then the medication is administered. Repeat samples of blood are drawn every thirty minutes or so for the next couple of hours. All the stimulated growth hormone levels must be less than 5 milligrams/liter (mg/L), to diagnose growth hormone deficiency. In children, however, a growth hormone level less than 10 mg/L is considered abnormal.

Pituitary Gland Testing

Growth hormone deficiency can be a clue to other pituitary gland hormone deficiency or excess. Anyone diagnosed with growth hormone deficiency should have a full pituitary gland evaluation, including thyroid, cortisol, testosterone, prolactin, estrogen, LH, FSH, and ACTH levels.

Lipid Profile

Growth hormone deficiency can cause higher LDL (bad) cholesterol and lower HDL (good) cholesterol. Cholesterol measurements are an important part of testing for growth hormone deficiency. Your doctor will monitor your lipid profile periodically if you are on growth hormone replacement therapy.

Blood Sugar Testing

Growth hormone deficiency is associated with insulin resistance, so it's important to measure blood sugar as part of the initial evaluation. Blood sugar and A_{1c} (chapter 6) should also be monitored regularly if you are taking growth hormone replacement.

Bone Density Testing

Growth hormone deficiency is an important causal factor in thinning of the bones (osteopenia or osteoporosis). If you have growth hormone deficiency I recommend that you have bone density testing performed. Dual-energy X-ray absorptiometry (DEXA) is the most accurate and advanced test available for measuring bone density. The test is quick and painless and gives very important information about the density of bones.

Magnetic Resonance Imaging

A magnetic resonance imaging (MRI) scan will give information about the structure of the pituitary gland as well as the presence of any tumors. Open MRI scanners are not very accurate for diagnosing pituitary gland problems, though. For the most accurate test, have a closed MRI scan.

Cancer Screening

Active tumor growth is a contraindication to the use of growth hormone. All patients who are considering starting growth hormone replacement should have a basic cancer screen with their primary care physician. Screen for cancer in the breast, cervix, prostate, and colon. I also recommend a total body skin exam to look for suspicious moles that could be early skin cancer.

Growth Hormone Replacement Therapy

In 1996, growth hormone therapy was approved for treatment of adult growth hormone deficiency. Despite the approval, treatment is still debated among endocrinologists. Most, however, agree that severe or symptomatic growth hormone deficiency should probably be treated. Growth hormone is given as a daily injection, though some patients take it less often. Injection pen devices are much easier to use than standard injection with a vial and syringe. Growth hormone comes as a powder that must be mixed with sterile water, and it comes in a premixed form. Aside from convenience factors, all brands of growth hormone are essentially equal.

The goals of growth hormone therapy are to lose fat, gain muscle (restore normal body composition), improve muscle and heart function, normalize cholesterol, increase energy, and improve quality of life. You should use growth hormone only under the supervision of a qualified endocrinologist.

How much is the right amount? Studies have reported a highly variable response to dosing of growth hormone. In the past, dosing of growth hormone was based on body weight. Today, most doctors start with a low dose and slowly increase the dose according to side effects and your response to therapy. This method is known as individualized dose titration. For many reasons, individuals respond differently to similar doses of growth hormone. Stress and illness, for example, cause growth hormone resistance, and higher doses may be required to overcome this resistance.

Some patients will respond to very low doses of growth hormone, but others require much higher doses. I usually have patients start on a dose of 0.2 milligrams (mg) at bedtime for a couple of months, then increase to 0.4 mg. The dose can be further increased every few months. Most patients with adult growth hormone deficiency rarely need more than 1.6 mg of growth hormone per day. Women who take estrogen medications such as hormone replacement therapy or birth control pills need higher doses of growth hormone, because

> ### Synthetic Growth Hormone Is Better Than Natural
>
> Until the 1980s, natural growth hormone was extracted from human cadaver pituitary glands. At the time, it was the only type of growth hormone available. Unfortunately, a rare and fatal brain disease known as Creutzfeldt-Jakob disease (similar to mad cow disease) was linked to natural growth hormone. In 1981, synthetic growth hormone was approved, which eliminates the risk of Creutzfeldt-Jakob disease, and synthetic is the kind used today.

estrogen cranks up the enzymes in the liver that break down growth hormone. Estrogen patches do not have the same effect as pills and are preferred for women who are on growth hormone replacement therapy. Bodybuilders and patients with AIDS may take doses of growth hormone as high as 6 mg per day. These mega doses are along the same lines of taking high doses of anabolic steroids.

No one can even agree on the perfect way of monitoring growth hormone therapy. Most doctors will follow IGF-1 levels as a marker of therapy. Accurate and correct dosing also depends on side effects. I generally start my patients with a very low dose, monitor IGF-1 levels, and slowly increase the dose over several months until the IGF-1 is normal for age. If side effects occur, I back off on the dose. To closely mimic your diurnal rhythms, I recommend taking the injection at bedtime. It may take as long as six months before you even begin to notice an effect.

Side Effects of Growth Hormone Replacement Therapy

Side effects occur more frequently in older patients and heavier patients. Side effects are related to the dose. If you lower your dose of growth hormone, side effects usually subside. The most common side effects of growth hormone therapy are muscle and joint aches and pains and fluid retention. High blood pressure, bloating, and edema can be due to the water and salt retention caused by growth hormone. Other side effects include headache, blurred vision, and carpal tunnel syndrome. Blood sugar problems and even diabetes can also occur as side effects of growth hormone replacement. You must have your blood sugar checked periodically if you are on growth hormone therapy. Nearly 10 percent of men and women have reported breast enlargement from growth hormone. There is a concern about cancer risk from growth hormone replacement. Any substance that causes cells to grow has the potential of causing cancer.

Optimize Your Body's Natural Growth Hormone

There are several ways of tapping into your body's natural supply of this mostly beneficial hormone.

Eat Healthy Food

The more body fat you have, the lower your growth hormone levels, and as you lose fat, your growth hormone levels will surge, helping you lose more fat. Fad diets, however, lower your growth hormone levels. The Hormonal Health Diet is the ideal diet for enhancing growth hormone levels.

Drink Water

You must drink enough water. I cannot emphasize this point enough. Drink at least eight 8-ounce glasses a day. Water is a major component of muscle. Without enough water, you can become dehydrated and your muscles suffer.

Consume Protein

Protein is critical to making the weight loss/growth hormone gain cycle work. Protein builds muscle. If you raise your growth hormone levels but are not eating enough protein, you won't see much good; you have to provide your body with all the tools. Eat the right amount of protein, though, because extra protein is easily converted into fat and stored in fat cells.

Engage in Physical activity

Physical activity is very important to lowering weight and raising growth hormone levels. Strenuous workouts are the best for growth hormone ones. Intensive exercise can make growth hormone levels surge. Once you start exercising, growth hormone will help you keep exercising, making your muscles stronger. The more you exercise, the stronger you get, which has long been known, but few realize growth hormone's role in this.

Get Enough Sleep

Growth hormone is released when you sleep. If you don't sleep well, you won't produce enough growth hormone.

Supplements

Growth hormone supplements aren't actual growth hormone. They are promoted to stimulate the pituitary gland to make growth hormone. Arginine and other amino acids, when taken in high enough doses, will stimulate the pituitary gland to make growth hormone. Amino acid supplements are touted as a "natural" way of enhancing growth hormone levels. When I test patients for growth hormone deficiency, I give them an intravenous infusion of arginine.

Over-the-counter growth hormone products are usually one or several amino acids combined with arginine, designed to boost the body's growth hormone production. I have seen several patients who have had very high growth hormone levels from taking amino acid supplements. Because of this, I don't recommend using supplements to boost growth hormone.

Acromegaly

For most of this chapter, I've talked about how growth hormone makes muscles grow, but I need now to discuss the dark side to this growth. Sometimes the pituitary gland develops a tumor that produces excessive amounts of growth hormone, a condition known as acromegaly. You've probably seen someone with acromegaly in the *Guinness Book of World Records* or on professional wrestling shows. If a child develops a growth hormone-producing pituitary tumor before puberty, he becomes a "giant," a condition given the obvious name gigantism. Today most of these children are diagnosed and treated. Victims of gigantism don't usually grow up to be basketball players or Herculean strongmen. Gigantism provides them with a whole new set of problems, particularly skeletal and muscular conditions. The human body isn't usually meant to be eight feet tall. For those who develop a problem with growth hormone excess after puberty, after growth has ceased, the situation is even worse.

After puberty, excessive growth hormones can cause acromegaly. The condition is much more common than people realize. Most patients who are diagnosed have had subtle symptoms for ten years or longer before being diagnosed. The symptoms can be very subtle, especially in the early years, but they progress. People with acromegaly end up with very large hands and feet—the name itself means *big extremity*—and a variety of problems. Besides the growth of the hands and feet, acromegaly causes the brow to thicken, the nose to broaden, the jaw to protrude, the teeth to space out, the tongue to grow, and the forehead to gain a large, deep furrowing. Andre the Giant, who had acromegaly, had a number of

Symptoms of Acromegaly	
Acanthosis nigricans (see chapter 6)	Growth of hands and feet
Arthritis	Heart disease
Cancer	High blood pressure
Carpal tunnel syndrome	High cholesterol
Change in facial appearance	Skin tags
Diabetes or elevated blood sugar	Weight gain

these features. Acromegaly can mimic insulin resistance. Why? When produced in high levels, growth hormone directly works against insulin, creating insulin resistance.

Acromegaly Treatment Options

What can you do if you have acromegaly? Fortunately, it's reversible. Surgery, radiation, and medications are all options, and all have been known to control—or even solve—the problem. Most endocrinologists recommend surgery as first-line therapy, but new and more effective medications are available for those who are not cured by surgery. Medications slow the production of growth hormone from the pituitary gland or block the receptor for growth hormone.

Chapter Review

Growth hormone deficiencies are often related to disorders of the pituitary gland. The disorders may be triggered or accelerated by a whole range of other causes, from head injuries to the process of aging to cancerous and noncancerous tumors growing in the gland to genetic or inherited tendencies; and, of course, the condition of simply being overweight.

The chapter noted the favorable impact of growth hormones on the body, including the potent muscle building and fat burning role. Anyone being treated for deficient growth hormone derives these positive benefits, plus better heart function, improved mood, and stronger bones. However, too much of the hormone in the body can have the exact opposite effect, including some cancer causing potential.

People with long-standing growth hormone deficiencies have very slow metabolisms because their muscles have wasted away and have been replaced by fat. Fatigue and muscle weakness are common complaints from those with growth hormone deficiencies. When obesity is involved, a destructive cycle is set up as metabolism slows in response to low levels of growth hormone and energy is sapped. Without the energy to exercise, the gain weight is a direct consequence. Stress can also disrupt normal growth hormone levels and lead to growth hormone resistance.

The chapter pointed out that a few blood-specific low growth hormone tests are available that measure a patient's blood sugar drop response when given an injection of insulin. Pituitary gland testing and conducting an MRI exam were also noted as two other available tests.

Finally, treatment options were covered, including growth hormone replacement therapy as well as natural options such as changes in diet, exercise patterns.

Practical Strategies for Intelligent Weight Loss

To lose weight and keep it off you have to have a plan. Eating right is an important part of losing weight, but it takes more than a healthy diet to achieve permanent weight loss. This section is about all the things you need to do in addition to eating right so that you balance your hormones and take the weight off for good. This section contains important information you'll need to lose weight intelligently.

Form Habits

Changing your lifestyle for the better requires committing to that change until it has become a habit, a way of life, and no longer a burden. Just like the habit of getting up in the morning and the systematic way that we prepare for work, so too will the habit of an improved diet and exercise become automatic. The key to success is that the change becomes a habit!

The best way to start a new habit is to slowly add healthy foods and behaviors to your lifestyle. You don't have to do everything all at once. I suggest starting with one or two healthy behaviors and slowly building. As you form new habits, they become part of your daily routine. It is normal for new things to feel unnatural or uncomfortable. Accept this uncomfortable feeling as part of growth and change. Change is usually difficult in the beginning, but you are probably reading this book because you are ready for a change.

Make This Your Last Diet

The hardest part of losing weight is keeping it off. This must be seen as your new way of life, not as a defined period in your life with a starting and stopping point. The fact that you have met your goal weight indicates motivation and success in forming new habits. This is the critical phase, the phase in which you must adhere stringently to your initial goals—this is now your way of life. It is not the quick fix for a special occasion. You've made the commitment to eat healthy and be more active. Now you need to continue to maintain these same habits.

- Are you ready to make a change? Your success is always at risk of being threatened by old habits and situations. Before you succumb to your former ways, be prepared to make a permanent life change when you first set out on this journey.

- Follow the plan. Reassure yourself that your diet plan is an integral part of your weight loss. Eat all the nutritionally balanced meals and snacks, and do not skip meals.

- Set a goal of exercising every day (or as many days as possible).

- Get enough good-quality sleep.

- Avoid chemicals that disrupt hormones.

- Be prepared. Stack the deck in your favor, and plan for the expected and the unexpected situations that threaten your success.

- Remain positive. A positive attitude will help you through the tough times, always reassuring you that you are making the right choices and changes in your life.

- Be flexible. You will always be changing and adjusting to accommodate your new lifestyle.

Planning for the Expected

Planning will keep you on your diet and will keep you successful. Don't let lack of preparation make you fail. By having the proper foods around all the time you've already won half the battle. Eating all these delicious foods is the easy part. You must have enough of the right foods around at all times. This means having lots of fresh fruits and vegetables throughout the week. I recommend shopping once a week from a list. With proper storage and preparation methods, you will have no problem keeping fruits and vegetables around. Plan on bringing your lunch with you instead of trying to find something healthy in a restaurant or cafeteria. Prepare snacks in advance.

Planning for the Unexpected

There will always be unplanned events. If your goals have not addressed these events you will not be adequately prepared for the foods that may be available or the choices you will have to make should the menu serve foods that you ordinarily consider off-limits. When such events occur, attempt to find out ahead of time the food that is available and make a note of what you will eat. Then when you arrive at the event you will be less likely to eat impulsively.

Preparing to Shop

The trip to the grocery store can be the initial link in the chain of events that determines how successful eating habits will be on subsequent days. If the choices made here follow the diet plan, then the meals prepared and eaten will be too. The following are guidelines to help you adhere to your goals.

- Shop only from a list.
- Do not be tempted by unhealthy items that are shelved conspicuously throughout the grocery store.
- Do not shop when hungry. Shopping on an empty stomach will only lead to compulsive buying and will likely include prepackaged foods that can be consumed quickly. Such foods are often laden with fat and salt and are unwise food choices.
- Prepare meals. Prepare as many meals as possible. The time it takes to prepare a meal can often prevent the impulsive, uncontrolled eating that occurs with fast foods.
- Shop as little as possible. The more frequent the trips, the more often the temptations. I recommend that you shop once a week. With the suggestions listed here, you will have fresh fruits and vegetables available for the entire week.
- Don't shop for the family favorites. These are likely to be your favorites too.
- Don't be tempted by the free food samples in the store as you shop.

See the Shopping List on pages 384–385 for a complete list of items.

Setting Goals

For every action you take, there must be a plan for guidance and a goal to define your achievement. You must determine how much weight loss is appropriate and how you will achieve it. Obviously that will require change in your eating habits and exercise. Your goals should be attainable. Set a goal of making a small improvement instead of doing everything perfectly. Don't get burned out by overloading yourself with too much all at once. You should continue to set new goals as you progress, and make new goals when necessary. You should be determined and focused on what it will take to achieve your goals, and plan for the challenges.

Practices that are vital to your success are

- **Put your goals in writing.** Writing down your goals will help you keep them in mind. Keep your list on the refrigerator or on the bathroom mirror. Continually review and update your goals.

- **Set a date for the completion of your goal.** Setting a date will help you to stay focused and motivated.

- **Set weight goals.** How much weight should you lose? This is a difficult decision. Many of us will have difficulty achieving a "normal" body weight. This does not mean that some weight loss will not be beneficial. In fact, many scientific studies have shown that weight loss as little as 5–10 percent of your initial body weight will help regulate hormones and improve medical problems caused by obesity, such as diabetes, high blood pressure, and arthritis.

- **Set exercise goals.** Be specific about the kind of exercise you will engage in. Determine your short-term goal for duration of exercise and a long-term goal that will be necessary for you to achieve your weight loss.

- **Set goals for behavior change.** This will be one of your biggest challenges. To be successful you must, in some way, change your behavior. You became overweight by engaging in specific behaviors that will require change. Perhaps you worked late into the evening, didn't have time to exercise, and ate fast food on the way home. You may now need to consider exercising in the morning before work, for example. To overcome a fast-food attraction, you may have to prepare meals and snacks at home to take to the office.

Achieving the Right Weight for Your Height

BMI, or body mass index, is the standard for adjusting weight for height, assigning a numerical value to this ratio. BMI is the standard used by scientists and doctors to study weight and health risk. The higher your BMI, the higher your risk of medical problems and death. BMI is used to determine whether you fall in the healthy range or you are overweight or obese. BMI is defined as body weight in kilograms divided by the square of height in meters (kg/m^2). This is a complicated metric formula that is easily converted to pounds and inches. You can calculate your own BMI by using a calculator on the Internet (http://www.nhlbisupport.com/bmi/) or use the following formula:

$$BMI = \frac{(\text{weight in pounds}) \times 703}{(\text{height in inches}) \times (\text{height in inches})}$$

For example, if you weigh 180 pounds and are 5 feet 6 inches

$$BMI = (180 \times 703) / (66 \times 66) = 29$$

A normal or healthy BMI range is between 18.5 and 25 kg/m^2. BMI values greater than 25 kg/m^2 are good indicators of degrees of excess fat and health risks. Overweight is defined as BMI 25 to 29.9 and obesity is defined as a BMI greater than 30.

BMI	Weight Category
18.5–24.9	Normal
25–29.9	Overweight
30–34.9	Class I Obesity
35–39.9	Class II Obesity
40–59.9	Class III Obesity
>60	Super-Obesity

How Much Should You Eat?

It is important to eat the right number of calories and have the right balance of nutrients. Your specific formula depends on several factors, including your current body weight, whether you are a man or a woman, and whether you are trying to lose weight or maintain your weight. As a general rule of thumb, to maintain your weight, most women need to eat 9–10 calories for every pound they weigh, and men need to eat 10–11 calories per pound. For example, if a 150-pound woman eats 1,500 calories daily, she will maintain her weight. To lose weight, the calories have to drop below this level. You can estimate that you will lose one pound for every 3,500 calories you save. So reducing your daily calories by 500 will result in losing one pound each week. The numbers are not exact, and studies have found that as we drop our calories, our metabolism slows a little bit. However, this doesn't take exercise into account. By exercising according to the guidelines in this section, you can lose weight faster and help keep your metabolism at a higher level.

Table R.1 on pages 332 and 333 is a general guide to the number of calories and the carbohydrates, protein, and fat you need to eat in a day to lose weight or maintain your weight. These numbers are to be used as a general guide for your nutrition. For more detailed advice regarding your specific needs, you should meet with a weight loss physician or registered dietitian.

Know What to Expect

Your weight loss results will depend on whether you are a novice or a veteran at attempting to lose weight. If this is your first attempt at weight loss, you may be more optimistic and a lot more confident in your attempts to succeed than someone who has attempted every diet designed. A positive attitude is critical, as is confidence in your ability to follow the diet plan and make the appropriate food choices as well as portion sizes.

Most of my patients lose 2 or 3 pounds per week, but that amount can vary considerably. Some of my patients lose as much as 5 or 10 pounds after one week on the diet. But weight loss tends to slow down after the first couple of weeks. Because there are so many factors that play a role in weight loss, you may feel like you are doing the exact same thing week to week and still experience different weight loss. Don't be misled by day-to-day weight fluctuations. Focus on the big picture and monitor your weekly weight loss, monthly weight loss, and total weight loss.

Your rate of weight loss depends upon multiple factors.

1. Are you ready to start a new lifestyle?
2. How closely are you following the plan? Are you eating enough healthy foods? Are you eating consistently throughout the day? Are you drinking enough water?
3. Are you exercising every day?
4. How do you view this effort in losing weight—as a diet or a lifestyle change?
5. What is your starting weight? People who are significantly overweight or obese tend to lose more weight in the initial phases of a diet. The heavier you are, the quicker the initial weight loss.

6. Are you on medications that may affect your weight?

7. Do you have hormonal imbalance or other medical problems that may affect the rate of weight loss?

Losing More Than Pounds

When I assess my patients' progress, I look at more than just their weight on the scale. Other factors such as body frame, waistline measurement, and body composition are important variables to consider when measuring health risk. Waist circumference is a measure of fat in the belly, which is more dangerous than other types of fat (see chapter 6). The waist circumference is an excellent way of determining whether you have central obesity. Men with a waist circumference more than 40 inches and women with a waist circumference of more than 35 inches have central obesity. Some of my patients measure their thighs, hips, stomach, arms, and neck and keep a tally of the number of inches they are losing.

Body fat analysis helps you to determine how much of your weight is lean tissue and how much is fat. There are many methods of measuring body composition, or your percentage of body fat, including underwater weighing, computed tomography (CT) scanning, ultrasound, bioimpedance analysis, body calipers, and Dual-energy X-ray absorptiometry (DEXA). Each of these methods has advantages and disadvantages. In general, tests that are easy to perform, such as bioimpedance analysis and body calipers, are less accurate (but easier and cheaper) than underwater weighing, CT scanning, and DEXA. Despite this, I believe that bioimpedance analysis or body calipers are an excellent way of keeping track of your body fat. Body fat analysis can be useful when you hit a plateau. Since lean tissue is denser than bone, it is possible to lose body fat and maintain your weight. Although your weight is the same, you are leaner and your clothes will be looser.

Eat a Healthy Diet

Keeping a Food Diary Doubles Your Weight Loss

Keeping a food diary is an important step to help you lose weight. A food diary is helpful because it helps bring awareness about the foods you eat from a broad perspective. It helps you have some accountability with yourself. Many of my patients have told me they have kept food diaries in the past, but they have given up on them. If you have kept a food diary and gave up because it didn't seem to work, there is a good reason to give it another try: a study in *American Journal of*

Table R.1   Guidelines for Weight Loss and Weight Maintenance

Men (Weight Loss)

Body Weight (pounds)	Under 150	150–175	175–200	200–225	225–250	250–275	275–300	300–325	325–350
Calories per day	1,100	1,200	1,400	1,600	1,800	2,000	2,200	2,400	2,600
Carbohydrates (grams per day)	110	120	140	160	180	200	220	240	260
Protein (grams per day)	84	90	104	120	134	150	164	180	194
Fat (grams per day)	38	40	46	54	60	66	72	80	86

Men (Weight Maintenance)

Body Weight (pounds)	Under 150	150–175	175–200	200–225	225–250	250–275	275–300	300–325	325–350
Calories per day	1,300	1,500	1,700	1,900	2,100	2,400	2,700	3,000	3,300
Carbohydrates (grams per day)	130	150	170	190	210	240	270	300	330
Protein (grams per day)	98	112	130	144	160	180	204	224	250
Fat (grams per day)	44	50	56	62	70	80	90	100	110

Table R.1   Guidelines for Weight Loss and Weight Maintenance

Women (Weight Loss)

Body Weight (pounds)	Under 125	125–150	175–200	175–200	225–250	200–225	225–250	250–275	325–350
Calories per day	1,000–1,100	1,100	1,200	1,400	1,600	1,800	2,000	2,200	2,400
Carbohydrates (grams per day)	100	110	120	160	180	200	220	240	260
Protein (grams per day)	76	84	90	120	134	150	164	180	196
Fat (grams per day)	32	36	40	52	60	66	72	80	86

Women (Weight Maintenance)

Body Weight (pounds)	Under 125	125–150	175–200	175–200	225–250	200–225	225–250	250–275	325–350
Calories per day	1,100–1,200	1,300	1,500	1,700	1,900	2,100	2,400	2,700	3,000
Carbohydrates (grams per day)	110	130	150	170	190	210	240	270	300
Protein (grams per day)	82	98	112	126	142	158	180	202	224
Fat (grams per day)	36	44	50	56	64	70	80	90	100

Preventive Medicine found that dieters who recorded everything they ate in a food diary lost twice as much weight as those who did not.

You must record everything you eat, bad or good, in your food diary. Use a small notebook or a smartphone app and keep it with you at all times. You can make it very detailed, documenting every calorie you eat, or simply write down the foods you eat as a list for the day. The idea is to document in writing everything you eat. Looking over your food diary every day helps you bring your notes back into your daily thinking and helps you make better decisions the next day. Awareness is paramount to changing habits.

A few tips on keeping a food diary:

- Record every item eaten.
- Record the amount of each item eaten.
- Record the times you eat during the day.
- Record where you eat and what you are doing.
- Do not wait to record your intake at the end of the day. It will be inaccurate.
- Record immediately after eating.
- Read over your diary periodically.

Maintain Your New Habits in Restaurants

It is easier to be in control of your eating habits when you are the person shopping for the food and preparing it. However, whether it is business or pleasure that takes you away, in restaurants you are faced with the task of maintaining your new habits in unfamiliar surroundings. Eating out can be a great challenge but can be simplified if you have a plan.

- Try to select from a menu versus all-you-can-eat buffets.
- Special-order items to be cooked with less oil or butter.
- Order a green salad with fat-free dressing before your meal.
- Order two extra sides of steamed vegetables and a side of fresh fruit.
- Avoid high-fat appetizers.
- Drink water throughout your meal.

- Order sauces and dressings on the side.
- When possible choose dishes that are steamed, poached, boiled, broiled, or grilled.
- Choose red sauces instead of creamed sauces for pasta dishes.
- Avoid filling up on bread before the meal; ask that the breadbasket be removed.
- Choose fresh fruit for dessert or at most share a dessert.
- Avoid alcoholic beverages.

Continue a Healthy Lifestyle When You Travel

Eating healthy food and getting regular exercise during travel for work or for pleasure can be particularly challenging. This doesn't mean that you have to stop being healthy when you travel.

Tips for healthy travel:

- Bring a cooler of healthy snacks such as fresh vegetables and fruit, yogurt, or other healthy foods.
- Take an empty water bottle to fill up after airport security.
- Look for healthy choices on restaurant menus.
- Always pack workout shoes and clothes.
- Stock up on healthy foods at a local grocery store.
- Work out at the hotel fitness center.
- Wear comfortable shoes in the airport and do some walking when you have extra time.
- Do not eat unhealthy snacks served on the plane.
- Bring healthy food with you on the plane.
- Have the hotel prepare a low-calorie lunch to take on the go.

Get Enough Exercise

Sitting Is Bad for Your Health

Prolonged time sitting, known as "habitual sedentary behavior," is now considered a risk factor for obesity and related diseases. It is clear that we need to cut out this new bad habit. According to the Centers for Disease Control (CDC) (see chapter 3 bibliography), we are in an epidemic of sitting.

Our places of work, schools, homes, and public areas have been designed in ways to enhance sitting and minimize movement and physical activity. Nowadays, you rarely need to walk and almost never need to run. Sitting has become the norm. We are not just sitting more . . . we are moving less.

Humans are designed to move. Our bodies have evolved over thousands of years to move and engage in physical labor throughout the day. The change in human lifestyle from a physically demanding life to a sedentary lifestyle over the past few decades has been relatively new, occurring just recently on the timeline of human existence. In 1970, 20 percent of Americans worked at desk jobs. Today more than 60 percent spend our entire workdays sitting. During the past twenty years, with computers, televisions, and video games, most of us spend significant amounts of time in front of a screen. TV watching time for the average American has quadrupled over the past forty years.

This increase in sitting has had detrimental effects on all of us, leading to a whole host of health problems. Research has focused our understanding on the health benefits of physical activity and how to incorporate daily physical activity so that we can emulate our ancestors. Physicians refer to people who sit too much as "sedentary." However, you can look at it two ways. There is either an excess of sitting behavior, or there is a lack of exercise. Either way, in order to be truly healthy, you must sit less and exercise more.

Researchers have categorized "nonexercise behavior" as either sedentary (sitting or lying, expending very little energy) or light-intensity activity (standing, self-care activities, or slow walking). Research from the U.S. National Health and Nutrition Examination Survey shows that the average person spends only 3 percent of their awake time exercising. One in four adults spends 70 percent of their time sitting, and 30 percent doing light activities, with almost no time exercising.

Exercise Is a Vital Element of Hormonal Balance

Even if you eat a healthy diet, your hormones won't be balanced unless you exercise.

Only 12 percent of people get enough exercise, according to the Centers for Disease Control. The National Weight Control Registry found that 94 percent of people who have successfully lost weight and kept it off reported doing at least sixty minutes of exercise on most days of the week. Regular daily exercise

Exercise Reverses the Effects of Aging

According to research done by Dr. Melov Tarnopopolsky at McMaster's University, exercise can prevent the body from aging. Moderate exercise can improve cellular function, reversing or decreasing the effects of aging.

is a surefire way to burn calories, increase metabolism, and alleviate both leptin and insulin resistance.

Exercise is even more important for maintaining weight loss than it is for losing weight. In fact, weight loss without exercise is almost always temporary. Consistent exercise does more than just help you lose weight. Studies have shown that people who exercise regularly have fewer health problems and report feeling better. Exercise reduces your risk for a multitude of ailments, including heart attacks, strokes, diabetes, hypertension, sleep apnea, and cancer. Exercise strengthens muscles, bones, and the immune system. In fact, people who exercise regularly get 40 percent fewer colds and upper respiratory infections, and they are less severe.

New guidelines from the American Society of Clinical Oncology recommend exercise as one of the best ways to fight cancer. Exercise has been shown to prevent cancer as well as improve survival rates, reduce fatigue, and improve quality of life. Having a healthy lifestyle can reduce the risk for a stroke by 80 percent. Thirty-four percent of cases of high blood pressure can be prevented by improving lifestyle. Exercise improves the function of the immune system. The amount of fat-burning substances in the body is increased by exercise.

Children who exercise have more brain cells and better brain connections than those who don't exercise. A study found that 10-minute exercise breaks during school led to higher test scores as well as higher activity levels outside of school. Physically fit children score higher on intelligence tests, have better attention spans, and better high brain functions coordinating complex thoughts, known as "executive control." College students who exercise regularly get better grades. Students with grade point averages of 3.5 or higher were three times more likely to exercise regularly than were those with lower grades.

As overweight people approach their forties and fifties, they experience a more pronounced and more rapid decline in brain function. A nine-year study published in the journal *Neurology* showed that walking just a mile each day can cut your risk of cognitive decline or dementia in half. Even small amounts of exercise can increase connections between brain circuits and can improve memory.

Exercise and Your Brain
Exercise makes you happier, calmer, and smarter. Exercise helps you stay fit not only below the collar but above as well. Exercise increases levels of a brain hormone called brain-derived neurotrophic factor. This substance acts like fertilizer in the brain, making neurons grow and thrive. Exercise alleviates depression, anxiety, and stress. There have been numerous studies showing the benefits of exercise on memory and academic performance.

Get Started with Daily Exercise

Getting started with an exercise program can feel overwhelming. Just getting started can be the hardest part. Many of my patients tell me they simply don't have time to exercise. I know it can be difficult to find the time to exercise, but I can tell you that the time you invest in exercise will give you a big payoff. You should start by setting a goal that is easy to attain. For example, exercise for 15 minutes twice a week. You don't have to be overwhelmed with exercise; you just have to get started. Once you get into the routine of exercising, start building on the time, frequency, and intensity. Any exercise you do is great; doing more is better. Set new goals that are challenging but attainable, with a long-term goal of exercising every day for 60 to 90 minutes. You can take a day off from exercising every once in a while, but for best results, I recommending making daily exercise a priority in your life.

You may think it seems unrealistic to plan on exercising every day. I challenge you to consider the reasons why *you can exercise every day.* Thousands of years ago, humans walked or ran 10 to 12 miles every day just to survive. Our bodies are meant to move. Our modern society makes exercise a luxury, not a necessity. But exercise is a necessity. And you need it to survive. I want you to have a plan for exercising that is realistic, so you shouldn't get overwhelmed. Start off slowly with a goal of doing something every day, even if it is only 5 minutes of exercise.

Move Your Body for 60 to 90 Minutes Every Day

Studies have shown that daily exercise is a critical factor for long-term weight loss. Most of your exercise should be moderate-intensity aerobic exercise like walking, slow jogging, an elliptical machine, or a stationary bike. According to

Make Sure Your Heart Is Ready for Exercise: See Your Doctor

If you are over the age of thirty-five or have other risk factors for heart disease, which include being overweight, you should see your doctor before beginning an exercise program. Although exercise is very healthy for your heart, you need to make sure you aren't at risk for having a heart attack before you get started. Your doctor should take a detailed history and perform a physical exam. Most doctors will also perform an electrocardiogram (EKG), which is an inexpensive way to screen for obvious heart problems but may miss subtle problems lurking under the surface. You may need to have a treadmill stress test, where you walk on a treadmill at an increasing pace while having a continuous EKG. This simulates the stress exercise places on the heart so that it can show up on the EKG. A treadmill stress test can be inaccurate at times, so doctors may order other heart tests as well, including a nuclear stress test, echocardiogram, and coronary calcium scoring. The idea is to get a general sense that it is safe for your heart to exercise.

the CDC, you can do moderate-intensity exercise for a sustained period of time. You should keep your heart rate between 100 and 140 beats per minute and feel winded but still have enough breath to carry on a conversation. Daily exercise at this level burns fat and alleviates insulin resistance and leptin resistance.

Set a goal of doing at least 6–8 hours of aerobic exercise weekly. Even if you don't do it all, do as much as you can. Continually push yourself to increase the duration of your exercise. The type of exercise you do is not as important as doing it consistently. It is helpful to do different types of aerobic exercises to keep things interesting. You should always have a backup plan for aerobic exercise in case of inclement weather.

You can substitute physical activity for some of your exercise. The definition of *physical activity* is moving your body through space. Physical activity counts for all those activities you can do that aren't formal exercise but still involve moving your body and burning calories. You can garden or mow the lawn, pace the room when on the phone, clean the house, walk the dog or wash your car, shop, and play with kids. All are great types of physical activity. You have

Aerobic Exercises

Active playing with kids	Fitness classes	Sports that require constant running or jogging
Biking	Hiking	
Calisthenics	Ice skating	Stair climbing
Carrying boxes	Jogging	Stationary bike
Car washing	Martial arts	Swimming
Chopping wood	Racquetball	Treading water
Circuit weight training	Roller skating	Walking
Cross-country skiing	Rowing	Walking in water
Dancing	Running	Water aerobics
Elliptical machine	Soccer	

probably heard every diet guru say take the stairs instead of the elevator. They all say it for a reason. The more physical activity you do, the better. If you have a desk job, you need to make an effort to get up from your desk and walk for at least one minute every hour. The point is to be more active all day long.

Increase Your Daily Activities

Formal exercise is not the only way you can burn calories. Any type of activity, from shopping to gardening, can burn calories. One of the reasons that obesity has reached epidemic proportions is that modern technology has almost eliminated the need to move your body. The car, telephone, elevator, electric garage door opener, and television with remote control are all contributors to this phenomenon. You can get rid of some of these "conveniences" and burn extra calories.

The following recommendations will increase physical activity in your life:

- Walk up stairs instead of taking the elevator or the escalator.
- Shop until you drop.
- Walk on the treadmill while watching TV.

Crunched on Time?

You can cut your workout time in half by doing more intense exercises, like running, swimming, biking, or any exercise that gets your heart rate up to 140–170 beats per minute so that you are breathing heavily. According to the Centers for Disease Control, one minute of vigorous exercise can count for two minutes of moderate-intensity exercise.

- Walk in place while talking on the phone.
- Throw away the remote control.
- Park your car a little farther away from your destination and walk the extra distance.
- Take a short walk around the block.
- Play actively with the kids.
- Mow the lawn.
- Pull the weeds.
- Clean out the garage.

Make Exercise a Habit

Some of my patients have told me that they quit exercising because they didn't see any results. This is not a reason to quit exercising. It is not uncommon to have a delayed response to exercise. Even if you feel tired after exercising or just don't feel like exercising, you should do it anyway. Treat exercise like brushing your teeth. In time, it will feel like a habit you can't go without. Exercise is a habit of my patients who have lost weight permanently. Many of my patients have changed their lives to make daily exercise a habit. If your schedule changes, you should plan ahead to make sure you can fit exercise in.

Exercise to Build Muscle

I recommend adding in some resistance exercises for 20 minutes two or three times each week. Resistance exercises build muscle and strength, alleviate insulin resistance, and boost metabolic rate. Resistance exercises are also referred to

Take Fitness Classes

A 2010 study published in the *Archives of Internal Medicine* concluded that patients who participated in supervised exercise classes had better outcomes than those who tried exercise on their own. The motivation, support, and structure of classes seem to help people exercise more frequently and at higher intensity.

as *anaerobic exercise.* Muscle-building exercises include weight lifting, calisthenics (push-ups and sit-ups), isometric exercises, resistance bands, yoga, gardening with shoveling, and moving heavy boxes. If you lift weights, you should rest at least one day between sessions to let your body rebuild muscle. Just 60 minutes of resistance exercises each week will make a big difference in your overall health and fitness level.

Exercise Early in the Day

When you exercise in the morning you are more likely to exercise consistently. There are fewer barriers to get in the way of exercise. It is easy to start the day with a plan to exercise in the evening, but it is just as easy to skip it when something else comes up. Make exercise a priority in your life by exercising early in the day.

Exercise Several Times in a Day

If you don't have a lot of time, try breaking your exercise into several small sessions throughout the day. You get the same benefit whether you do all your exercise at once or you break it up into multiple small bouts throughout the day. Both are just as good at boosting metabolism and burning calories. Make plans so that you can get in your exercise during the day. When you get in a little exercise when you have time, it makes it more likely you will reach your goal of exercising 60–90 minutes every day. Exercising all day long also keeps your metabolism higher.

Make Exercise Fun and Enjoyable

Exercise activates reward centers in the brain, especially when it makes you feel good. Choose activities that you enjoy doing, because you will be more likely to do them consistently. Studies have shown that exercising with a friend or

Combine Aerobic and Resistance Training

A 2010 study published in the *Archives of Internal Medicine* concluded that patients who participated in supervised exercise classes had better outcomes than those who tried exercise on their own. The motivation, support, and structure of classes seem to help people exercise more frequently and at higher intensity.

taking a class you enjoy will also increase the likelihood that you will exercise consistently. On the other hand, people who exercise alone are not as likely to exercise regularly. Making exercise fun gives your brain a non-food reward and helps you get addicted to exercise. This is the kind of addiction that you can benefit from. The good feeling you get from exercise activates dopamine reward circuits in the brain, which I discuss in chapter 5.

Push Yourself to Work Out Harder

Even with regular exercise, it is important to challenge yourself. As you push your body harder, you will become stronger and healthier. Each time you work out, try to go a little further or faster.

- Add 5–10 minutes of extra exercise to your daily workout.
- Add in a few short sprints.
- Increase the elevation on the treadmill.
- Increase treadmill speed.
- Play a team sport.
- Power-walk up hills.
- Take a boot camp class.
- Use a trainer who pushes you a little harder.
- Work out with a competitive friend.
- Work out twice on the weekends.
- Add a few pounds of extra weight to your resistance routine.
- Add an extra mini-workout at lunch.

Get Enough Sleep

Your Internal Clock

The body has a built-in biological time clock that influences most of our basic functions, including the sleep and wake cycle. The hypothalamus, which regulates hormone production through the pituitary gland, also contains the master circadian clock. Organs throughout the body, including fat cells, the stomach and intestines, liver, heart, eyes, and the immune system, have their own circadian clocks. Glands like the thyroid gland, adrenal gland, testicles, and ovaries also have their own clocks that are responsible for the natural rhythms of hormones throughout the day. A healthy balance of hormones requires all of the body's clocks to be synchronized. Anything that disturbs the biological timekeeping system can have a detrimental impact on hormones, metabolism, and weight.

Many people who work outside of traditional hours have a disrupted sleep/ wake cycle. When there are chronic or episodic periods of disturbed sleep, the circadian rhythm is affected, causing a misalignment between the brain and the body. Hormonal problems leading to weight gain and slow metabolism can occur when the biological clock is out of sync. The hypothalamus synchronizes the brain with the body, maintaining the proper ebb and flow of various hormones throughout the day and night.

Melatonin and cortisol are two hormones important in the sleep/wake cycle. Melatonin, produced by the pineal gland in the brain, increases about two hours before bedtime and decreases shortly before waking. So normally, melatonin levels are low during the day and higher at night. If sleep or waking up occurs at the wrong time, melatonin can be too high or too low. The circadian clock must be reset on a daily basis. Melatonin, light, and darkness help keep biological rhythms in sync. Cortisol is discussed in chapter 11.

Poor Sleep Makes You Hungry

It is well known that when people don't get enough sleep, they eat more calories than when they're well rested and not under stress. Poor-quality sleep stimulates the hungry hormones neuropeptide Y (chapter 5) and ghrelin (chapter 5), boosting appetite and increasing cravings for unhealthy "comfort foods" like ice cream and fast food. Sleep problems also cause insulin resistance (chapter 6), especially in brain cells. Glucose can't get into brain cells, which leads to sugar cravings. Chronic stress increases cortisol (chapter 11), further stimulating appetite and slowing metabolism. Studies have also shown that stress can lead to overeating

Stress and Your Sleep

Stress affects every aspect of your life, including your appetite, your mood, your energy level, your level of anxiety, and your sleep. A study by Kaiser Permanente Center for Health Research highlights the importance of stress and sleep on your weight. Researchers found that getting six to eight hours of sleep and reducing stress increases the likelihood of weight loss success. The study examined 472 adults in their fifties who attended group counseling sessions, followed a healthy diet, and exercised regularly. After six months, the majority of the participants had lost weight, but the most successful dieters reported that they had better sleep and lower levels of stress. Those who slept more than eight hours or less than six hours each night had less success losing weight. Weight loss was linked to reductions in depression and stress over time.

high-fat, high-sugar foods as a form of coping. These foods trigger the same regions of the brain as drugs—meaning that these foods can be addictive.

Get Better Sleep to Decrease Appetite and Cravings

Seventy million Americans either don't get enough sleep or have difficulty sleeping. A good night's sleep is one the best things you can do to balance your hormones and achieve permanent weight loss. Make it a priority to get seven to nine hours of quality sleep every night. Make it a habit to get to bed on time.

If you struggle with insomnia, you don't need to take a sleeping pill to get to sleep. Nondrug therapy, known as sleep hygiene, is the best approach to better sleep. The first step is to establish healthy sleep habits and to adhere to a regular sleep and wake schedule. Having healthy sleep habits is just as important as eating healthy foods and exercising regularly.

- Keep a regular sleep and wake cycle.

- Start winding down two hours before bedtime.

- Take a hot bath or a shower in the evening.

- Get to bed on time.

- Reserve your bedroom for sleeping and do other activities in another room.

- Keep your bedroom cool and dark.
- Avoid turning on lights if you wake up in the night.
- Exercise regularly, but not two hours before bedtime.
- Don't drink caffeinated beverages after noon.
- Don't take naps.

When Sleep Hygiene Isn't Enough

Because having quality sleep is so vital for your health and hormonal balance, I sometimes recommend medications if traditional sleep hygiene doesn't get the desired results.

Melatonin

Melatonin is a supplement that can be helpful for sleep because when taken before bedtime it can help reset a misaligned circadian clock. The usual dose is 1–6 milligrams (mg) taken one to two hours before bedtime. Side effects can include headache and drowsiness in the morning. There isn't convincing evidence that putting melatonin under your tongue is better than swallowing it. Melatonin seems to work when natural melatonin levels are low. If the body is already making enough melatonin, taking more will have little influence on sleep. The main side effects of melatonin are nausea, fatigue, and sleepiness.

Ramelteon (Rozerem)

Ramelton is a medication that mimics the effects of melatonin. It can be helpful when medications are needed because it doesn't seem to cause sedation or affect weight. Ramelteon is not like a regular sleeping pill. It takes several weeks to start working and must be taken every night at bedtime.

Sleeping Pills

Although pills are not the first choice for treating sleeping problems, they can be helpful for some people. Short-acting medications are preferred, because longer-acting medications can lead to sedation during the day.

Alcohol Disturbs Sleep

Many people use alcohol to help them fall asleep, but this can backfire. If you have a nightcap or drink a glass of wine before bedtime, you may drift off to sleep and then wake up suddenly around 2:00 or 3:00 A.M. when the drink wears off.

Dim the Lights in the Evening and Use Bright Lights in the Morning

Light has a powerful influence on the human timekeeping system. Light exposure throughout the day and darkness at night help maintain circadian rhythms. The timing, intensity, and color of light all have influences. Bright lights close to bedtime can shift the circadian clock, leading to insomnia or poor-quality sleep. Research from Harvard University Medical School has shown that keeping the lights on before bedtime can suppress levels of melatonin, leading to poor sleep and other health problems. Melatonin is a hormone known to regulate sleep, but it also has influences on blood pressure, blood sugar, and body temperature. Dimming the lights for an hour or two before bedtime can enhance melatonin levels significantly. Brighter light in the morning, particularly blue light, signals the internal clock that it is time to wake up. Several studies have shown that 15–20 minutes of bright light exposure in the morning can improve mood and alertness and can help reset a misaligned circadian clock.

Avoid Antihistamine Sleeping Pills

Most over-the-counter sleeping pills are antihistamine medications that have a side effect of making you sleepy. These medications tend to cause weight gain and can lead to excessive daytime sedation.

Do You Have a Sleep Disorder?

If you have a sleep disorder, you can diet and exercise and you still might not lose weight. I have worked with many patients who struggled with losing even a single pound because an underlying sleep disorder was preventing them from losing weight. In fact, sleep disorders are a leading cause of weight gain. Many studies have linked sleep disorders, especially sleep apnea, to weight gain, increased hunger, and sugar cravings.

Sleep disorders cause disrupted sleep and are a major cause of weight gain. If you feel tired all the time, have unrestful sleep, or have been told that you snore, you should see your physician right away.

The Epworth Sleepiness Scale

If you have excessive daytime sleepiness, you could have sleep apnea. The Epworth Sleepiness Scale is a test to determine how sleepy you are. It is a validated way to measure your degree of sleepiness. The questionnaire describes eight everyday situations for which you rate your chances of dozing off or falling asleep on a scale of 0 to 3.

0   Would never doze
1   Slight chance of dozing
2   Moderate chance of dozing
3   High chance of dozing

Situation	Score
Sitting and reading	0 1 2 3
Watching television	0 1 2 3
Sitting inactive in a public place—for example, a theater or meeting	0 1 2 3
Lying down to rest in the afternoon when circumstances permit	0 1 2 3
Sitting and talking to someone	0 1 2 3
Sitting quietly after lunch without alcohol	0 1 2 3
In a car, while stopped for a few minutes in traffic	0 1 2 3
As a passenger in a car for an hour without a break	0 1 2 3
TOTAL SCORE	_ _ _ _

An ESS score of 10 or more suggests that you have excessive daytime sleepiness, which may be caused by a sleep disorder. Any score of 10 or above requires evaluation by your physician.

Sleep Apnea

Sleep apnea is a serious, possibly life-threatening condition that is caused by closure of the airway during sleep, resulting in frequent short episodes of waking up, which then leads to excessive daytime sleepiness. A person with sleep apnea is usually not aware of the condition, except for the symptoms that linger on into the day. The main symptoms of sleep apnea are severe fatigue and daytime sleepiness. The fatigue and sleepiness can be severe enough to cause one

Do You Have Shift-Work Disorder?

One in five Americans works outside of normal hours, which causes disruptions in normal circadian rhythms. Many people who work at night or start their days early in the morning have insomnia or excessive sleepiness that can contribute to increased appetite and decreased metabolism. Features of shift-work disorder include:

Working shifts or outside of a traditional work schedule

Difficulty staying awake when you should be awake

Difficulty staying asleep when you should be asleep

Negative impact on your work, home, or social life

In shift-work disorder, the circadian clock is unable to adapt to the work and sleep schedule. This misalignment results in excessive sleepiness and lower metabolism and increases the risk for heart disease, depression, gastrointestinal disorders, infertility, and some cancers. Animal studies have shown dramatic increases in obesity when they are subjected to simulated shift work schedules.

to fall asleep at the wheel while driving. Symptoms may include loud snoring, awakening with gasping, choking, or breath holding, weight gain, depression, anxiety, memory loss, sexual dysfunction, and restless legs. Headaches, especially in the morning, are common. Sleep apnea is linked to high blood pressure, heart rhythm disturbances, heart attack, and stroke and sudden death. Sleep is not restful, and it is hard to wake up in the morning. People with sleep apnea commonly say that they are too tired to exercise.

The risk of sleep apnea is three times higher in men than in women, but the gender gap decreases after women reach menopause. Pregnant women are also at increased risk for sleep apnea. Having insulin resistance, elevated cortisol, low thyroid, high growth hormone, or increased belly fat increases the risk for sleep apnea. Sinus problems, allergies, smoking, and drinking alcohol can contribute to sleep apnea. Sleep apnea increases the risk for heart disease, lung disease, high blood pressure, and sudden death. Many of my patients with sleep apnea are hungry all the time and too tired to exercise. They gain more and more weight, further worsening sleep apnea. Sleep apnea has been linked to blood sugar abnormalities and even diabetes. In one study, patients who were treated for sleep apnea showed dramatic changes in body weight and diabetes control.

Sleep apnea is diagnosed by a sleep study or polysomnography. This test is conducted in a sleep lab, where simultaneous measurements of heart, brain, muscle, and breathing activity are monitored and measured. Treatment for sleep apnea includes weight loss, sleeping on your side or stomach, dental appliances, and various breathing devices such as CPAP, BiPAP, or AutoPap. Modafinil (Provigil) and armodafinil (Nuvigil) are nonamphetamine wakefulness-promoting agents used to treat excessive sleepiness in patients with sleep apnea, narcolepsy, and shift-work disorder. They tend to cause modest weight loss. Other side effects include headache and risk for allergic reaction. Surgery is also an option for patients with severe sleep apnea, but in my experience, without weight loss, sleep apnea surgery has a low success rate.

Reduce Your Exposure to Chemicals That Disrupt Hormones

We are being exposed to an increasing number of chemicals. In the past two decades scientists have begun to develop an understanding of how these chemicals can interfere with hormonal balance. The U.S. Environmental Protection Agency has labeled a hormone-disrupting chemical as any "exogenous agent that interferes with . . . natural blood-borne hormones that are present in the body." Endocrine-disrupting chemicals were formally recognized as a public health concern by Congress in 1996 with the Food Quality Protection Act and Safe Drinking Water Act. Despite this, currently there is no comprehensive approach to regulation of endocrine-disrupting chemicals in the United States.

Hormone-disrupting chemicals work in different ways, many of which can cause increased appetite, fat cell growth, and weight gain. These chemicals can interfere with virtually every hormone, including thyroid hormone, estrogen, testosterone, and insulin. Endocrine-disrupting chemicals contaminate and concentrate in food during storage. They are contained in household products that accumulate in dust and can be absorbed through the skin. Chemicals can even be inhaled.

We know that eating too much food and not getting enough exercise is the main cause of weight gain. But hormone-disrupting chemicals play a role in making you more susceptible to gaining weight by increasing appetite, lowering metabolism, and stimulating fat cells to grow larger and multiply. Experts

Endocrine-Disrupting Chemicals Are Everywhere

Drinking water can contain trace amounts of chemicals and pharmaceuticals.

Food can be contaminated with pesticides and other chemicals.

Meat can contain polychlorinated biphenyls (PCBs) and animal hormones.

Seafood can contain mercury and other obesity-promoting chemicals.

Preservatives, additives, and food colorings can disrupt hormones.

Cans and plastic containers leach out bisphenol A (BPA) and other contaminants.

Pollution and secondhand smoke have been linked to obesity.

Antibacterial soap contains chemicals that can interfere with thyroid hormone.

call these chemicals "obesogens" because they make people gain weight. In our society, it is impractical to completely stay away from chemicals. However, there is a lot you can do to reduce your exposure.

Toxins Accumulate in Body Fat

Environmental toxins concentrate in body fat and accumulate over time. Losing weight will release these toxins back into your body. This can result in feeling lousy, like having the flu or feeling very tired. Metabolism may slow down, and your weight loss momentum may stall. The best way to eliminate built-up toxins is to drink plenty of water, at least 2 quarts daily, and to exercise regularly. Drinking more water will help dilute the toxins and get them out of your body more quickly. Exercise also helps your body eliminate toxins faster.

Natural Endocrine Disruptors

Although most endocrine disruptors are synthetic chemicals, natural compounds can also interfere with hormones. Vegetables like broccoli, cabbage, and radishes contain a compound that can block thyroid function (see chapter 7). Soy contains compounds that can inhibit thyroid hormones in addition to disrupting male and female hormone balance.

Lead

Lead paint was banned in the 1970s, and leaded gasoline has been banned for many years. However, lead contamination remains a serious concern. Many buildings built before the 1970s still contain lead paint. Today, 1.4 percent of children have high amounts of lead in their blood. Lead toxicity is a major concern for children because it can cause brain damage and other neurological problems.

BPA and Phthalates Cause Weight Gain and Other Hormone Disruptions

Bisphenol A and phthalates are hormone-disrupting chemicals found in plastics, plasticizers, dental fillings, cash register receipts, and other products. These compounds are most notorious for mimicking the effects of estrogen and blocking the effects of testosterone. Even products labeled as BPA-free can contain similar chemicals that do just as much harm. According to the National Health and Nutrition Examination Survey, more than 90 percent of Americans have detectable BPA their urine.

These substances are also known obesogens and have been linked to weight gain, insulin resistance, and diabetes. BPA and phthalates have also been linked to infertility, early puberty (see chapter 8), attention deficit/hyperactivity disorder, autism, cardiovascular disease, liver disease, breast cancer, and prostate cancer. There is some conflicting data about the effect of BPA. A study from China, for example, did not confirm a previously reported association between urinary BPA levels and type 2 diabetes.

BPA and phthalates contaminate food and beverages when foods and beverages are stored in cans and plastic containers. Avoid plastic containers by storing perishables in glass or stainless steel containers. One can now purchase

Your Drinking Water Should Be Free of Contaminants

Although most drinking water is clean, it can be contaminated with hundreds of chemicals and pharmaceuticals. I recommend drinking filtered water that has been stored in a glass container.

BPA-free plastics, and some companies are using BPA-free linings for their cans; however, little is known about the endocrine-disrupting potential of these new products. It is possible they have the same or even more potential to disrupt the endocrine system. Studies have shown that eating fresh foods will reduce BPA levels by more than 50 percent. Fresh vegetables wrapped in plastic wrap ironically also contain a lot of BPA. Whenever possible, buy fresh vegetables that aren't wrapped in plastic. Never microwave in plastic containers. Heating a plastic container increases the amount of chemicals leached into food. Automatic coffee makers may have BPA in the tubing. Use an old-fashioned percolator or a French press instead. BPA is in dust that settles on countertops and cookware. Always rinse knives and cookware with running water before using them. You should wipe off countertops frequently. Thermal cash register receipts also contain BPA. You should throw them away instead of keeping them around. Scan them or photocopy them if you need a record.

Tributyltin Is a Weight Gain Chemical in Seafood and Drinking Water

Tributyltin is a chemical that is well known to cause weight gain. It is found in fungicidal paint used on the bottoms of boats and in polyvinyl chloride (PVC) pipe. Studies have found that tributyltin stimulates fat cells to grow larger and multiply, in addition to increasing appetite, blocking estrogen, and raising cortisol production. No one really knows how much tributylin from the bottoms of boats is contaminating the seafood we eat. And we aren't sure whether the tributyltin in PVC pipe truly poses a risk. However, there is cause for concern, because even tiny amounts of this potent obesogen can cause weight gain.

Pesticides Contaminate Fruits and Vegetables

Organophosphates are chemicals used in insecticides and pesticides that can contaminate vegetables and fruits. Green leafy vegetables as well as fruits and vegetables with thin skins absorb the most toxins. Washing does not remove all the toxins. Therefore, I recommend buying organic vegetables and fruits whenever practical. Whether organic or not, make sure to wash all vegetables and fruits thoroughly.

Hormones in Meat and Dairy Products

There is widespread use of hormones in cattle and other animals to make them produce more milk or meat. Animal hormones are thought to be specific to a certain species. But no one really knows whether animal hormones may have a

Worst and Best Fruits and Vegetables for Pesticide Contamination

The Dirty Dozen: The Worst

Apples	Grapes (imported)	Nectarines	Spinach
Blueberries	Kale/collard greens	Peaches	Strawberries
Celery	Lettuce	Potatoes	Sweet bell peppers

Vegetables and Fruits Lowest in Pesticides: The Best

Asparagus	Eggplant	Mushrooms	Sweet peas
Avocados	Grapefruit	Onions	Sweet potatoes
Cabbage	Kiwi	Pineapples	Watermelon
Cantaloupe	Mangoes	Sweet corn	

Source: Environmental Working Group

small effect in people. You should reduce your exposure to animal hormones by eating lean, hormone-free meat and dairy products.

PCBs Are Still a Concern

Even though polychlorinated biphenyls were banned in the 1970s, they remain in our environment. For fifty years PCBs were widely used as lubricants and solvents and were used in electrical equipment, lighting, insulation, oil-based paint, and floor finish. PCBs cause a variety of hormone disruptions, including causing insulin and leptin resistance. PCBs increase inflammation and directly stimulate appetite centers in the brain. They have been shown in numerous

MSG Makes You Hungry

A study from the University of North Carolina at Chapel Hill found that monosodium glutamate (MSG) caused weight gain. Scientists don't know why MSG causes weight gain but suspect that the flavor-enhancing properties of MSG boost appetite and cause leptin resistance.

Worst and Best Fruits and Vegetables for Pesticide Contamination

High Mercury

Mackerel (King)	Shark	Swordfish	Tilefish

Intermediate Mercury

Chilean bass	Halibut	Mackerel (Spanish)	Tuna
Grouper	Lobster	Orange roughy	

Low Mercury

Anchovies	Crawfish	Pollock	Tilapia
Catfish	Haddock	Salmon	Trout
Clams	Herring	Scallops	
Cod	Oysters	Shrimp	
Crab	Perch	Squid	

Source: Adapted from www.fda.gov

studies to make fat cells to grow larger and cause other cells to turn into fat cells. People who are exposed to PCBs are at increased risk for type 2 diabetes and cardiovascular disease.

If you live or work in an older building, you should make sure you don't go near any old electrical equipment, especially old fluorescent light ballasts, which can contain PCBs. However, it turns out that the main way most people get exposed to PCBs is by eating fatty meat. PCBs are in our environment. Animals, especially grazing cattle, consume PCBs, which primarily concentrate in their fat. People who eat less fatty meat are known to have lower PCB levels in their blood.

Eat Low-Mercury Seafood

There has been a lot of concern about mercury in fish. For most people, eating fish is the main way the body is exposed to mercury. The mercury in fish is a potent neurotoxin. It is best to eat less fish with high mercury content, like mackerel, shark, and swordfish, and to eat more seafood with lower mercury content. A good rule of thumb is the larger the fish, the higher the mercury content.

> ## Pollution and Secondhand Smoke Linked to Obesity
>
> Researchers from the University of Southern California, Los Angeles, have found that breathing air pollution from cars and trucks as well as breathing secondhand smoke increases the risk for obesity. They speculate that pollutants in smoke increase inflammation, leading to leptin resistance and insulin resistance.

Fiber Helps Rid the Body of Chemicals

Eating high-fiber foods will decrease your exposure and help you eliminate toxins and chemicals from your body. A high-fiber diet helps your bowels move more efficiently, so that the chemicals in food have less time to be absorbed. Eating more fresh fruits and vegetables and other high-fiber foods has been shown to increase excretion of toxins. A high-fiber diet reduces the risk many other ailments, including colon cancer. You don't need to purchase supplements to cleanse your body. To flush out chemicals, eat a lot of high-fiber foods like fruits, vegetables, and whole grains. High-fiber cereals can be helpful as well. You should eat around 25–35 grams of fiber daily.

Wash Your Hands with Regular Soap

A study from Boston University School of Public Health found that washing the hands for 20 seconds under lukewarm running water at least four times daily reduced levels of chemicals in the bloodstream. The chemical triclosan, found in antibacterial soap and some brands of toothpaste, acts as an endocrine disruptor by decreasing production of thyroid hormone, estrogen, and testosterone. Regular soap is just as effective in killing the germs on your hands without the endocrine-disrupting effect.

Hormone Disorders
A Guide to Symptoms

The table following is designed to help you determine whether your symptoms are associated with a particular hormone problem. A single symptom can be nonspecific and may be associated with a variety of possible problems.

The following is a key to the abbreviations used in the chart:

DM	Type 2 diabetes (Chapter 6)
IR	Insulin resistance (Chapter 6)
RH	Reactive hypoglycemia (Chapter 3)
IN	Insulinoma (Chapter 3)
MH	Male hypogonadism (Chapter 10)
PCOS	Polycystic ovary syndrome (Chapter 8)
VIR	Virilism (Chapter 8)
MP	Menopausal or perimenopausal (Chapter 9)
HT	Hypothyroidism (Chapter 7)
CS	Cushing's syndrome (Chapter 11)
PC	Pseudo-Cushing's (Chapter 11)
GHD	Growth hormone deficiency (Chapter 12)
ACR	Acromegaly (Chapter 12)

Hormone Disorder Symptom Table	DM	IR	RH	IN	MH	PCOS	VIR	MP	HT	CS	PC	GHD	ACR
Acanthosis nigricans	X	X				X	X			X	X		X
Aches and pains								X	X			X	X
Acne	X	X				X	X			X	X		
Aggressiveness							X			X			
Allergies/Hives									X				
Anemia					X				X			X	
Anger				X	X	X	X						X
Anxiety			X	X	X	X		X	X	X	X	X	
Appetite, decreased									X				
Appetite, increased	X	X	X	X		X				X	X		X
Attention deficit disorder									X				
Binge eating	X	X				X				X	X		X
Bloating						X		X	X	X	X		
Blood clots	X	X					X			X			X
Body odor, excessive							X						X
Bone problems					X			X		X		X	X
Breast milk production					X	X		X	X				X
Bruising									X				
Buffalo hump										X	X		
Carbohydrate cravings	X	X	X			X				X	X		
Cardiovascular disease	X	X	X	X	X	X	X	X	X	X	X	X	X
Carpal tunnel syndrome	X								X				X
Cheeks red								X		X			
Cheeks round	X	X								X	X		
Circulation problems	X	X						X		X			X
Colon cancer	X	X				X		X					X
Concentration problems			X	X				X		X		X	X
Confusion				X									
Constipation									X				

Hormone Disorder Symptom Table	DM	IR	RH	IN	MH	PCOS	VIR	MP	HT	CS	PC	GHD	ACR
Decreased endurance					X			X	X	X		X	
Decreased quality of life	X	X	X	X	X	X	X	X	X	X	X	X	X
Decreased sense of well being	X	X	X	X	X	X	X	X	X	X	X	X	X
Depression					X	X	X	X	X	X	X	X	X
Deterioration in work performance				X	X			X	X	X	X	X	X
Diabetes	X	X	X			X		X		X			X
Difficulty concentrating				X	X			X	X	X	X	X	X
Difficulty relating to others					X			X	X	X	X	X	
Dry skin					X			X	X			X	
Edema								X	X	X			X
Eyebrows thinner									X				
Face round (moon face)	X	X								X	X		
Facial puffiness									X	X	X		
Family history of diabetes	X	X				X					X		
Family history of heart disease		X				X							
Family history of high blood pressure		X				X							
Family history of thyroid problems									X				
Fat over the collar bones										X	X		
Fatigue	X	X	X	X	X	X	X	X	X	X	X	X	X
Feeling cold									X			X	
Fingernails brittle									X				
Fluid retention									X	X	X		
Flushing					X			X					
Fractures					X			X		X		X	
Gaps between teeth													X
Goiter									X				X
Gout	X	X									X		
Growth of hands or feet													X
Hair falling out (body)					X				X				

Hormone Disorder Symptom Table	DM	IR	RH	IN	MH	PCOS	VIR	MP	HT	CS	PC	GHD	ACR
Hair falling out (head)								X	X	X	X		
Hair thin					X			X					
Head injury					X				X			X	
Headaches			X	X	X		X			X		X	
Heart disease	X	X				X		X		X	X	X	X
Heart failure									X			X	X
Heart palpitations			X	X									
Heartburn										X			
High blood pressure	X	X				X	X	X	X	X	X		X
High carb food preference	X	X	X			X					X		
High fat food preference	X	X				X					X		
High LDL (bad) cholesterol	X	X				X	X	X	X	X	X		X
High stress	X	X	X			X		X			X		
High triglycerides	X	X				X	X	X		X	X		
Hot flashes					X			X					
Hunger, excessive	X	X	X	X		X				X	X		X
Inability to lose weight	X	X	X	X	X	X	X	X	X	X	X	X	X
Increased body fat	X	X		X	X	X		X	X	X	X	X	
Increased fat in the belly	X	X			X	X		X		X	X	X	
Infections, frequent	X									X			
Infertility	X	X		X	X	X	X	X	X	X			X
Insomnia								X		X			X
Irritability				X				X	X			X	
Joint aches								X	X			X	X
Kidney disease	X	X				X	X			X			X
Kidney stones										X			
Libido, decreased					X		X	X		X		X	X
Liver disease						X	X			X	X	X	X
Loss of consciousness				X									
Loss of zest for life					X			X	X	X	X	X	

Hormone Disorder Symptom Table	DM	IR	RH	IN	MH	PCOS	VIR	MP	HT	CS	PC	GHD	ACR
Low HDL (good) cholesterol	X	X				X	X	X		X	X	X	X
Low potassium	X						X			X			
Memory loss				X				X	X	X		X	X
Mood swings					X	X	X	X	X	X	X		
Muscle wasting					X					X		X	
Muscle weakness					X				X	X		X	
Nausea				X									
Numbness or tingling	X			X						X			
Osteoporosis or osteopenia					X			X		X		X	
Overeating	X	X								X			X
Peripheral vascular disease	X	X						X					X
Personality changes				X			X	X		X			X
Poor general health	X	X			X	X	X	X	X	X	X	X	X
Poor wound healing	X						X			X			
Premature aging					X				X			X	
Protein in the urine	X	X			X								X
Sedentary lifestyle	X	X			X						X		
Seizure				X									
Sense of well-being, decreased					X			X				X	
Skin tags	X	X			X					X	X		X
Skin, darker	X	X			X					X	X		
Skin, pale					X				X			X	
Skin, red									X	X			
Skin, thin									X	X		X	
Skin, yellow									X				
Sleep apnea									X	X	X		X
Sleeping too much					X			X	X			X	
Slow reflexes									X				
Sluggishness in the afternoons	X	X	X					X		X	X	X	
Sluggishness in the morning								X		X			

Hormone Disorder Symptom Table	DM	IR	RH	IN	MH	PCOS	VIR	MP	HT	CS	PC	GHD	ACR
Smoke cigarettes		X						X					
Snoring									X	X	X		X
Social isolation					X	X						X	
Stomach ulcers										X			
Stretch marks, pink or white										X	X		
Stretch marks, red or purple										X			
Stretch marks, wider than 1/2 inch											X		
Strokes	X	X						X					X
Stuffy nose									X				
Sweating, decreased										X			
Sweating, increased									X		X	X	
Thin arms and legs										X	X		
Thirst, excessive	X									X			
Unrestful sleep								X					
Urinary incontinence								X					
Urination, frequent	X									X			
Vision problems	X									X			X
Vision, blurred	X			X									
Voice, deeper							X		X				
Weight gain	X	X	X	X	X	X	X	X	X	X	X	X	X
Weight loss					X		X					X	
Female Only													
Balding							X			X			
Birth to child over 10 pounds	X	X											
Breast cancer	X	X				X							X
Breast shrinkage							X			X			
Enlargement of the clitoris							X			X			
Extensive muscle growth							X			X			

Hormone Disorder Symptom Table	DM	IR	RH	IN	MH	PCOS	VIR	MP	HT	CS	PC	GHD	ACR
Hirsutism	X	X				X	X	X		X	X		
Infections, urinary	X							X		X			
Infections, yeast	X									X			
Menstrual problems	X	X				X	X	X	X	X	X		
Neck circumference more than 13½ inch	X	X				X				X	X		
Pain with intercourse						X	X	X					
PMS						X	X	X	X	X	X		
Pregnancy, weight gain (excessive)	X	X				X							
Premature menopause									X				
Uterine cancer	X	X				X							X
Vaginal dryness								X					
Waistline greater than 35 inches	X	X				X	X			X	X		
Male Only													
Breast growth					X					X	X	X	
Decreased sexual performance	X	X							X	X	X	X	X
Erectile dysfunction					X					X			
Infertility					X					X			
Less body hair					X								
Neck circumference more than 14½ inches	X	X								X	X		
Prostate cancer	X	X											X
Shaving less					X								
Softening of the testicles					X								
Softening of the voice					X								
Waistline greater than 40 inches	X	X								X	X		

7-Day Meal Plan

For precise calories and quantities, see chapter 4.

The asterisked (*) items are included in the recipes in the next section.

Day 1

Breakfast

1 slice whole grain bread

1 ounce low-fat cheese

1 hardboiled egg (or 2 hardboiled egg whites)

1 cup Greek yogurt

2 cups strawberries

Lunch

Chicken with Broccoli*

1/2 cup whole grain pasta

1 banana

Mid-Afternoon Snack

2 ounces cut-up chicken breast

Supper

4 ounces lean turkey burger

1/2 cup brown rice

2 cups of mixed vegetables

Large green salad

Creamy Herb Dressing*

Dessert

1 cup fresh pineapple cubes

Day 2

Breakfast

1 cup whole-grain protein cereal

1/2 cup skim milk (pour on cereal)

1 large apple

2 scrambled egg whites

Lunch

1 large green salad

4 ounces grilled lean chicken or steak

Herb Vinaigrette*

1 cup steamed broccoli

1 cup berries

Mid-Afternoon Snack

Protein smoothie with fruit

Supper

Baked Salmon in Parchment with
    Lime and Cilantro*

1 small baked potato with skin

Steamed zucchini and onions

Steamed carrots

Large green salad

Creamy Herb Dressing*

Dessert

1 cup of cubed cantaloupe

Day 3

Breakfast

Egg white omelet with chopped
    vegetables

1 grapefruit

1 slice whole grain bread

Lunch

Black beans

1/2 cup brown rice

Grilled mushrooms, onions, and
    peppers

Mid-Afternoon Snack

2 hardboiled egg whites

Supper

Wild Rice and Chicken Salad with
    Broccoli Cole Slaw*

1 cup each steamed cauliflower and
    green beans

Large green salad

Dessert

1 cup protein breakfast cereal

1/2 cup skim milk (pour on cereal)

Day 4

Breakfast

1 cup steel-cut oatmeal or protein
    oatmeal

1 ounce chopped nuts

1/2 cup fat-free cottage cheese

1 cup blueberries

Lunch

Middle Eastern Salad with Lemon
    Garlic Dressing*

4 ounces grilled chicken

Mid-Afternoon Snack

Can of tuna (packed in water)

Supper

Honey-Orange Chicken*

1/2 cup pasta

Vegetarian Pasta Sauce*

Large green salad

Herb Vinaigrette*

Dessert

Low calorie frozen dessert (Skinny
    Cow, WeightWatchers, and
    so on)

Day 5

Breakfast

Egg white scramble with chopped
    vegetables

1 small pita bread or bagel thin

2 ounces lean chicken sausage or
    turkey sausage

1 cup honeydew cubes

Lunch

Vegetable soup

One-half sandwich:
    1 slice whole grain bread
    1 ounce low-fat cheese
    2 ounces turkey
    Lettuce and tomato
    Mustard

Red Cabbage and Apples*

Mid-Afternoon Snack

Cucumber rounds with Sour Cream
    and Chutney*

Supper

Charbroiled Tuna with Oregano
    Mango Sauce*

1/2 cup brown rice

Large green salad

Herb Vinaigrette*

1 cup steamed spinach

Dessert

1 cup grapes

Day 6

Breakfast

1 cup unsweetened cereal

1/2 cup skim milk

1 banana

1 hardboiled egg (or 2 hardboiled egg
  whites)

Lunch

4 ounces grilled chicken or fish

Roasted Red Pepper Sauce*

Green Beans with Dill*

1/2 cup brown rice

1 pear

Mid-Afternoon Snack

Boiled shrimp

Supper

4 ounces grilled tuna

1/2 cup quinoa

Sautéed Sugar Snap Peas*

Large green salad

1 cup Greek yogurt

Dessert

2 peaches

Day 7

Breakfast

1 cup fat-free cottage cheese

1 apple

1 slice Canadian bacon

1 cup Greek yogurt

Lunch

4 ounces grilled fish

Beans (black, pinto, navy, and so on)

1/2 cup wild rice

Mid-Afternoon Snack

Protein fruit smoothie

Supper

4–6 ounces lean grilled beef, chicken,
  or pork

Roasted Asparagus with Mushrooms
  and Onions*

1 baked sweet potato with skin

Sautéed Sugar Snap Peas*

Large green salad

Dessert

1 cup berries

Recipes

Chicken with Broccoli

Yield: Makes 4 servings

2	Whole chicken breasts, skinned and boned
2	Egg yolks
1½ cups	Chicken broth
1 Tablespoon	Olive oil
1 clove	Garlic, minced (optional)
8 stalks	Broccoli
1 teaspoon	Sea salt
	Fresh ground black pepper
1 Tablespoon	Lemon juice (optional)
2	Lemons, quartered
8 ounces	Chicken broth

1. Slice chicken breasts into 4 lengthwise strips.

2. Beat egg yolks in a non-metal bowl with chicken broth. Stir together. Coat chicken with this egg mixture.

3. Heat olive oil and garlic (optional) to foaming in a sauté pan or skillet. Add chicken strips and cook over medium heat until golden brown on all sides. This will take about 4 minutes.

4. With a chef's knife cut the tops off the broccoli (2-inch florets). Chop coarsely.

5. Remove chicken from pan to a warm dish; put broccoli into pan over medium heat, stir in remaining chicken broth and lemon juice (optional). Catch all the cooked bits in the pan with your spoon. Cook broccoli for about 5 minutes. Season to taste.

6. Place chicken and broccoli together on plates. Pour sauce from pan over broccoli and garnish with quartered lemons.

Nutritional Analysis

Per serving: 190 calories. 7 g fat, 18 g protein, 16 g carbohydrates

---

Creamy Herb Dressing

Yield: Makes 6 servings

1/2 cup	Low-calorie mayonnaise
1/4 cup	Plain nonfat yogurt
1/4 cup	Parsley, minced
1 teaspoon	Chives, minced
2 Tablespoons	Apple cider vinegar
1 dash	Sea salt
1 dash	Black pepper
1/2 Tablespoon	Fresh basil, minced
1 clove	Garlic, minced

Blend all the ingredients until smooth. Makes about 1¼ cups.

Note: Snappy and low in calories. This dressing is also good on coleslaw or broccoli slaw.

Nutritional Analysis

Per serving: 70 calories. 6 g fat, 1 g protein, 3 g carbohydrates

---

Herb Vinaigrette

Yield: Makes 4 servings

3 Tablespoons	Balsamic vinegar
1 Tablespoon	Rice vinegar
2 Tablespoons	Lemon juice
3 Tablespoons	Extra virgin olive oil
2 Tablespoons	Water
1 teaspoon	Dijon mustard

1 Tablespoon	Cilantro, minced
1 Tablespoon	Fresh basil, minced
1 Tablespoon	Fresh oregano, minced
1	Garlic clove, minced
Dash	Sea salt
Dash	Fresh ground pepper

1. Pour vinegars, lemon juice, and water into a small bowl.

2. Stir in mustard, herbs, and seasonings. Adjust seasonings to taste.

3. Pour in olive oil and mix.

4. Refrigerate at least one day for best results.

5. Remove from refrigerator 1 hour before using.

Nutritional Analysis

Per serving: 46 calories. 4 g fat, 0.5g protein, 2 g carbohydrates

---

Baked Salmon in Parchment
with Lime and Cilantro

Yield: Makes 4 servings

1/2 teaspoon	Safflower oil, to grease parchment
2 pounds	Salmon fillets, cut into 4 pieces
1	Garlic clove, minced
2 Tablespoons	White wine
1 Tablespoon	Lime juice
1 teaspoon	Lime zest
2 Tablespoons	Fresh cilantro
1 teaspoon	Dark sesame oil

1. Preheat oven to 350 degrees F. Lightly oil 4 sheets of parchment paper.

2. Place 1 salmon fillet on the center of each sheet.

3. In a small bowl, combine garlic, white wine, lime juice, lime zest, cilantro, and sesame oil. Spoon equal amount over each salmon fillet.

4. Roll edges of the parchment paper together to form a packet around the salmon. Bake for 12 minutes.

5. To serve, unroll parchment packets and gently slide the salmon onto plates. Spoon poaching liquid over the salmon and serve immediately.

Note: You can marinate the fish in the poaching liquid overnight before cooking. Fillets of red snapper, cod, flounder, or orange roughy also can be used with this recipe.

Nutritional Analysis

Per serving: 86 calories. 2 g fat, 16 g protein, 1 g carbohydrates

---

Wild Rice and Chicken Salad with Broccoli Cole Slaw

Yield: Makes 4 servings

Chicken salad

1/2 cup	Wild rice
1 pound	Chicken breast
1	Scallion, sliced
1 cup	Broccoli slaw
3/4 cup	Granny Smith apple, diced

Dressing

1 teaspoon	Olive oil
1½ Tablespoons	Cider vinegar
1 clove	Garlic, minced
1 teaspoon	Dijon mustard
	Salt and pepper, to taste

Broccoli slaw

1/4 cup	Fat-free sour cream
1/4 cup	2 percent buttermilk
2 Tablespoons	Cider vinegar
1 cup	Broccoli slaw
1	Granny Smith apple, large, grated
1 clove	Garlic, minced
1/2 teaspoon	Salt

1/4 teaspoon	White pepper
2 Tablespoons	Pine nuts, toasted and chopped

1. Combine broth and wild rice in a small sauce pan. Bring to a boil. Cover and simmer over medium-low heat until rice is tender and liquid is absorbed—about 50 minutes. Transfer to medium-sized glass bowl. Cover and refrigerate until well chilled.
2. Add diced cooked chicken, broccoli coleslaw, apple, scallion, and garlic to the wild rice.
3. Whisk dressing ingredients together. Pour dressing over the wild rice mixture and toss well. Season to taste with salt and pepper. Toss until coated. Sprinkle with pine nuts.

Note: Broccoli slaw mix, which consists of shredded broccoli stems, carrots, and red cabbage, is available packaged in many supermarkets. If you can't find it, you can make your own.

Nutritional Analysis

Per serving: 178 calories. 6.5 g fat, 5 g protein, 25 g carbohydrates

---

Middle Eastern Salad with Lemon Garlic Dressing

Yield: Makes 4 servings

Salad

2	Navel or Valencia oranges
1	Onion
1	Green pepper
16	Mediterranean black olives

Lemon garlic dressing

1 clove	Garlic
1 teaspoon	Paprika
1 teaspoon	Hot pepper sauce
1 Tablespoon	Lemon juice
1/4 teaspoon	Ground cumin
1/4 teaspoon	Salt
3 Tablespoons	Extra virgin olive oil

1. Grate zest from half an orange. Peel the oranges and cut them into approximately 1/4-inch-thick slices.
2. Cut the onion into thin slices. Seed and cut the green pepper into thin slices.
3. Pit the olives.
4. Combine the oranges, onion, green pepper slices, and the olives in a bowl and refrigerate until 1/2 hour before serving.

Lemon-garlic dressing preparation

Lightly crush the garlic. In a bowl, whisk together crushed garlic, paprika, hot pepper sauce, lemon juice, cumin, and salt . Gradually add olive oil, whisking constantly. Recipe can be prepared to this point several hours ahead.

Note: Pour dressing over orange and vegetable mixture and stir gently. Let stand at room temperature for 30 minutes. Remove garlic. Serve salad on lettuce and garnish with grated orange zest.

Nutritional Analysis (Salad)

Per serving: 80 calories. 2 g fat, 1.5 g protein, 14 g carbohydrates

Nutritional Analysis (Dressing)

Per serving: 95 calories. 10 g fat, 0.1 g protein, 1 g carbohydrates

---

Red Cabbage and Apples

Yield: Makes 4 servings

1/2 Tablespoon	Olive oil
2	Unpeeled yellow apples
2 cups	Chopped red cabbage
1/8 cup	Red wine

1. Heat olive oil over low heat in a sauté pan or skillet; slice apples into pan and add cabbage, stirring.
2. Cook 5 minutes over medium heat. Stir in wine.
3. Cover pan and cook 6–7 minutes.

Nutritional Analysis

Per serving: 74 calories. 2 g fat, 1 g protein, 13 g carbohydrates

Honey-Orange Chicken

Yield: Makes 4 servings

1 Tablespoon	Cornstarch
1/4 teaspoon	Salt
1/4 teaspoon	Pepper
4	Chicken breasts, halves, boneless and skinless
1½ teaspoons	Olive oil
1/4 cup	Chicken broth
1 teaspoon	Frozen orange juice concentrate
1/2 teaspoon	Dijon mustard
1/4 teaspoon	Honey
1 Tablespoon	Fresh parsley, minced
4	Orange slices

1. In a small paper bag, combine the cornstarch, salt, and pepper. Shake to mix. Add the chicken. Shake to coat evenly.

2. Remove the chicken from the bag. Save the excess cornstarch mixture.

3. In a large skillet, heat 1 Tablespoon olive oil over medium heat. Add chicken breasts and brown on one side, about 5 minutes. If needed add the remaining 1/2 Tablespoon of olive oil. Brown the second side. Transfer to a warm plate and set aside.

4. Dissolve the remaining cornstarch in the chicken broth. Whisk in orange juice concentrate, mustard, and honey. Pour in a large skillet. Bring to a boil over a medium heat, stirring often.

5. Add the chicken. Reduce the heat to low and cover the skillet. Cook until the chicken is tender.

6. Divide the chicken and sauce among 4 plates. Sprinkle with parsley and garnish with orange slices.

Nutritional Analysis

Per serving: 275 calories. 3.5 g fat, 35 g protein, 26 g carbohydrates

Vegetarian Pasta Sauce

Yield: Makes 8 servings

1 Tablespoon	Olive oil
1	Medium onion, diced
1 cup	Carrots, diced
1/2 cup	Celery, diced
1 cup	Mushrooms, sliced
1/4 cup	Green bell pepper, diced
1/4 cup	Red wine
3/4 cup	Tomato paste
3 cups	Tomatoes, chopped (fresh or canned)
3 cloves	Garlic, minced
2 Tablespoons	Fresh basil (1 Tablespoon dried)
1 Tablespoon	Fresh oregano (1/2 Tablespoon dried)
1 Tablespoon	Fresh thyme (1/2 Tablespoon dried)
1 teaspoon	Brown sugar
	Black pepper, to taste
	Salt, to taste

1. Sauté onion in olive oil until clear, add carrots, celery, and mushrooms with olive oil. Sauté for about 5 more minutes, stirring frequently.

2. Add green bell pepper and the rest of the ingredients. Simmer for 30 minutes.

3. If sauce is too thick, add water. Cook 15 minutes more, and salt and pepper to taste.

Note: Carrots, celery, and mushrooms make this tomato sauce as hearty as a meat sauce. Best if prepared one day in advance.

Serve over pasta. Can also spoon sauce over boneless chicken breast and bake.

Nutritional Analysis

Per serving: 102 calories. 4 g fat, 2.5 g protein, 14 g carbohydrates

Cucumber Rounds with Sour Cream and Chutney

Yield: Makes 4 servings

2	Cucumbers
2 Tablespoons	Lemon juice
	Sea salt
2 teaspoons	Fat-free sour cream
1 teaspoon	Chutney

1. Slice cucumbers crosswise about 1/4-inch thick.

2. Sprinkle with lemon juice. Lightly salt.

3. Top each slice with sour cream and chutney.

Note: This is a simple recipe that will help lessen the burden of coming up with that perfect little something before dinner. Place on a bed of greens to serve as a salad.

Nutritional Analysis

Per serving: 53 calories. 0.5 g fat, 2 g protein, 10 g carbohydrates

Charbroiled Tuna with Oregano Mango Sauce

Yield: Makes 4 servings

1½ pounds	Tuna steaks
Salt	
2 cloves	Garlic, minced
1	Lime, juiced
1	Mango, peeled
1 cup	2 percent milk
1/4 cup	Sherry
Lemon juice	
1 Tablespoon	Fresh oregano, minced

1. Preheat broiler.

2. Season tuna with a little salt and fresh crushed garlic. Sprinkle with lime juice. Broil for about 2 minutes on each side.

3. Blend mango into a pureé. In a saucepan, reduce milk to about half. Add mango, sherry, lemon juice, and oregano. Boil for 2 minutes.

4. Pour mango sauce over tuna. Broil 3 minutes. Serve immediately.

Nutritional Analysis

Note: Mango sauce can be stored in a glass container, refrigerated for 3 days. Per serving: 306 calories. 10 g fat, 43 g protein, 11 g carbohydrates

---

Roasted Red Pepper Sauce

Yield: Makes 6 servings

2 medium	Red bell peppers
1 Tablespoon	Olive oil
1 medium	Onion, diced
1 Tablespoon	White balsamic vinegar
2 Tablespoons	Dry white wine
1 cup	Chicken broth
1 Tablespoon	Fresh oregano, minced
1 clove	Garlic, minced
1 teaspoon	Salt
1/2 teaspoon	White pepper

1. Roast bell peppers over a gas flame, under the broiler, or on the grill, until skins blacken and blister. Cool, peel, seed, and chop bell peppers coarse; set aside.

2. Heat oil in a medium skillet. Add onions and bell peppers; sauté until onions soften, about 3 minutes. Add vinegar, simmer until vinegar evaporates, about 1 minutes. Add wine; simmer until liquid reduces to 1 tablespoon, about 2 minutes. Add broth; simmer until liquid reduces to 1/2 cup, about 10 minutes.

3. Cool slightly, then transfer to a food processor; add oregano, 1 teaspoon salt, and 1/2 teaspoon pepper; purée until smooth. Set sauce aside. (Can be cooled, covered, and refrigerated up to three days.)

To serve: Warm over low heat. Spoon a portion of sauce onto each warm dinner plate. Arrange a portion of meat or roasted veal in each pool of sauce and serve immediately.

Nutritional Analysis

Per serving: 47 calories. 2.5 g fat, 1 g protein, 5 g carbohydrates

---

Green Beans with Dill

Yield: Makes 16 servings

2 pounds	Whole green beans
1 teaspoon	Cayenne pepper powder
4 cloves	Garlic
1/4 teaspoon	Salt
4 sprigs	Fresh dill
2½ cups	Water
2 cups	Cider vinegar

1. Trim ends on the green beans.
2. Pack beans lengthwise into jars, leaving 1/4 inch head space.
3. To each pint, add 1/4 teaspoon Cayenne powder, 1 clove of garlic, and 1 sprig of dill.
4. Combine remaining ingredients and bring to boil. Pour, boiling hot, over beans, leaving 1/4-inch head space.
5. Cook 10 minutes in boiling water bath. Pour water off. Let stand covered and refrigerated 2 weeks to allow flavor to develop.

Note: Makes a terrific appetizer or snack. Also serve as a vegetable side dish.

Nutritional Analysis

Per serving: 28 calories. 0 g fat, 1 g protein, 6 g carbohydrates

Roasted Asparagus with Mushrooms and Onions

Yield: Makes 4 servings

1/2 pound	Asparagus
1	Medium white onion, sliced
4 cloves	Garlic, sliced
	Salt
	Pepper
1/2 pound	Shittake mushrooms
1/2 Tablespoon	Olive oil
1/4 cup	Balsamic vinegar

1. Preheat oven to 350 degrees F.

2. Wash and dry asparagus.

3. Evenly distribute asparagus in oblong roasting dish.

4. Top asparagus with sliced onion, mushrooms, and sliced garlic cloves. Season with salt and pepper.

5. Drizzle olive oil over the vegetables.

6. Bake in 350-degree oven for 30 minutes. Remove from oven when done.

7. Sprinkle with balsamic vinegar.

Nutritional Analysis

Per serving: 130 calories. 1 g fat, 4 g protein, 26 g carbohydrates

Sautéed Sugar Snap Peas

Yield: Makes 4 servings

2 teaspoons	Olive oil
1 pound	Sugar snap peas
2	Scallions, sliced
1 pinch	Sugar
	Salt, to taste
	Freshly ground pepper, to taste

1. In a large skillet over medium heat, heat olive oil; add sugar snap peas and scallions. Sauté, stirring frequently until tender, about 3 to 4 minutes.

2. Season to taste with sugar, salt, and pepper.

Note: Sugar snap peas remain succulent and colorful with this quick preparation.

Nutritional Analysis

Per serving: 72 calories. 2 g fat, 3.5g protein, 10 g

Shopping List

Fresh Vegetables and Fruits[1]

Apples

Artichokes

Asparagus

Bananas

Beets

Bell peppers

Blueberries

Broccoli

Brussels sprouts

Cabbage

Cantaloupe

Carrots

Cauliflower

Celery

Cherries

Cucumber

Eggplant

Grapefruit

Grapes

Green beans

Honeydew melon

Lemons

Lettuce

Mango

Mushrooms

Okra

Onions

Oranges

Peaches

Pears

Pineapple

Plums

Raspberries

Spinach

Strawberries

Tomatoes

Watermelon

Yellow squash

Zucchini

Grains and Starches

Corn

High-protein breakfast cereal

Lentils

Peas

Potatoes

Quinoa

Sweet potatoes

Steel-cut oatmeal (not instant)

Whole-grain bread

Wild rice

---

[1]Choose organic whenever possible. Purchase enough to have at least 35–70 servings per person per week. Frozen fruits and vegetables can be substituted for fresh. Canned vegetables and fruits are acceptable but not preferred, even if they're in BPA-free cans and without added sugar. Do not eat dried fruit.

Spices and Condiments

Basil	Garlic	Olive oil
Black pepper	Ginger	Oregano
Chili powder	Hot sauce	Rosemary
Cinnamon	Mint	Turmeric
Dark chocolate	Mustard	Vinegar

Lean Protein[2]

Beans	Fish	Shrimp
Chicken breast	Lean beef	Turkey breast
Chickpeas	Lentils	
Eggs	Powdered smoothie mix	

Low-Fat Dairy Products

Fat-free cottage cheese	Greek yogurt	String cheese
Fat-free sour cream	Low-fat frozen yogurt	Skim milk
Frozen dessert treats	Low-fat mozzarella	

Beverages

Coffee

Sparkling water

Tea

---

[2]Choose organic or hormone-free whenever possible.

Health and Nutrition Websites

Aetna Intelihealth   (www.intelihealth.com)
American Academy of Family Physicians   (www.familydoctor.org)
American Academy of Pediatrics   (www.aacap.org)
American Association of Retired Persons   (www.aarp.org/health)
American Diabetes Association   (www.diabetes.org)
American Heart Association   (www. americanheart.org)
Asthma and Allergy Foundation of America   (www.aafa.org)
Calorie King   (www.calorieking.com)
Centers for Disease Control and Prevention   (www.cdc.gov/healthyweight)
Cooking Light   (www.cookinglight.com)
Eating Well   (www.eatingwell.com)
eMedicine Health   (www.emedicinehealth.com)
Fruits and Vegetables Matter   (www.fruitsandveggiesmatter.gov)
Health   (www.health.com)
Hormone Foundation   (www.hormone.org)
Jillian Michaels   (www.jillianmichaels.com)
Joy Bauer   (www.joybauer.com)
Mayo Clinic   (www.mayoclinic.com)
Medline Plus   (www.nlm.nih.gov/medlineplus)
My Fitness Pal   (www.myfitnesspal.com)
National Cancer Institute   (www.cancer.gov)
National Digestive Diseases Information Clearinghouse
     (www.digestive.niddk.nih.gov)
National Heart, Lung, Blood Institute   (www.nhlbi.nih.gov)
National Institute on Aging   (www.nia.nih.gov)
National Institutes of Health   (http://health.nih.gov)
Nutrition.gov   (www.nutrition.gov)
Prevention   (www.prevention.com)
Shape   (www.shape.com)
The Cleveland Clinic   (http://my.clevelandclinic.org/health)
U.S. Department of Health and Human Services   (www.healthfinder.gov)

Bibliography

Chapter 1

Albu JB, Bray GA, Despres MJP, Pi-Sunyer FX. Obesity: Is It a Disease? If So, How Should It Be Treated? *Medical Crossfire*. 1999;Oct:35–43.

Bender R, Jockel KH, Truatner C, Spraul M, Berger M. Effect of Age on Excess Mortality in Obesity. *Journal of the American Medical Association*. 1999;281:1498–1504.

Bjorntorp P. The Regulation of Adipose Tissue Distribution in Humans. *International Journal of Obesity and Related Metabolic Disorders*. 1996;20:291–302.

Bray GA. The Epidemic of Obesity and Changes in Food Intake: The Fluoride Hypothesis. *Physiology and Behavior* 2004;Aug;82(1):115–121.

Davidson MH, Hauptman J, DiGirolamo, M, et al. Weight Control and Risk Factor Reduction in Obese Subjects Treated for Two Years with Orlistat. *Journal of the American Medical Association*. 1999;281:235–279.

Hill, J. Quoted on CNN "Study: Americans Fatter Than Ever and Getting Even Fatter." May 28, 1998. Available at: http://articles.cnn.com/1998-05-28/health/9805_28_obesity_1_obesity-highfat-foods-new-diet-drug?_s=PM:HEALTH.

Kushner R. The Treatment of Obesity: A Call for Prudence and Professionalism. *Archives of Internal Medicine*. 1997;157:602–604.

Leach HM. Popular Diets and Anthropological Myths. *New Zealand Medical Journal*. 1989;102:474–477.

Ross R, Dagnone D, Jones PJH, et al. Reduction in Obesity and Related Comorbid Conditions after Diet-Induces Weight Loss or Exercise-Induced Weight Loss in Men: A Randomized, Controlled Trial. *Annals of Internal Medicine*. 2000;133:92–103.

Trivedi AN, et al. Increased Ambulatory Care Copayments and Hospitalizations among the Elderly. *New England Journal of Medicine*. 2010;Jan 28;362(4):320–328.

Willett WC, Dietz WH, Colditz GA. Guidelines for Healthy Weight. *New England Journal of Medicine*. 1999;341:427–434.

Wright SM, Aronne LJ. Obesity in 2010: The Future of Obesity Medicine: Where Do We Go from Here? *National Review of Endocrinology*. 2011;Feb;7(2):69–70.

www.diabetes.org/diabetes-basics/diabetes-statistics/.

Chapter 2

Bantam Medical Dictionary. Bantam Medical Books, 1981.

Collins English Dictionary, Complete and Unabridged. HarperCollins, 2003.

Cypess AM, et al. Identification and Importance of Brown Adipose Tissue in Adult Humans. *New England Journal of Medicine.* 2009;Apr 9;360(15):1509–1517.

Lee P, et al. High Prevalence of Brown Adipose Tissue in Adult Humans. *Journal of Clinical Endocrinology and Metabolism.* 2011;Aug;96(8):2450–2455.

Lee P, et al. Inducible Brown Adipogenesis of Supraclavicular Fat in Adult Humans. *Endocrinology.* 2011;Oct;152(10):3597–3602.

Richard D, et al. Determinants of Brown Adipocyte Development and Thermogenesis. *International Journal of Obesity (London).* 2010;Dec;34 Suppl 2:S59–S66.

Richard D, Picard F. Brown Fat Biology and Thermogenesis. *Frontiers in Bioscience.* 2011;Jan 1;16:1233–1260.

Ruderman N, Chisholm D, Pi-Sunyer X, Schneider S. The Metabolically Obese, Normal-Weight Individual Revisited. *Diabetes.* 1998;47:35–48.

van Marken Lichtenbelt WD. Cold-Activated Brown Adipose Tissue in Healthy Men. *New England Journal of Medicine.* 2009;Apr 9;360(15):1500–1508.

Virtanen KA, et al. Functional Brown Adipose Tissue in Healthy Adults. *New England Journal of Medicine.* 2009;Apr 9;360(15):1518–1525.

Zingaretti MC, et al. The Presence of UCP1 Demonstrates That Metabolically Active Adipose Tissue in the Neck of Adult Humans Truly Represents Brown Adipose Tissue. *Federation of American Societies for Experimental Biology Journal.* 2009;Sep;23(9):3113–3120.

Chapter 3

Aronne L. *The Skinny on Losing Weight without Being Hungry.* New York: Broadway Books, 2009.

Baron JA, Schori A, Crow B, et al. A Randomized Controlled Trial of Low Carbohydrate and Low Fat/High Fiber Diets for Weight Loss. *American Journal of Public Health.* 1986;76:1293–1296.

Calle-Pascual AL, Gomez V, Leon E, Bordiu E. Foods with a Low Glycemic Index Do Not Improve Glycemic Control of Both Type 1 and Type 2 Diabetic Patients After One Month of Therapy. *Diabète & Métabolisme.* 1988;14:629–633.

Cham BE, Roeser HP, Linton I, Gaffney T. Effect of a High Energy, Low Carbohydrate Diet on Serum Levels of Lipids and Lipoproteins. *Medical Journal of Australia.* 1981;1:237–240.

Chandalia M, et al. Beneficial Effect of High Dietary Fiber Intake in Patients with Type 2 Diabetes Mellitus. *New England Journal of Medicine.* 2000;342:1392–1398.

Forster H. Is the Atkins Diet Safe in Respect to Health? *Fortschr Med.* 1978;96:1697–1702.

Hollenbeck CB, Coulston AM. The Clinical Utility of the Glycemic Index and Its Application to Mixed Metals. *Canadian Journal of Physiology and Pharmacology.* 1991;69:100–107.

Hu FB, Stampfer MJ, Rimm EB, et al. A Prospective Study of Egg Consumption and Risk of Cardiovascular Disease in Men and Women. *Journal of the American Medical Association*. 1999;281:1387–1394.

International Table of Glycemic Index.

Isaacs S, Vagnini F. *Overcoming Metabolic Syndrome*. Omaha, NE: Addicus Books, 2009.

Jenkins DJ, Wolever TM, Kalmusky J, et al. Low-Glycemic Index Diet in Hyperlipidemia: Use of Traditional Starchy Foods. *American Journal of Clinical Nutrition*. 1987;46:66–71.

Jenkins DJA, Jenkins AL. Nutrition Principles and Diabetes: A Role for "Lente Carbohydrate"? *Diabetes Care*. 1995;18:1491–1498.

Lichenstein AH, Ausman LM, Jalbert SM, Schaefer EJ. Effecta of Different Forms of Dietary Hydrogenated Fats on Serum Lipoprotein Cholesterol Levels. *New England Journal of Medicine*. 1999;340:1933–1998.

Ludwig DS, Perieira MA, Kroenke CH, et al. Dietary Fiber, Weight Gain and Cardiovascular Disease Risk Factor in Young Adults. *Journal of the American Medical Association*. 1999;282:1539–1546.

Michaels J. *Master Your Metabolism*. New York: Crown, 2009.

Mickelsen O, Makdani DD, Cotton RH, et al. Effects of a High Fiber Bread Diet on Weight Loss in College-Age Males. *American Journal of Clinical Nutrition*. 1979;32:1703–1709.

Natt N, Service FJ. The Highway to Insulinoma: Road Signs and Hazards. *Endocrinologist*. 1997;7:89–96.

Phinney SD, Bistrian BR, Wolfe RR, Blackburn GL. The Human Metabolic Response to Chronic Ketosis without Caloric Restriction: Physical and Biochemical Adaptation. *Metabolism*. 1983;32:757–768.

Pi-Sunyer, FX, et al. The Practical Guide: Identification, Evaluation, and Treatment of Overweight and Obesity in Adults. NHLBI Obesity Education Initiative Expert Panel on the Identification, Evaluation, and Treatment of Overweight and Obesity in Adults, September 1998.

Raben A, Jensen ND, Marckmann P, et al. Spontaneous Weight Loss during 11 Weeks' Ad Libitum Intake of a Low Fat/High Fiber Diet in Young, Normal Weight Subjects. *International Journal of Obesity*. 1995;19:916–923.

Rendell M. Dietary Treatment of Diabetes Mellitus. *New England Journal of Medicine*. 2000;342:1440–1441.

Rolls BJ. Carbohydrates, Fats, and Satiety. *American Journal of Clinical Nutrition*. 1995;61(Suppl 4):960S–967S.

Rolls BJ. Is the Low-Fat Message Giving People a License to Eat More? *Journal of the American College of Nutrition*. 1997;16:535–543.

Seinfeld J. *Deceptively Delicious*. New York: Morrow, 2008.

Stevens, J. Does Dietary Fiber Affect Food Intake and Body Weight? *Journal of the American Dietetic Association*. 1988;88:939–945.

Stubbs RJ, Prentice AM, James WPT. Carbohydrates and Energy Balance. *Annals of the New York Academy of Sciences*. 1997;May 23;819:44-69.

Vogel RA. The Mediterranean Diet and Endothelial Function: Why Some Dietary Fats May Be Healthy. *Cleveland Clinic Journal of Medicine*. 2000;67:232–236.

Wolever TM, Jenkins DJA, Vuksan V, et al. Beneficial Effect of Low-Glycemic Index Diet in Overweight NIDDM Subjects. *Diabetes Care*. 1992;15:562–564.

Yang MU, Van Itallie TB. Composition of Weight Lost during Short-Term Weight Reduction: Metabolic Responses of Obese Subjects to Starvation and Low-Calorie Ketogenic and Nonketogenic Diets. *Journal of Clinical Investigation*. 1976;58:722–730.

Zambon D, Sabate J, Munoz S, et al. Substituting Walnuts for Monounsaturated Fat Improves the Serum Lipid Profile of Hypercholesterolemic Men and Women. *Annals of Internal Medicine*. 2000;132:538–546.

Chapter 4

Agostoni C, et al. Role of Dietary Factors and Food Habits in the Development of Childhood Obesity: A Commentary by the ESPGHAN Committee on Nutrition. *Journal of Pediatric Gastroenterology and Nutrition*. 2011;Jun;52(6):662–669.

Anderson JW, et al. Health Benefits of Dietary Fiber. *Nutrition Review*. 2009;Apr;67(4):188–205.

Anderson JW, et al. Soy Compared to Casein Meal Replacement Shakes with Energy-Restricted Diets for Obese Women: Randomized Controlled Trial. *Metabolism*. 2007 Feb;56(2):280–288.

Aronne L. *The Skinny on Losing Weight without Being Hungry.* New York: Broadway Books, 2009.

Behme MT, Dupre J. All Bran vs Corn Flakes: Plasma Glucose and Insulin Responses in Young Females. *American Journal of Clinical Nutrition*. 1989 Dec;50(6):1240–1243.

Blatt AD, Roe LS, Rolls BJ. Hidden Vegetables: An Effective Strategy to Reduce Energy Intake and Increase Vegetable Intake in Adults. *American Journal of Clinical Nutrition*. 2011;Apr;93(4):756–763.

Blom WA, et al. Effect of a High-Protein Breakfast on the Postprandial Ghrelin Response. *American Journal of Clinical Nutrition*. 2006 Feb;83(2):211–220.

Coppinger T, Jeanes YM, Hardwick J, Reeves S. Body Mass, Frequency of Eating and Breakfast Consumption in 9–13-Year-Olds. *Journal of Human Nutrition and Dietetics*. 2011;Jun 8. doi: 10.1111/j.1365–277X.2011.01184.x.

Davis LM, et al. Efficacy of a Meal Replacement Diet Plan Compared to a Food-Based Diet Plan after a Period of Weight Loss and Weight Maintenance: A Randomized Controlled Trial. *Nutrition Journal*. 2010;Mar 11;9:11.

de Jong E. et al. Behavioural and Socio-Demographic Characteristics of Dutch Neighbourhoods with High Prevalence of childhood obesity. *International Journal of Pediatric Obesity*. 2011 Aug;6(3–4):298–305.

Farshchi HR, Taylor MA, Macdonald IA. Deleterious Effects of Omitting Breakfast on Insulin Sensitivity and Fasting Lipid Profiles in healthy lean women. *American Journal of Clinical Nutrition*. 2005 Feb;81(2):388–396.

Hamdy O, Zwiefelhofer D, Weight Management Using a Meal Replacement Strategy in type 2 Diabetes. *Current Diabetes Reports*. 2010;Apr;10(2):159–164.

Hill BR, De Souza MJ, Williams NI. Characterization of the Diurnal Rhythm of Peptide YY and Its Association with Energy Balance Parameters in Normal Weight Premenopausal Women. *American Journal of Physiology—Endocrinology and Metabolism*. 2011 Aug;301(2):E409–E415.

Holt SH, Delargy HJ, Lawton CL, Blundell JE. The Effects of High-Carbohydrate vs High-Fat Breakfasts on Feelings of Fullness and Alertness, and Subsequent Food Intake. *International Journal of Food Sciences and Nutrition*. 1999 Jan;50(1):13–28.

Jakubowicz D. *The Big Breakfast Diet: Eat Big before 9 A.M. and Lose Big for Life*. New York: Workman, 2009.

Jones JM, Anderson JW. Grain Foods and Health: A Primer for Clinicians. *Physician and Sportsmedicine*. 2008;Dec;36(1):18–33.

Kaplan GD, Stifler LT. Very Low-Calorie Diets for Obesity. *Journal of the American Medical Association*. 1994 Jan 5;271(1):24–25.

Kim JY, Kim JH, Lee da H, Kim SH, Lee SS. Meal Replacement with Mixed Rice Is More Effective Than White Rice in Weight Control, While Improving Antioxidant Enzyme Activity in Obese Women. *Nutrition Research*. 2008;Feb;28(2):66–71.

Kral TV, Kabay AC, Roe LS, Rolls BJ. Effects of Doubling the Portion Size of Fruit and Vegetable Side Dishes on Children's Intake at a Meal. *Obesity (Silver Spring)*. 2010;Mar;18(3):521–527.

Leahy KE, Birch LL, Rolls BJ. Reducing the Energy Density of an Entrée Decreases Children's Energy Intake at Lunch. *Journal of American Dietetic Association*. 2008;Jan;108(1):41–48.

Leahy KE, Birch LL, Rolls BJ. Reducing the Energy Density of Multiple Meals Decreases the Energy Intake of Preschool-Age Children. *American Journal of Clinical Nutrition*. 2008;Dec;88(6):1459–1468.

Levitsky DA, Pacanowski C. Losing Weight without Dieting: Use of Commercial Foods as Meal Replacements for Lunch Produces an Extended Energy Deficit. *Appetite*. 2011 Oct;57(2):311–317.

Makris AP, et al. The Individual and Combined Effects of Glycemic Index and Protein on Glycemic Response, Hunger, and Energy Intake. *Obesity (Silver Spring)*. 2011;Jun 30. doi: 10.1038/oby.2011.145.

Marmonier C, Chapelot D, Louis-Sylvestre J. Effects of Macronutrient Content and Energy Density of Snacks Consumed in a Satiety State on the Onset of the Next Meal. *Appetite*. 2000 Apr;34(2):161–168.

National Weight Control Registry. http://www.nwcr.ws/Research/default.htm.

Osterholt KM, Roe LS, Rolls BJ. Incorporation of Air into a Snack Food Reduces Energy Intake. *Appetite*. 2007 May;48(3):351–358.

Pombo-Rodrigues S, Calame W, Re R. The Effects of Consuming Eggs for Lunch on Satiety and Subsequent Food Intake. *International Journal of Food Science and Nutrition*. 2011 Sep;62(6):593-9.

Poole CN, et al. The Combined Effects of Exercise and Ingestion of a Meal Replacement in Conjunction with a Weight Loss Supplement on Body Composition and Fitness Parameters in College-Aged Men And Women. *Journal of Strength and Conditioning Research*. 2011;Jan;25(1):51–60.

Purslow LR, et al. Energy Intake at Breakfast and Weight Change: Prospective Study of 6,764 Middle-Aged Men and Women. *American Journal of Epidemiology.* 2008; Jan 15;167(2):188–192.

Ratliff J, et al. Consuming Eggs for Breakfast Influences Plasma Glucose and Ghrelin, While Reducing Energy Intake during the Next 24 hours in Adult Men. *Nutrition Research.* 2010;Feb;30(2):96–103.

Rodríguez-Rodríguez E, et al. An Adequate Calcium Intake Could Help Achieve Weight Loss in Overweight/Obese Women Following Hypocaloric Diets. *Annals of Nutrition & Metabolism* 2010;57(2):95–102.

Rolls BJ. The Relationship between Dietary Energy Density and Energy Intake. *Physiology & Behavior.* 2009; Jul 14;97(5):609–615.

Rolls BJ, Drewnowski A, Ledikwe JH. Changing the Energy Density of the Diet as a Strategy for Weight Management. *Journal of American Dietetic Association.* 2005 May;105(5 Suppl 1):S98–S103.

Rolls BJ, Roe LS, Beach AM, Kris-Etherton PM. Provision of Foods Differing in Energy Density Affects Long-Term Weight Loss. *Obesity Research.* 2005 Jun;13(6):1052–1060.

Rolls BJ, Roe LS, Meengs JS. Portion Size Can Be Used Strategically to Increase Vegetable Consumption in Adults. *American Journal of Clinical Nutrition.* 2010;Apr;91(4):913–922. Epub 2010;Feb 10.

Rolls BJ, Roe LS, Meengs JS. Reductions in Portion Size and Energy Density of Foods Are Additive and Lead to Sustained Decreases in Energy Intake. *American Journal of Clinical Nutrition.* 2006 Jan;83(1):11–17.

So HK, et al. Breakfast Frequency Inversely Associated with BMI and Body Fatness in Hong Kong Chinese Children Aged 9–18 Years. *British Journal of Nutrition.* 2011;May 3:1–10.

Spill MK, Birch LL, Roe LS, Rolls BJ. Eating Vegetables First: The Use of Portion Size to Increase Vegetable Intake in Preschool Children. *American Journal of Clinical Nutrition.* 2010;May;91(5):1237–1243.

Spill MK, Birch LL, Roe LS, Rolls BJ. Serving Large Portions of Vegetable Soup at the Start of a Meal Affected Children's Energy and Vegetable Intake. *Appetite.* 2011;Aug;57(1):213–219.

Treyzon L, et al. A Controlled Trial of Protein Enrichment of Meal Replacements for Weight Reduction with Retention of Lean Body Mass. *Nutrition Journal.* 2008;Aug 27;7:23.

Vander Wal JS, et al. Short-Term Effect of Eggs on Satiety in Overweight and Obese Subjects. *Journal of the American College of Nutrition.* 2005. 24(6):510–515.

Vander Wal JS, Gupta A, Khosla P, Dhurandhar NV. Egg Breakfast Enhances Weight loss. *International Journal of Obesity (London).* 2008;Oct;32(10):1545–1551.

Chapter 5

Ando, H. Impairment of Peripheral Circadian Clocks Precedes Metabolic Abnormalities in Ob/Ob Mice. *Endocrinology.* 2011;Feb 1;doi: 10.1210/en.2010-1028.

Barth S, et al. Expression of Neuropeptide Y, Omentin and Visfatin in Visceral and Subcutaneous Adipose Tissues in Humans: Relation to Endocrine and Clinical Parameters. *Obesity Facts*, 2010;Aug. PMID 20823688.

Beck B. Neuropeptide Y in Normal Eating and in Genetic and Dietary-Induced Obesity. *Philosophical Transactions of the Royal Society of London B Biological Sciences*. 2006;Jul 29;361(1471):1159–1185.

Blom WA, et al. Effect of a High-Protein Breakfast on the Postprandial Ghrelin Response. *American Journal of Clinical Nutrition*. 2006;Feb;83(2):211–220.

Blum K, Liu Y, Shriner R, Gold MS. Reward Circuitry Dopaminergic Activation Regulates Food and Drug Craving Behavior. *Current Pharmaceutical Design*. 2011;17(12):1158–1167.

Crespillo A, et al. Expression of the Cannabinoid System in Muscle: Effects of a High-Fat Diet and CB1 Receptor Blockade. *Biochemical Journal*. 2010;Dec 15;433(1):175–185.

Crum AJ, et al. Mind over Milkshakes: Mindsets, Not Just Nutrients, Determine Ghrelin Response. *Health Psychology*. 2011;Jul;30(4):424-9;discussion 430–431.

Després JP. The Endocannabinoid System: A New Target for the Regulation of Energy Balance and Metabolism. *Critical Pathways in Cardiology*. 2007;Jun;6(2):46–50.

Di Marzo V, et al. Leptin-Regulated Endocannabinoids Are Involved in Maintaining Food Intake. *Nature*. 2001;Apr 12;410(6830):822–825.

Dickson SL, et al. The Role of the Central Ghrelin System in Reward from Food and Chemical Drugs. *Molecular Cell Endocrinology*. 2011;Jun 20;340(1):80–87. Epub 2011;Feb 24.

Disse E, et al. Systemic Ghrelin and Reward: Effect of Cholinergic Blockade. *Physiology and Behavior*. 2011;Mar 28;102(5):481–484. Epub 2010;Dec 1.

Enriori PJ, et al. Diet-Induced Obesity Causes Severe but Reversible Leptin Resistance in Arcuate Melanocortin Neurons. *Cell Metabolism*. 2007 Mar;5(3):181–194.

Exner C, et al. Leptin Suppresses Semi-Starvation Induced Hyperactivity in Rats: Implications for Anorexia Nervosa. *Molecular Psychiatry*. 2000;Sep;5(5):476–481.

Fehm HL, et al. The Selfish Brain: Competition for Energy Resources. *Progress in Brain Research*. 2006;153:129–140.

Fernández-Sánchez A, et al. Inflammation, Oxidative Stress, and Obesity. *International Journal of Molecular Sciences*. 2011;12(5):3117–3132.

Francès F, et al. The 1258 G>A Polymorphism in the Neuropeptide Y Gene Is Associated with Greater Alcohol Consumption in a Mediterranean Population. *Alcohol*. 2011;Mar. PMID 21303710.

Fulton S, Appetite and Reward. *Frontiers in Neuroendocrinology*. 2010;Jan;31(1):85–103.

Gerson, W.T. Less Sleep, Childhood Obesity Linked. *Endocrine Today*. 2011;Feb;9(2).

Gutierrez-Aguilar R, et al. Expression of New Loci Associated with Obesity in Diet-Induced Obese Rats: From Genetics to Physiology. *Obesity (Silver Spring)*. 2011;Jul 21. doi: 10.1038/oby.2011.236.

Guy EG, Choi E, Pratt WE. Nucleus Accumbens Dopamine and mu-Opioid Receptors Modulate the Reinstatement of Food-Seeking Behavior by Food-Associated Cues. *Behavioural Brain Research*. 2011;Jun 1;219(2):265–272.

Hammond RA. Complex Systems Modeling for Obesity Research. *Preventing Chronic Disease*. 2009;Jul;6(3):A97.

Hanson ES, Dallman MF. Neuropeptide Y (NPY) May Integrate Responses of Hypothalamic Feeding Systems and the Hypothalamo-Pituitary-Adrenal Axis. *Journal of Neuroendocrinology*. 1995;Apr;7 (4):273–279.

Hartocollis, A. Diet Plan with Hormone Has Fans and Skeptics. *New York Times*, March 7, 2011. http://www.nytimes.com/2011/03/08/nyregion/08hcg.html?pagewanted=all.

Hill AJ. The Psychology of Food Craving. *Proceedings of the Nutrition Society*. 2007;May;66(2):277–285.

Hofmann W, et al. As Pleasure Unfolds: Hedonic Responses to Tempting Food. *Psychological Science*. 2010;Dec 1;21(12):1863–1870. Epub 2010;Nov 24.

Howard JK, et al. Leptin Protects Mice from Starvation-Induced Lymphoid Atrophy and Increases Thymic Cellularity in Ob/Ob Mice. *Journal of Clinical Investigation*. 1999;Oct;104(8):1051–1059.

Ilhan A, et al. Plasma Neuropeptide Y Levels Differ in Distinct Diabetic Conditions. *Neuropeptides*. 2010;Dec. PMID 20832114.

Jeon, JY, et al. Leptin Response to Short-Term Fasting in Sympathectomized Men: Role of the SNS. *American Journal of Physiology—Endocrinology and Metabolism*. 2003;Mar;284(3):E634–E640.

Jéquier E. Leptin Signaling, Adiposity, and Energy Balance. *Annals of the New York Academy of Sciences*. 2002;Jun;967:379–388.

Karhunen LJ, et al. Serum Leptin, Food Intake and Preferences for Sugar and Fat in Obese Women. *International Journal of Obesity* and *Related Metabolic Disorders*. 1998 Aug;22(8):819–821.

Klein, S, et al. Leptin Production during Early Starvation in Lean and Obese Women. *American American Journal of Physiology—Endocrinology and Metabolism*. 2000;Feb;278(2):E280–E284.

Komatsu S. Rice and Sushi Cravings: A Preliminary Study of Food Craving among Japanese Females. *Appetite*. 2008;Mar–May;50(2–3):353–358. Epub 2007;Sep 20.

Kuo, LE, et al. Neuropeptide Y Acts Directly in the Periphery on Fat Tissue and mediates Stress-Induced Obesity and Metabolic Syndrome. *Nature Medicine*. 2007;13:803–811.

Lafrance V, Inoue W, Kan B, Luheshi GN. Leptin Modulates Cell Morphology and Cytokine Release in Microglia. *Brain, Behavior, and Immunity*. 2010;Mar;24(3):358–365. Epub 2009;Nov 14.

Lee YB, Nagai A, Kim SU. Cytokines, Chemokines, and Cytokine Receptors in Human Microglia. *Journal of Neuroscience Research*. 2002;Jul 1;69(1):94–103.

Leibowitz SF. The Role of Serotonin in Eating Disorders. *Drugs*. 1990;39 Suppl 3:33–48.

Lenard NR, Berthoud HR. Central and Peripheral Regulation of Food Intake and Physical Activity: Pathways and Genes. *Obesity (Silver Spring)*. 2008;Dec;16 Suppl 3:S11–S22.

Lowe MR, Butryn ML. Hedonic Hunger: A New Dimension of Appetite? *Physiology & Behavior*. 2007 Jul 24;91(4):432–439.

Naleida, AM, et al. Ghrelin Induces Feeding in the Mesolimbic Reward Pathway between the Ventral Tegmental Area and the Nucleus Accumbens. *Peptides*. 2005;Nov;26(11):2274–2279.

Pan W, et al. Astrocytes Modulate Distribution and Neuronal Signaling of Leptin in the Hypothalamus of Obese Avy Mice. *Journal of Molecular Neuroscience*. 2011;Mar;43(3):478–484.

Pandit R, et al. Neurobiology of Overeating and Obesity: The Role of Melanocortins and Beyond. *European Journal of Pharmacology*. 2011;Jun 11;660(1):28–42.

Park J, Scherer PE. Leptin and Cancer: From Cancer Stem Cells to Metastasis. *Endocrine-Related Cancers*. 2011;Jul 11;18(4):C25–C29. Print 2011 Aug.

Peters A, et al. Causes of Obesity: Looking beyond the Hypothalamus. *Progress in Neurobiology*. 2007;Feb;81(2):61–88. Epub 2007;Jan 5.

Polivy J, Coleman J, Herman CP. The Effect of Deprivation on Food Cravings and Eating Behavior in Restrained and Unrestrained Eaters. *International Journal of Eating Disorders*. 2005;Dec;38(4):301–309.

Prior LJ, Armitage JA. Neonatal Overfeeding Leads to Developmental Programming of Adult Obesity: You Are What You Ate. *Journal of Physiology*. 2009;Jun 1;587(Pt 11):2419.

Rada P, Avena NM, Hoebel BG. Daily Bingeing on Sugar Repeatedly Releases Dopamine in the Accumbens Shell. *Neuroscience*. 2005;134(3):737–744.

Raffaella F, et al. Reduced Leptin Levels in Starvation Increase Susceptibility to Endotoxic Shock. *American Journal of Pathology*. 2000;156:1781–1787.

Reece AS. Hypothalamic Opioid-Melanocortin Appetitive Balance and Addictive Craving. *Medical Hypotheses*. 2011;Jan;76(1):132–137.

Rejeski WJ, et al. State Craving, Food Availability, and Reactivity to Preferred Snack Foods. *Appetite*. 2010;Feb;54(1):77–83. Epub 2009;Sep 25.

Rodrigues AL, et al. Postnatal Early Overnutrition Changes the Leptin Signaling Pathway in the Hypothalamic-Pituitary-Thyroid Axis of Young and Adult Rats. *Journal of Physiology*. 2009;Jun 1;587(Pt 11):2647–2661. Epub 2009;Apr 29.

Rogers PJ, Smit HJ. Food Craving and Food Addiction: A Critical Review of the Evidence from a Biopsychosocial Perspective. *Pharmacology Biochemistry* and *Behavior*. 2000;May;66(1):3–14.

Sahu A. Minireview: A Hypothalamic Role in Energy Balance with Special Emphasis on Leptin. *Endocrinology*. 2004;Jun;145(6):2613–2620. Epub 2004;Mar 24.

Sclafani A, Touzani K, Bodnar RJ. Dopamine and Learned Food Preferences. *Physiology* and *Behavior*. 2011;Jul 25;104(1):64–68.

Sellayah, D et al. Orexin Is Required for Brown Adipose Tissue Development, Differentiation, and Function. *Cell Metabolism*. 2011;Oct 5;14(4):478–490.

Skibicka KP, et al. Role of Ghrelin in Food Reward: Impact of Ghrelin on Sucrose Self-Administration and Mesolimbic Dopamine and Acetylcholine Receptor Gene Expression. *Addiction Biology*. 2011;Feb 11. doi: 10.1111/j.1369-1600.2010.00294.x.

Surmi BK, Hasty AH. Macrophage Infiltration into Adipose Tissue: Initiation, Propagation and Remodeling. *Future Lipidology.* 2008;3(5):545–556.

Tanaka M, et al. Role of Central Leptin Signaling in the Starvation-Induced Alteration of B-Cell Development. *Journal of Neuroscience.* 2011;Jun 8;31(23):8373–8380.

van Dijk G. The Role of Leptin in the Regulation of Energy Balance and Adiposity. *Journal of Neuroendocrinology.* 2001;Oct;13(10):913–921.

Volkow ND, Wang GJ, Baler RD. Reward, Dopamine and the Control of Food Intake: Implications for Obesity. *Trends in Cognitive Sciences.* 2011;Jan;15(1):37–46.

Wang H, et al. Effects of Dietary Fat Types on Body Fatness, Leptin, and ARC Leptin Receptor, NPY, and AgRP mRNA Expression. *American Journal of Physiology—Endocrinology and Metabolism.* 2002;Jun;282(6):E1352–E1359.

Wang J, et al. Neuropeptide Y in Relation to Carbohydrate Intake, Corticosterone and Dietary Obesity. *Brain Research.* 1998;Aug 17;802(1–2):75–88.

Wang, GJ, et al. Brain Dopamine and Obesity. *Lancet.* 2001;Feb 3;9253:354–357.

Wauman J, Tavernier J. Leptin Receptor Signaling: Pathways to Leptin Resistance. *Frontiers of Bioscience.* 2011;Jun 1;17:2771–2793.

Weingarten HP, Elston D. The Phenomenology of Food Cravings. *Appetite.* 1990;Dec;15(3):231–246.

White BD, He B, Dean RG, Martin RJ. Low Protein Diets Increase Neuropeptide Y Gene Expression in the Basomedial Hypothalamus of Rats. *Journal of Nutrition.* 1994;Aug;124(8):1152–1160.

Yanovski S. Sugar And Fat: Cravings and Aversions. *Journal of Nutrition.* 2003;Mar;133(3):835S–837S.

Young SN. How to Increase Serotonin in the Human Brain without Drugs. *Journal of Psychiatry and Neuroscience.* 2007;Nov;32(6):394–349.

Yu Y, et al. Obese Reversal by a Chronic Energy Restricted Diet Leaves an Increased Arc NPY/AgRP, But No Alteration in POMC/CART, mRNA Expression in diet-Induced Obese Mice. *Behavioural Brain Research.* 2009;Dec 14;205(1):50–56.

Zheng H, et al. Appetite Control and Energy Balance Regulation in the Modern World: Reward-Driven Brain Overrides Repletion Signals. *International Journal of Obesity (London).* 2009;Jun;33 Suppl 2:S8–S13.

Zupancic ML, Mahajan A. Leptin as a Neuroactive Agent. *Psychosomatic Medicine.* 2011;Jun;73(5):407–414.

Chapter 6

Alemzadeh R, Kichler J, Babar G, Calhoun M. Hypovitaminosis D in Obese Children and Adolescents: Relationship with Adiposity, Insulin Sensitivity, Ethnicity, and Season. *Metabolism.* 2008;Feb;57(2):183–191.

Ather, A. Chromium Effects on Glucose Tolerance and Insulin Sensitivity in Persons at Risk for Diabetes Mellitus. *Endocrine Practice.* 2011;17:16–25.

Barth RJ. Insulin Resistance, Obesity and the Metabolic Syndrome. *South Dakota Medicine.* 2011;Spec No:22–27.

Bastard JP, et al. Recent Advances in the Relationship between Obesity, Inflammation, and Insulin Resistance. *European Cytokine Network.* 2006;Mar;17(1):4–12.

Brown BG, Does ENHANCE Diminish Confidence in Lowering LDL or in Ezetimibe? *New England Journal of Medicine.* 2008;358:1504–1507.

Buse JB, Ginsberg HN, Bakris GL, Clark NG, Costa F, Eckel R, Fonseca V, Gerstein H, Grundy S, Nesto RW, Pignone MP, Plutzky J, Porte D, Redberg R, Stitzel KF, Stone NJ. Primary Prevention of Cardiovascular Diseases in People with Diabetes Mellitus: A Scientific Statement from the American Heart Association and the American Diabetes Association. *Circulation.* 2007;115:114–126.

Center for Disease Control. *National Diabetes Fact Sheet.* 2011. www.cdc.gov/diabetes/pubs/factsheet11.htm.

Després JP, et al. Abdominal Obesity and the Metabolic Syndrome: Contribution to Global Cardiometabolic Risk. *Arteriosclerosis, Thrombosis, and Vascular Biology.* 2008;Jun;28(6):1039–49.

Drazen JM. Ezetimibe and Cancer: An Uncertain Association. *New England Journal of Medicine* 2008;359:1398–1399.

Duvnjak L, Duvnjak M. The Metabolic Syndrome: An Ongoing Story. *Journal of Physiology and Pharmacology.* 2009;Dec;60 Suppl 7:19–24.

El-Khatib F. Valproate, Weight Gain and Carbohydrate Craving: A Gender Study. *Seizure.* 2007;Apr;16(3):226–32. Epub 2007;Jan 8.

Gallagher, EJ. The Pathway from Diabetes and Obesity to Cancer, on the Route to Targeted Therapy. *Endocrine Practice.* 2010;16:864–873.

Gerstein HC, Miller ME, Byington RP, Goff DC Jr, Bigger JT, Buse JB, Cushman WC, Genuth S, IsmailBeigi F, Grimm RH Jr, Probstfield JL, Simons-Morton DG, Friedewald WT. Effects of Intensive Glucose Lowering in Type 2 Diabetes. *New England Journal of Medicine.* 2008;358:2545–2559.

Giordano D, et al. Effects of Myo-Inositol Supplementation in Postmenopausal Women with Metabolic Syndrome: A Perspective, Randomized, Placebo-Controlled Study. *Menopause: The Journal of the North American Menopause Society.* 18(1):102–104.

Guay AT. The Emerging Link between Hypogonadism and Metabolic Syndrome. *Journal of Andrology.* 2009;Jul–Aug;30(4):370–6. Epub 2008;Sep 4.

Healy, GN. Sedentary Time and Cardio-Metabolic Biomarkers in US Adults: NHANES 2003–06. *European Heart Journal* (2011) doi: 10.1093/eurheartj/ehq451.

Hofeldt FD. Reactive Hypoglycemia. *Endocrinology and Metabolism Clinics of North America.* 1989;Mar;18(1):185–201.

Holman RR, Paul SK, Bethel MA, Matthews DR, Neil HAW. 10-Year Follow-Up of Intensive Glucose Control in Type 2 Diabetes. *New England Journal of Medicine.* 2008;359:1577–1589.

Insull W Jr. Clinical Utility of Bile Acid Sequestrants in the Treatment of dyslipidemia: A Scientific Review. *Southern Medical Journal* 2006;99:257–73.

Jellinger, P. Prediabetes Must Be Identified, Treated. *Clinical Endocrinology News.* 6(2).

Jialal I, Devaraj S. Vitamin E Supplementation and Cardiovascular Events in High-Risk Patients. *New England Journal of Medicine.* 2000; Jun 22;342(25):1917–8.

Kastelein JJ, Akdim F, Stroes ESG, et al. Simvastatin with or without Ezetimibe in Familial Hypercholesterolemia. *New England Journal of Medicine.* 2008;358:1431–1443.

Keech A, et al. (FIELD study investigators). Effects of Long-Term Fenofibrate Therapy on Cardiovascular Events in 9795 People with Type 2 Diabetes Mellitus (The FIELD Study): Randomised Controlled Trial *Lancet.* 2005 Nov 26;366(9500):1849–61.

Kirkham S, Akilen R, Sharma S, Tsiami A. The Potential of Cinnamon to Reduce Blood Glucose Levels in Patients with Type 2 Diabetes and Insulin Resistance. *Diabetes, Obesity and Metabolism.* 2009;Dec;11(12):1100–13.

Kristensen M, et al. Wholegrain vs. Refined Wheat Bread and Pasta: Effect on Postprandial Glycemia, Appetite, and Subsequent Ad Libitum Energy Intake in Young Healthy Adults. *Appetite.* 2010;Feb;54(1):163–9. Epub 2009;Oct 27.

Levy AP, et al. Haptoglobin Phenotype and Vascular Complications in Patients with Diabetes. *New England Journal of Medicine.* 2000 Sep 28;343(13):969–70.

Love TJ, et al. Prevalence of the Metabolic Syndrome in Psoriasis: Results from the National Health and Nutrition Examination Survey. 2003–2006, *Archives of Dermatology.* 2011;Apr;147(4):419–24.

Marsh KA, et al. Effect of a Low Glycemic Index Compared with a Conventional Healthy Diet on Polycystic Ovary Syndrome. *American Journal of Clinical Nutrition.* 2010;Jul;92(1):83–92.

McCarty MF, et al. Regular Thermal Therapy May Promote Insulin Sensitivity While Boosting Expression of Endothelial Nitric Oxide Synthase: Effects Comparable to Those of Exercise Training. *Medical Hypotheses.* 2009;Jul;73(1):103–5.

Mozaffarian D et al. Trans-Palmitoleic Acid, Metabolic Risk Factors, and New-Onset Diabetes in U.S. Adults. *Annals of Internal Medicine* 2010;153: 790–799.

MRC/BHF Heart Protection Study of Cholesterol-Lowering Therapy and of Antioxidant Vitamin Supplementation in a Wide Range of Patients at Increased Risk of Coronary Heart Disease Death: Early Safety and Efficacy Experience. *European Heart Journal* 1999;20:725–741.

Patel A, et al. (ADVANCE Collaborative Group). Intensive Blood Glucose Control and Vascular Outcomes in Patients with Type 2 Diabetes. *New England Journal of Medicine.* 2008 Nov 20;358:2560–2572.

Pedersen TR. Effect of Simvastatin on Ischemic Signs and Symptoms in the Scandinavian Simvastatin Survival Study (4S). *American Journal of Cardiol.* 1998 Feb 1;81(3):333–5.

Ridker PM, JUPITER Study Group. Rosuvastatin to Prevent Vascular Events in Men and Women with Elevated C-Reactive Protein. *New England Journal of Medicine.* 2008;359:2195–2207. November 20, 2008.

Ros Pérez M, Medina-Gómez G. Obesity, Adipogenesis and Insulin Resistance. *Endocrinología y nutrición (Madrid).* 2011; Jul 19.

Roussel AM, et al. Antioxidant Effects of a Cinnamon Extract in People with Impaired Fasting Glucose That Are Overweight or Obese. *Journal of the American College of Nutrition.* 2009;Feb;28(1):16–21.

Skyler, Jay S. et al. Intensive Glycemic Control and the Prevention of Cardiovascular Events: Implications of the ACCORD, ADVANCE, and VA Diabetes Trials. *Diabetes Care.* 2009;January;32(1): 187–192. doi: 10.2337/dc08-9026.

Smith, J. Diabetes Prevalence Keeps Climbing in U.S. *Clinical Endocrinology News.* 6, No. 2.

Smith, KM, et al. Relationship between Fish Intake, n-3 Fatty Acids, Mercury and Risk Markers of CHD. *Public Health Nutrition.* 2009;12:1261.

Taylor AJ, Villines TC, Stanek EJ, et al. Extended-Release Niacin or Ezetimibe and Carotid Intima-Media Thickness. *New England Journal of Medicine.* 2009;361:2113–2122.

Tremblay A, Gilbert JA. Milk Products, Insulin Resistance Syndrome and Type 2 Diabetes. *Journal of the American College of Nutrition* 2009;Feb;28 Suppl 1:91S–102S.

Tzotzas, T. Rising Serum 25 Hydroxy-Vitamin D Levels after Weight Loss in obese Women Correlate with Improvements in Insulin Resistance. *Journal of Clinical Endocrinology and Metabolism* 2010, 95:4251–4257.

Chapter 7

Anselmo J, Cesar R. Resistance to Thyroid Hormone: Report of Two Kindreds with 35 Patients. *Endocrine Practice.* 1998;4:368–374.

Appelhof BC, et al. Combined Therapy with Levothyroxine and Liothyronine in Two Ratios, Compared with Levothyroxine Monotherapy in Primary Hypothyroidism: A Double-Blind, Randomized, Controlled Clinical Trial. *Journal of Clinical Endocrinology and Metabolism.* 2005 May;90(5):2666–74.

Baskin HJ, et al. American Association of Clinical Endocrinologists Medical Guidelines for Clinical Practice for the Evaluation and Treatment of Hyperthyroidism and Hypothyroidism. *Endocrine Practice.* 2002 Nov–Dec;8(6):457–69.

Bolk N, Visser TJ, Kalsbeek A, van Domburg RT, Berghout A. Effects of Evening vs Morning Thyroxine Ingestion on Serum Thyroid Hormone Profiles in Hypothyroid Patients. *Clinical Endocrinology (Oxford).* 2007 Jan;66(1):43–8.

Bolk, Nienke MD, et. al. Effects of Evening vs Morning Levothyroxine Intake: A Randomized Double-Blind Crossover Trial. *Archives of Internal Medicine.* 2010;170(22).

Brennan MD, Bahn RS. Thyroid Hormones and Illness. *Endocrine Practice.* 1998;4:396–402.

Bunevicius R, Kazanavicius G, Zalinkevicius R, Prange AJ. Effects of Thyroxine as Compared with Thyroxine plus Triiodothyronine in Patients with Hypothyroidism. *New England Journal of Medicine.* 1999;340:424–429.

Canaris GJ, Manowitz NR, Mayor G, Ridgway EC. The Colorado Thyroid Disease Prevalence Study. *Archives of Internal Medicine.* 2000;160:526–534.

Clyde PW, Harari AE, Getka EJ, Shakir KM. Combined Levothyroxine Plus Liothyronine Compared with Levothyroxine Alone in Primary Hypothyroidism: A Randomized Controlled Trial. *Journal of the American Medical Association.* 2003 Dec 10;290(22):2952–8.

Crawford BA, et al. Iodine Toxicity from Soy Milk and Seaweed Ingestion. *Medical Journal of Australia.* 2010;Oct 4;193(7):413–5.

Cushing GW. Subclinical Hypothyroidism: Understanding Is the Key to Decision Making. *Postgraduate Medicine.* 1993;94:1–7.

Doerge DR, Chang HC, Inactivation of Thyroid Peroxidase by Soy Isoflavones, in Vitro and in Vivo. *Journal of Chromatography B. Analytical Technologies in the Biomedical and Life Sciences.* 2002 Sep 25;777(1–2):269–79.

Doerge DR, Sheehan DM. Goitrogenic and Estrogenic Activity of Soy Isoflavones. *Environmental Health Perspectives.* 2002 Jun;110 Suppl 3:349–53.

Duntas LH, Biondi B. New Insights into Subclinical Hypothyroidism and Cardiovascular Risk. *Seminars in Thrombosis and Hemostasis.* 2011;Feb;37(1):27–34.

Endocrine Society: http://www.hormone.org/Public/upload/Wilsons-Syndrome-Web.pdf.

Escobar-Morreale HF, et al. Review: Treatment of hypothyroidism with Combinations of Levothyroxine Plus Liothyronine. *Journal of Clinical Endocrinology and Metabolism.* 2005 Aug;90(8):4946–54.

Escobar-Morreale HF, et al. Thyroid Hormone Replacement Therapy in Primary Hypothyroidism: A Randomized Trial Comparing L-Thyroxine Plus Liothyronine With L-Thyroxine Alone. *Annals of Internal Medicine.* 2005 Mar 15;142(6):412–24.

Farwell AP. Thyroid Hormone Therapy Is Not Indicated in the Majority of Patients with the Sick Euthyroid Syndrome. *Endocrine Practice.* 2008;Dec;14(9):1180–7.

Ferretti E, Persani L, Jaffrain-Rea ML, et al. Evaluation of the Adequacy of Levothyroxine Replacement Therapy in Patients with Central Hypothyroidism. *Journal of Clinical Endocrinology and Metabolism.* 1999;84:924–929.

Gordon MB and Gordon MS. Variations in Adequate Levothyroxine Replacement Therapy in Patients with Different Casues of Hypothyroidism. *Endocrine Practice.* 1999;5:233–301.

Hak E, Huibert APP, Visser TJ, et al. Subclinical Hypothyroidism Is an Independent Risk Factor for Atherosclerosis and Myocardial Infarction in Elderly Women: The Rotterdam Study. *Annals of Internal Medicine.* 2000;132:270–278.

Helfand M, Redfern CC, Sox HC. Screening for Thyroid Disease. *Annals of Internal Medicine.* 1998;129:141–158.

Monzani F, Del Guerra P, Caraccio N, et al. Subclinical Hypothyroidism: Neurobehavioral Features and Beneficial Effect of L-thyroxine Treatment. *Clinical Investigator.* 1993;71:367–371.

Herrick B. Subclinical Hypothyroidism, *American Family Physician.* 2008;Apr 1;77(7):953–5.

Kapustin JF. Hypothyroidism: An Evidence-Based Approach to a Complex Disorder. *Nurse Practitioner.* 2010;Aug;35(8):44–53.

Karmisholt J, Andersen S, Laurberg P. Variation in Thyroid Function in Subclinical Hypothyroidism: Importance of Clinical Follow-Up and Therapy. *European Journal of Endocrinology.* 2011;Mar;164(3):317–23.

Lania A, Persani L, Beck-Peccoz P. Central Hypothyroidism. *Pituitary.* 2008;11(2):181–6.

Laurberg P, Andersen S, Bülow Pedersen I, Carlé A. Hypothyroidism in the elderly: pathophysiology, diagnosis and treatment. *Drugs and Aging.* 2005;22(1):23–38.

Leung AM, Iodine Status and Thyroid Function of Boston-Area Vegetarians and Vegans. *Journal of Clinical Endocrinology and Metabolism.* 2011 Aug;96(8):E1303-7.

Li Y, Nishihara E, Kakudo K. Hashimoto's Thyroiditis: Old Concepts and New Insights. *Current Opinion in Rheumatology.* 2011;Jan;23(1):102–7.

Ma C, et al. Thyroxine Alone or Thyroxine Plus Triiodothyronine Replacement Therapy for Hypothyroidism. *Nuclear Medicine Communications.* 2009;Aug;30(8):586–93.

McDermott MT. In the Clinic: Hypothyroidism. *Annals of Internal Medicine.* 2009;Dec 1;151(11):ITC61.

McIver B, Gorman CA. Euthyroid Sick Syndrome: An Overview. *Thyroid.* 1997 Feb;7(1):125–32.

McMillan M, Spinks EA, Fenwick GR. Preliminary Observations on the Effect of Dietary Brussels Sprouts on Thyroid Function. *Human Toxicology.* 1986 Jan;5(1):15–9.

Mortoglou A, Candiloros H. The Serum Triiodothyronine to Thyroxine (T3/T4) ratio in Various Thyroid Disorders and after Levothyroxine Replacement Therapy. *Hormones (Athens).* 2004 Apr–Jun;3(2):120–6.

Mufti TS, Jielani A. Deranged Thyroid Hormone Status in Non-Thyroid Illnesses: Sick Euthyroid Syndrome. Journal of Ayub Medical College Abbottabad. 2006 Oct–Dec;18(4):1–3.

Palmieri EA, Fazio S, Lombardi G, Biondi B. Subclinical Hypothyroidism and Cardiovascular Risk: A Reason to Treat? *Treatments in Endocrinology.* 2004;3(4):233–44.

Peplow M. Chernobyl's Legacy. *Nature.* 2011;Mar 31;471(7340):562–5.

Polikar R, Burger AG, Scherrer U and Nicod P. The Thyroid and the Heart. *Circulation.* 1993;87:1435–1441.

Saravanan P, et al. Twenty-Four-Hour Hormone Profiles of TSH, Free T3 and Free T4 in Hypothyroid Patients on Combined T3/T4 Therapy. *Experimental and Clinical Endocrinology and Diabetes.* 2007 Apr;115(4):261–7.

Sathyapalan T, et al. The Effect of Soy Phytoestrogen Supplementation on Thyroid Status and Cardiovascular Risk Markers in patients with Subclinical Hypothyroidism: A Randomized, Double-Blind, Crossover Study. *Journal of Clinical Endocrinology and Metabolism.* 2011;May;96(5):1442–9.

Sehgal VN. Vitiligo and Alopecia Areata Associated with Subclinical/Clinical Hypothyroidism. *Skinmed.* 2011;May–Jun;9(3):192–4.

Siegmund W, et al. Replacement Therapy with Levothyroxine Plus Triiodothyronine (Bioavailable Molar Ratio 14 : 1) Is Not Superior to Thyroxine Alone to Improve Well-Being and Cognitive Performance in Hypothyroidism. *Clinical Endocrinology (Oxford).* 2004 Jun;60(6):750–7.

Singer PA, Cooper DS, Levy EG, et al. Treatment Guidelines for Patients with Hyperthyroidism and Hypothyroidism. *Journal of the American Medical Association.* 1995;273:808–812.

Sosi-Jurjevi B, et al. Suppressive Effects of Genistein and Daidzein on Pituitary-Thyroid Axis in Orchidectomized Middle-Aged Rats. *Experimental Biology and Medicine (Maywood).* 2010;May;235(5):590–8.

St. Germain DL. Selenodeiodinases: Preceptor Regulators of Thyroid Action. *Thyroid Today*. 1999;22:1–11.

Stabouli S, Papakatsika S, Kotsis V. Hypothyroidism and Hypertension. *Expert Review of Cardiovascular Therapy*. 2010;Nov;8(11):1559–65.

Tadi K, 3,3′-Diindolylmethane: A Cruciferous Vegetable Derived Synthetic Anti-Proliferative Compound in Thyroid Disease. *Biochemical and Biophysical Research Communications*. 2005 Nov 25;337(3):1019–25.

Toft AD. Thyroxine Therapy. *New England Journal of Medicine*. 1994;331:174–180.

Verhoeven DT, et al. Epidemiological Studies on Brassica Vegetables and Cancer Risk. *Cancer Epidemiology, Biomarkers and Prevention*. 1996 Sep;5(9):733–48.

Ward LS. The Difficult Patient: Drug Interaction and the Influence of concomitant diseases on the Treatment of hypothyroidism. *Arquivos Brasileiros de Endocrinologia & Metabologia*. 2010;54(5):435–42.

Woeber KA. Subclinical Thyroid Dysfunction. *Archives of Internal Medicine*. 1997;157:1065–1068.

Yamada M, Mori M. Mechanisms Related to the Pathophysiology and Management of Central Hypothyroidism. *Nature Clinical Practice Endocrinology & Metabolism*. 2008;Dec;4(12):683–94.

Chapter 8 References

Aghajanova L, Giudice LC. Effect of Bisphenol A on Human Endometrial Stromal Fibroblasts in Vitro. *Reproductive BioMedicine Online*. 2011;Mar;22(3):249–56.

Arase S, et al. Endocrine Disrupter Bisphenol A Increases in Situ Estrogen Production in the Mouse Urogenital Sinus. *Biology of Reproduction*. 2011;Apr;84(4):734–42.

Arlt W, Callies FC, Van Viljmen JC, et al. Dehydroepiandrosterone Replacement in Women with Adrenal Insufficiency. *New England Journal of Medicine*. 1999;341:1013–1020.

Artini PG, et al. Best Methods for Identification and Treatment of PCOS. *Minerva Ginecologica*. 2010;Feb;62(1):33–48.

Ayala C, Steinberger E, Smith KD, et al. Serum Testosterone Levels and Reference Ranges in Reproductive-Age Women. *Endocrine Practice*. 1999;5:322–329.

Azziz R, et al. The Androgen Excess and PCOS Society Criteria for the polycystic Ovary Syndrome: The Complete Task Force Report. *Fertility and Sterility*. 2009;Feb;91(2):456–88.

Azziz R, Hincapie LA, Knochenhauer ES, et al. Screening for 21-Hydroxylase Deficient Non-Classic Adrenal Hyperplasia Among Hyperandrogenic Women: A Prospective Study. *Fertility and Sterility*. 1999;72:915–925.

Azziz R. Adrenal Androgen Excess in the Polycystic Ovary Syndrome. *Endocrinologist*. 2000;10:245–254.

Azziz R. Polycystic Ovary Syndrome is a Family Affair. *Journal of Clinical Endocrinology and Metabolism*. 2008;May;93(5):1579–1581.

Berenson, AB, Effect of Injectable and Oral Contraceptives on Glucose and Insulin Levels. *Obstetrics & Gynecology*. 2011;117:41–47.

Bertanza G, et al. Effect of Biological and Chemical Oxidation on the Removal of Estrogenic Compounds (NP and BPA) from Wastewater: An Integrated Assessment Procedure. *Water Research* 2011;Apr;45(8):2473–84.

Birdsall MA, Farquhar CM, and White HD. Association between Polycystic Ovaries and Extent of Coronary Artery Disease in Women Having Cardiac Catherization. *Annals of Internal Medicine*. 1997;126:32–35.

Bruce Jancin. Blood Type, Ovarian Reserve Linked. *Clinical Endocrinology News*. 6, 2, February 2011.

Branhardt KT, Freeman E, Grisso JA, et al. The Effect of Deydroepiandrosterone Supplementation to Symptomatic Perimenopausal Women on Serum Endocrine Profiles, Lipid Parameters, and Health Related Quality of Life. *Journal of Clinical Endocrinology and Metabolism*. 1999;84:3896–3901.

Buccola JM, Reynolds EE. Polycystic Ovary Syndrome: A Review for Primary Providers. *Journal of Primary Care and Community Health*. 2003 Dec;30(4):697–710.

Casson PR, Buster JE. DHEA Replacement after Menopause: HRT 2000 or Nostrum of the 90s? *Contemporary OB/GYN*. 1997;119–133.

Chen MJ, et al. High Serum Dehydroepiandrosterone Sulfate Is Associated with Phenotypic Acne and a Reduced Risk of Abdominal Obesity in Women with Polycystic Ovary Syndrome. *Human Reproduction*. 2011;Jan;26(1):227–234.

Chocano-Bedoya PO, et al. Dietary B Vitamin Intake and Incident Premenstrual Syndrome. *American Journal of Clinical Nutrition*. 2011;May;93(5):1080–6.

Crinnion WJ. Toxic Effects of the Easily Avoidable Phthalates and Parabens. *Alternative Medicine Review*. 2010;Sep;15(3):190–6.

Duranteau L, et al. Should Physicians Prescribe Metformin to Women with Polycystic Ovary Syndrome PCOS? *Annales d'Endocrinologiel (Paris)*. 2010;Feb;71(1):25–7.

Edelman A, et al. Combined Oral Contraceptives and Body Weight: Do Oral Contraceptives Cause Weight Gain? A Primate Model. *Human Reproduction*. 2011;Feb;26(2):330–6.

Foidart JM, Faustmann T. Advances in Hormone Replacement Therapy: Weight Benefits of Drospirenone, A 17alpha-Spirolactone-Derived Progestogen. *Gynecological Endocrinology*. 2007 Dec;23(12):692-9.

Franks S. Polycystic Ovary Syndrome. *New England Journal of Medicine*. 1995;333:853–860.

Fruzzetti F, Bitzer J. Review of Clinical Experience with estradiol in Combined Oral Contraceptives. *Contraception* 2010;81:8–15.

Geisthovel F, Olbrich M, Frorath B, et al. Obesity and Hypertestosteronaemia Are Independently and Synergistically Associated with Elevated Insulin Concentrations and Dyslipidaemia in Pre-Menopausal Women. *Human Reproduction*. 1994;9:610–616.

Giallauria F, et al. Cardiovascular Risk in Women with Polycystic Ovary Syndrome. *Journal of Cardiovascular Medicine (Hagerstown)*. 2008;Oct;9(10):987–92.

Glueck CJ, et al. Sex Hormone-Binding Globulin, Oligomenorrhea, Polycystic Ovary Syndrome, and Childhood Insulin at Age 14 Years Predict Metabolic Syndrome and Class III Obesity at Age 24 Years. *Journal of Pediatrics*. 2011;Aug;159(2):308–313.e2.

Gollenberg AL, et al. Perceived Stress and Severity of Perimenstrual Symptoms: The BioCycle Study. *Journal of Women's Health (Larchmont)*. 2010;May;19(5):959–67.

Hart R. PCOS and Infertility. *Panminerva Medica*. 2008;Dec;50(4):305–14.

Jick SS, Hernandez RK. Risk of Non-Fatal Venous Thromboembolism in Women Using Oral Contraceptives Containing Drospirenone Compared with Women Using Oral Contraceptives Containing Levonorgestrel: Case-Control Study Using United States Claims Data. *British Medical Journal*. 2011;Apr 21;342:d2151. doi: 10.1136/bmj.d2151.

Kandaraki E, et al. Endocrine Disruptors and Polycystic Ovary Syndrome (PCOS): Elevated Serum Levels of Bisphenol A in Women with PCOS. *Journal of Clinical Endocrinology and Metabolism*. 2011;Mar;96(3):E480–4.

Ketel IJ, et al. Obese but Not Normal-Weight Women with Polycystic Ovary Syndrome Are Characterized by Metabolic and Microvascular Insulin Resistance. *Journal of Clinical Endocrinology and Metabolism*. 2008;Sep;93(9):3365–72.

Knox SS, et al. Implications of Early Menopause in women exposed to Fluorocarbons. *Journal of Clinical Endocrinology and Metabolism*. 2011;Jun;96(6):1747–53.

Kulie T, et al. Obesity and Women's Health: An Evidence-Based Review. *Journal of American Board of Family Medicine*. 2011;Jan–Feb;24(1):75–85.

Legro RS. Impact of Metformin, Oral Contraceptives, and Lifestyle Modification on Polycystic Ovary Syndrome in Obese Adolescent Women: Do We Need a New Drug? *Journal of Clinical Endocrinology and Metabolism*. 2008;Nov;93(11):4218–20.

Lobo RA and Carmina E. The Importance of Diagnosing the Polycystic Ovary Syndrome. *Annals of Internal Medicine*. 2000;132:989–993.

Mlynarcikova A, Fickova M, Scsukova S. Ovarian Intrafollicular Processes as a Target for Cigarette Smoke Components and Selected Environmental Reproductive Disruptors. *Endocrine Regulations*. 2005 Jan;39(1):21–32.

Mogensen, SS, et al. Diagnostic Work-Up of 449 Consecutive Girls Who Were Referred to Be Evaluated for Precocious Puberty. *Journal of Clinical Endocrinology and Metabolism*, Feb 23, 2011;doi:10.1210/jc.2010-2745.

Mouritsen A, et al. Hypothesis: Exposure to Endocrine-Disrupting Chemicals May Interfere with Timing of Puberty. *International Journal of Andrology*. 2010;Apr;33(2):346–59.

Nestler JE and Jakubowicz DJ. Decreases in Ovarian Cytochrome P450c17? Activity and Serum Free Testosterone after Reduction of Insulin Secretion in Polycystic Ovary Syndrome. *New England Journal of Medicine*. 1996;335:617–623.

Nestler JE, Jakubowicz DJ, Evans WS, Pasquali R. Effects of Metformin on Spontaneous and Clomiphene-Induced Ovulation in the Polycystic Ovary Syndrome. *New England Journal of Medicine*. 1998;338:1876–1880.

Nitsche K, Ehrmann DA. Obstructive Sleep Apnea and Metabolic Dysfunction in Polycystic Ovary Syndrome. *Best Practice & Research Clinical Endocrinology & Metabolism*. 2010;Oct;24(5):717–30.

Norman RJ, et al. Subjects with polycystic ovaries without Hyperandrogenaemia Exhibit Similar Disturbances in Insulin and Lipid Profiles as Those with Polycystic Ovary Syndrome. *Human Reproduction*. 1995 Sep;10(9):2258–61.

Poppe K, Velkeniers B, Glinoer D. Thyroid Disease and Female Reproduction. *Clinical Endocrinology (Oxford)*. 2007 Mar;66(3):309–21.

Reubinoff BE, et al. Effects of Low-Dose Estrogen Oral Contraceptives on weight, Body Composition, and Fat Distribution in Young Women. *Fertility and Sterility*. 1995 Mar;63(3):516–21.

Riu A, et al, Peroxysome Proliferator-Activated Receptor-*y* Is a Target for Halogenated Analogues of Bisphenol-A. *Environmental Health Perspectives*. 2011;May 11.

Rocha Filho EA, et al. Essential Fatty Acids for Premenstrual Syndrome and Their Effect on Prolactin and Total Cholesterol Levels: A Randomized, Double Blind, Placebo-Controlled Study. *Reproductive Health*. 2011;Jan 17;8(1):2.

Roy JR, Chakraborty S, Chakraborty TR. Estrogen-Like Endocrine Disrupting Chemicals Affecting Puberty in Humans: A Review. *Medical Science Monitor*. 2009;Jun;15(6):RA137–45.

Rudel RA, et al. Food Packaging and Bisphenol a and Bis(2-ethyhexyl)phthalate Exposure: Findings from a Dietary Intervention. *Environmental Health Perspectives*. 2011;Jul;119(7):914–20.

Salawu, AA. Effect of the Juice of Lime on Estrous Cycle and Ovulatation of Sprague-Dawley Rats. *Endocrine Practice*. 16,. 4 July/August 2010, 561–565.

Schmidt PJ, et al. Depression in Women with Spontaneous 46, XX primary Ovarian Insufficiency. *Journal of Clinical Endocrinology and Metabolism*. 2011;Feb;96(2):E278–87.

Schoeters G, et al. Endocrine Disruptors and Abnormalities of Pubertal Development. *Basic & Clinical Pharmacology & Toxicology*. 2008;Feb;102(2):168–75.

Sheehan MT. Polycystic Ovarian Syndrome: Diagnosis and Management. *Clinical Medicine & Research*. 2004 Feb;2(1):13–27.

Szabo, Liz. Keeping Her a Kid as Long as Possible. *USA Today*. April 11, 2011.

Tabb MM, Blumberg B. New modes of Action for Endocrine-Disrupting Chemicals. *Molecular Endocrinology*. 2006 Mar;20(3):475–82.

Teede H, Deeks A, Moran L. Polycystic Ovary Syndrome: A Complex Condition with Psychological, Reproductive and Metabolic Manifestations That Impacts on Health across the Lifespan. *BMC Medicine*. 2010;Jun 30;8:41.

Thomson RL, et al. The Effect of a Hypocaloric Diet with and without Exercise Training on Body Composition, Cardiometabolic Risk Profile, and Reproductive Function In Overweight and Obese Women with Polycystic Ovary Syndrome. *Journal of Clinical Endocrinology and Metabolism*. 2008;Sep;93(9):3373–80.

Verma S, Mather K, Dumont AS, and Anderson TJ. Pharmacological Modulation of Insulin Resistance and Hyperinsulinemia in Polycystic Ovary Syndrome: The Emerging Role. *Endocrinologist*. 1998;8:418–424.

vom Saal FS, Hughes C. An Extensive New Literature Concerning Low-Dose Effects of Bisphenol A Shows the Need for a New Risk Assessment. *Environmental Health Perspectives*. 2005 Aug;113(8):926–33.

Welshons WV, Nagel SC, vom Saal FS. Large effects from Small Exposures. III. Endocrine Mechanisms Mediating Effects of Bisphenol A at Levels of Human Exposure. *Endocrinology*. 2006 Jun;147(6 Suppl):S56–69.

Chapter 9

Cirillo D, et al. Leptin Signaling in Breast Cancer: An Overview. *Journal of Cellular Biochemistry*. 2008;Nov 1;105(4):956–64.

Clarke BO, Smith SR. Review of "Emerging" Organic Contaminants in Biosolids and Assessment of International Research Priorities for the Agricultural Use of Biosolids. *Environment International* 2011;Jan;37(1):226–47.

Crinnion WJ. Toxic Effects of the Easily Avoidable Phthalates and Parabens. *Alternative Medicine Review*. 2010;Sep;15(3):190–6.

Davis M, et al. The Psychosocial Transition Associated with Spontaneous 46,XX Primary Ovarian Insufficiency: Illness Uncertainty, Stigma, Goal Flexibility, and Purpose in Life as Factors in Emotional Health. *Fertility and Sterility*. 2010;May 1;93(7):2321–9.

Diamanti-Kandarakis E, et al. Endocrine-Disrupting Chemicals: An Endocrine Society Scientific Statement. *Endocrinology Review*. 2009;Jun;30(4):293–342.

Doherty LF, et al. In Utero Exposure to Diethylstilbestrol (DES) or Bisphenol-A (BPA) Increases EZH2 Expression in the Mammary Gland: An Epigenetic Mechanism Linking Endocrine Disruptors to Breast Cancer. *Hormones and Cancer*. 2010;Jun;1(3):146–55.

Friedman, E. J. et al. Efficacy of Escitalopram for Hot Flashes in Healthy Menopausal Women. *Journal of the American Medical Association*, 2010:305:267–74.

Hermansen K, et al. Beneficial Effects of a soy-Based Dietary Supplement on Lipid Levels and Cardiovascular Risk Markers in Type 2 Diabetic Subjects. *Diabetes Care*. 2001 Feb;24(2):228–33.

Jardé T, et al. Molecular Mechanisms of Leptin and Adiponectin in Breast Cancer. *European Journal of Cancer*. 2011;Jan;47(1):33–43.

Jayagopal V, et al. Beneficial Effects of Soy Phytoestrogen Intake in Postmenopausal Women with Type 2 Diabetes. *Diabetes Care*. 2002 Oct;25(10):1709–14.

Kim MH, et al. Genistein and Daidzein Repress Adipogenic Differentiation of Human Adipose Tissue-Derived Mesenchymal Stem Cells via Wnt/?-Catenin Signaling or Lipolysis. *Cell Proliferation.* 2010;Dec;43(6):594–605. doi: 10.1111/j.1365–2184.2010.00709.x.

Laliberte F, et al. Does the route of administration for Estrogen Hormone Therapy Impact the Risk of Venous Thromboembolism? Estradiol Transdermal System versus Oral Estrogen-Only Hormone Therapy. *Menopause*. 2011 Oct;18(10):1052–1059.

Langdon KA, et al. Selected Personal Care Products and Endocrine Disruptors in Biosolids: An Australia-Wide Survey. *Science of the Total Environment*. 2011;Feb 15;409(6):1075–81.

Lee J, Hopkins V. *What Your Doctor May Not Tell You about Menopause*. New York: Warner, 2004.

McTiernan, A. Exercise and Breast Cancer—Time to Get Moving? *New England Journal of Medicine*. 1997;336(18):1311–1312.

McTiernan, A. Physical Activity, Weight, Diet and Breast Cancer Risk Reduction. *Archives of Internal Medicine*. 170(20), Nov 8, 2010, 1792–1793.

Naaz A, et al. The Soy Isoflavone Genistein Decreases Adipose Deposition in Mice. *Endocrinology*. 2003 Aug;144(8):3315–20.

Paz-Filho G, et al. Associations between Adipokines and Obesity-Related Cancer. *Frontiers in Bioscience*. 2011;Jan 1;16:1634–50.

Penza M, et al. Genistein Affects Adipose Tissue Deposition in a Dose-Dependent and Gender-Specific Manner. *Endocrinology*. 2006 Dec;147(12):5740–51.

PubMed.gov. U.S. National Library of Medicine, National Institutes of Health.

Relic B, et al. Genistein Induces Adipogenesis but Inhibits Leptin Induction in Human Synovial Fibroblasts. *Laboratory Investigation*. 2009;Jul;89(7):811–22.

2009;Rose DP, et al. Obesity, Adipocytokines, and Insulin Resistance in Breast Cancer. *Obesity Review*. 2004 Aug;5(3):153–65.

Rose DP, Gilhooly EM, Nixon DW. Adverse Effects of Obesity on Breast Cancer Prognosis, and the Biological Actions of Leptin (Review). *International Journal of Oncology*. 2002 Dec;21(6):1285–92.

Rossouw JE, et al. Risks and Benefits of Estrogen Plus Progestin in Healthy Postmenopausal Women: Principal Results from the Women's Health Initiative Randomized Controlled Trial. *Journal of the American Medical Association*. 2002 Jul 17;288(3):321–33.

Surmacz E. Obesity Hormone Leptin: A New Target in Breast Cancer? *Breast Cancer Research*. 2007;9(1):301.

Thune I. Physical Activity and the Risk of Breast Cancer. *New England Journal of Medicine*. 1997;336(18):1269–1275.

Yang YJ, et al. Bisphenol A Exposure Is Associated with Oxidative Stress and Inflammation in Postmenopausal Women. *Environmental Research*. 2009;Aug;109(6):797–801.

Chapter 10

Bassil N, Alkaade S, Morley JE. The Benefits and Risks of Testosterone Replacement Therapy: A Review. *Journal of Therapeutic and Clinical Risk Management*. 2009;Jun;5(3):427–48.

Berglund LH, et al. Testosterone Levels and Psychological Health Status in Men From A General Population: The Tromsø Study. *Aging Male*. 2011;Mar;14(1):37–41.

Corona G. et al. Hypogonadism, ED, Metabolic Syndrome and Obesity: A Pathological Link Supporting Cardiovascular Diseases. *International Journal of Andrology*. 2009;Dec;32(6):587–98.

Cortés-Gallegos V, et al. Sleep Deprivation Reduces Circulating Androgens in Healthy Men. *Archives of Andrology*. 1983 Mar;10(1):33–7.

Dandona P, et al. Hypogonadotrophic Hypogonadism in Type 2 Diabetes, Obesity and the Metabolic Syndrome. *Current Molecular Medicine*. 2008;Dec;8(8):816–28.

Dandona, P and Dhindsa, S. Update: Hypogonadotropic Hypogonadism in Type 2 Diabetes and Obesity. *Journal of Clinical Endocrinology and Metabolism*. September 2011, 96(9):2643–2651.

Ginzburg E, et al. Long-Term Safety of Testosterone and Growth Hormone Supplementation: A Retrospective Study of Metabolic, Cardiovascular, and Oncologic Outcomes. *Journal of Clinical Medicine and Research*. 2010;Aug 18;2(4):159–66.

Gopal, RA. Treatment of Hypogonadism with Testosterone in Patients with Type 2 Diabetes Mellitus. *Endocrine Practice*. 16, 4 July/August 2010, 570–576.

Gruenewald DA, Matsumoto AM. Testosterone Supplementation Therapy for older Men: Potential Benefits and Risks. *Journal of American Geriatrics Society*. 2003 Jan;51(1):101–15;discussion 115.

Guay AT. The Emerging Link between Hypogonadism and Metabolic Syndrome. *Journal of Andrology*. 2009;Jul–Aug;30(4):370–6.

Leproult R, Van Cauter E. Effect of 1 Week of Sleep Restriction on testosterone levels in Young Healthy Men. *Journal of the American Medical Association*. 2011;Jun 1;305(21):2173–4.

Moncada I. Testosterone and Men's Quality of Life. *Aging Male*. 2006 Dec;9(4):189–93.

Morales A. et al. A Practical Guide to Diagnosis, Management and Treatment of Testosterone Deficiency for Canadian Physicians. *Canadian Urological Association Journal*. 2010;Aug;4(4):269–75.

Morley JE, et al. Validation of a Screening Questionnaire for Androgen Deficiency in Aging Males. *Metabolism*. 2000 Sep;49(9):1239–42.

Olsen S, et al. Creatine Supplementation Augments the Increase in Satellite Cell and Myonuclei Number in Human Skeletal Muscle Induced by Strength Training. *Journal of Physiology*. 2006 Jun 1;573(Pt 2):525–34.

Raynaud JP. Prostate Cancer Risk in Testosterone-Treated Men. *Journal of Steroid Biochemistry and Molecular Biology*. 2006 Dec;102(1–5):261–6.

Rosner W, Vesper H on behalf of the Endocrine Society and Centers for Disease Control. Toward Excellence in Testosterone Testing: A Consensus Statement. *Journal of Clinical Endocrinology and Metabolism*, October 2010, 95(10);4542–4548.

Rosner, W, et al. Utility, Limitations, and Pitfalls in Measuring Testosterone an Endocrine Society Position Statement. *Journal of Clinical Endocrinology and Metabolism*, 2007 92:405–413.

Rosner, W, et al. CDC Workshop Report on Improving Steroid Hormone Measurements in Patient Care and Research Translation. *Steroids*. 2008;73:1285–1352.

Schroeder ET. et al. Treatment with Oxandrolone and the Durability of Effects in Older Men. *European Journal of Applied Physiology*. 2004 Mar;96(3):1055–62.

Seftel A. Male Hypogonadism. Part II: Etiology, Pathophysiology, and Diagnosis. *International Journal of Impotence Research* 2006;18(3):223–228.

Travison TG, et al. Changes in Reproductive Hormone Concentrations Predict the Prevalence and progression of the Frailty Syndrome in Older Men: The Concord Health and Aging in Men Project. *Journal of Clinical Endocrinology and Metabolism*. 2011;Aug;96(8):2464–74.

Trinick TR, et al. International Web Survey Shows High Prevalence of Symptomatic Testosterone Deficiency in Men. *Aging Male*. 2011;Mar;14(1):10–5.

Vesper, HW, et al. 2009;Interlaboratory Comparison Study of Serum Total Testosterone [Corrected] Measurements Performed by Mass Spectrometry Methods. *Steroids* [Erratum (2009) 74:791] 74: 498–503.

Chapter 11

Adam TC, Epel ES. Stress, Eating and the Reward System. *Physiology and Behavior*. 2007 Jul 24;91(4):449–58.

Anagnostis P, et al. Clinical Review: The Pathogenetic Role of Cortisol in the Metabolic Syndrome: A Hypothesis. *Journal of Clinical Endocrinology and Metabolism*. 2009;Aug;94(8):2692–701.

Asensio C, et al. Role of Glucocorticoids in the Physiopathology of Excessive Fat Deposition and insulin resistance. *International Journal of Obesity and Related Metabolic Disorders*. 2004 Dec;28 Suppl 4:S45–52.

Beauregard C, et al. Classic and Recent Etiologies of Cushing's Syndrome: Diagnosis and Therapy. *Treatments in Endocrinology*. 2002;1(2):79–94.

Bertagna X, et al. Cushing's Disease. Best Pract Res *Clinical Endocrinology and Metabolism*. 2009;Oct;23(5):607–23.

Bose M, et al. Stress and Obesity: The Role of the Hypothalamic-Pituitary-Adrenal Axis in Metabolic Disease. *Current Opinion in Endocrinology, Diabetes and Obesity*. 2009;Oct;16(5):340–6.

Brown ES, et al. Association of Depression with Medical Illness: Does Cortisol Play A Role? *Biological Psychiatry*. 2004 Jan 1;55(1):1–9.

Bruno OD, et al. In What Clinical Settings Should Cushing's Syndrome Be Suspected? *Medicina (Buenos Aires)*. 2009;69(6):674–680.

Chaput JP, et al. Do all sedentary activities lead to weight gain: sleep does not. *Current Opinion in Clinical Nutrition & Metabolic Care*. 2010;Nov;13(6):601–7.

Chiodini I. Clinical Review: Diagnosis and Treatment of Subclinical Hypercortisolism. *Journal of Clinical Endocrinology and Metabolism*. 2011;May;96(5):1223–36.

Chubinskaya, K. et al. Myth vs. Fact: Adrenal Fatigue. *Endocrine Society Fact Sheet*. www.hormone.org. August 2010.

Coelho JS, et al. Inaccessible Food Cues Affect Stress and Weight Gain in Calorically-Restricted and Ad Lib Fed Rats. *Appetite*. 2010;Feb;54(1):229–32.

Dallman MF, et al. Feast and Famine: Critical Role of Glucocorticoids with Insulin in Daily Energy Flow. *Frontiers in Neuroendocrinology*. 1993 Oct;14(4):303–47.

Drake AJ, et al. Reduced Adipose Glucocorticoid Reactivation and Increased Hepatic Glucocorticoid Clearance as an Early Adaptation to High-Fat Feeding in Wistar Rats. *Endocrinology*. 2005 Feb;146(2):913–9.

Fontana L. Neuroendocrine Factors in the Regulation of Inflammation: Excessive Adiposity and Calorie Restriction. *Experimental Gerontology*. 2009;Jan–Feb;44(1–2):41–5.

Gade W, et al. Beyond Obesity: The Diagnosis and Pathophysiology of Metabolic Syndrome. *Clinical Laboratory Science*. 2010;Winter;23(1):51–61.

Gagliardi L, et al. Corticosteroid-Binding Globulin: The Clinical Significance of Altered Levels and Heritable Mutations. *Molecular and Cellular Endocrinology.* 2010;Mar 5;316(1):24–34.

Gathercole LL, Stewart PM. Targeting the Pre-Receptor Metabolism of Cortisol as a Novel Therapy in Obesity and Diabetes. *Journal of Steroid Biochemistry and Molecular Biology.* 2010;Oct;122(1–3):21–7.

Gross BA, et al. Diagnostic Approach to Cushing Disease. *Neurosurgical Focus.* 2007;23(3):E1.

Hinkelmann K, et al. Cognitive Impairment in Major Depression: Association with Salivary Cortisol. *Biological Psychiatry.* 2009;Nov 1;66(9):879–85.

Kiecolt-Glaser JK, Glaser R. Chronic Stress and Mortality among Older Adults. *Journal of the American Medical Association.* 1999 Dec 15;282(23):2259–60.

Kivimäki M, et al. Work Stress, Weight Gain and Weight Loss: Evidence for Bidirectional Effects of Job Strain on Body Mass Index in the Whitehall II Study. *International Journal of Obesity (London).* 2006 Jun;30(6):982–7.

Korkeila M, et al. Predictors of Major Weight Gain in Adult Finns: Stress, Life Satisfaction and Personality Traits . *International Journal of Obesity and Related Metabolic Disorders.* 1998 Oct;22(10):949–57.

Kuo LE, et al. Chronic Stress, Combined with a High-Fat/High-Sugar Diet, Shifts Sympathetic Signaling toward Neuropeptide Y and Leads to Obesity and the Metabolic Syndrome. *Annals of the New York Academy of Sciences.* 2008;Dec;1148:232–7.

Labeur M, et al. New Aspects in the Diagnosis and Treatment of Cushing Disease. *Frontiers of Hormone Research.* 2006;35:169–78.

Leproult R, Van Cauter E. Role of Sleep and Sleep Loss in Hormonal Release and Metabolism. *Endocrine Development.* 2010;17:11–21.

London E, Castonguay TW. Diet and the Role of 11beta-Hydroxysteroid Dehydrogenase-1 on Obesity. *Journal of Nutritional Biochemistry.* 2009;Jul;20(7):485–93.

Mann JN, Thakore JH. Melancholic Depression and Abdominal Fat Distribution: A Mini-Review. *Stress.* 1999 Aug;3(1):1–15.

Mattsson C, Olsson T. Estrogens and Glucocorticoid Hormones in Adipose Tissue Metabolism. *Current Medicinal Chemistry.* 2007;14(27):2918–24.

Messerli FH, et al. The President and the Pheochromocytoma. *American Journal of Cardiology.* 2007 May 1;99(9):1325–9.

Michel C, et al. Stress Facilitates Body Weight Gain in Genetically Predisposed Rats on Medium-Fat Diet. *American Journal of Physiology—Regulatory, Integrative and Comparative Physiology.* 2003 Oct;285(4):R791–9.

Morton NM. Obesity and Corticosteroids: 11beta-Hydroxysteroid Type 1 as a cause and Therapeutic Target in Metabolic Disease. *Molecular and Cellular Endocrinology.* 2010;Mar 25;316(2):154–64.

Müssig K, et al. Brief Review: Glucocorticoid Excretion in Obesity. *Journal of Steroid Biochemistry and Molecular Biology.* 2010;Aug;121(3–5):589–93.

Nieuwenhuizen AG, Rutters F. The Hypothalamic-Pituitary-Adrenal-Axis in the regulation of Energy Balance. *Physiology & Behavior.* 2008;May 23;94(2):169–77.

O'Brien JT, et al. A Longitudinal Study of Hippocampal Volume, Cortisol Levels, and cognition in Older Depressed Subjects. *American Journal of Psychiatry.* 2004 Nov;161(11):2081–90.

Overgaard D, et al. Psychological Workload and Body Weight: Is There an Association? A Review of the Literature. *Occupational Medicine (London).* 2004 Jan;54(1):35–41.

Pankevich DE, et al. Caloric Restriction Experience Reprograms Stress and Orexigenic Pathways and Promotes Binge Eating. *Journal of Neuroscience.* 2010;Dec 1;30(48):16399-407.

Park, A. Men vs. Women: Who Gains More Weight after Marriage and Divorce? *Time,* August 22, 2011. http://healthland.time.com/2011/08/22/men-vs-women-who-gains-more-weight-after-marriage-and-divorce/.

Pasquali R, et al. Sex-Dependent role of Glucocorticoids and Androgens in the Pathophysiology of Human Obesity. *International Journal of Obesity (London).* 2008;Dec;32(12):1764–79.

Pasquali R, et al. The Hypothalamic-Pituitary-Adrenal Axis Activity in Obesity and the Metabolic Syndrome. *Annals of the New York Academy of Sciences.* 2006 Nov;1083:111-28.

Reynolds RM. Corticosteroid-Mediated Programming and the Pathogenesis of Obesity and Diabetes. *Journal of Steroid Biochemistry and Molecular Biology.* 2010;Oct;122(1–3):3–9.

Terzolo M, et al. Subclinical Cushing's Syndrome. *Arquivos Brasileiros de Endocrinologia & Metabologia (São Paulo).* 2007 Nov;51(8):1272–1279.

Terzolo M, et al. Subclinical Cushing's Syndrome. *Pituitary.* 2004;7(4):217–223.

Torres SJ, Nowson CA. Relationship between Stress, Eating Behavior, and Obesity. *Nutrition.* 2007 Nov–Dec;23(11–12):887–94.

Tritos NA, et al. Management of Cushing Disease. *Nature Reviews Endocrinology.* 2011;May;7(5):279–89.

van Jaarsveld CH, et al. Perceived Stress and Weight Gain in adolescence: A Longitudinal Analysis. *Obesity (Silver Spring).* 2009;Dec;17(12):2155–61.

Velez DA, et al. Cyclic Cushing Syndrome: Definitions and Treatment Implications. *Neurosurgical Focus.* 2007;23(3):E4;discussion E4a.

Yildiz BO, Azziz R. The Adrenal and Polycystic Ovary Syndrome. *Reviews in Endocrine and Metabolic Disorders.* 2007 Dec;8(4):331–42.

Chapter 12

Allen DB. Lessons Learned from the hGH Era. *Journal of Clinical Endocrinology and Metabolism.* 2011 Oct;96(10):3042-7.

Al-Regaiey KA, et al. Long-Lived Growth Hormone Receptor Knockout Mice: Interaction of Reduced Insulin-Like Growth Factor i/Insulin Signaling and Caloric Restriction. *Endocrinology.* 2005 Feb;146(2):851–860.

al-Shoumer KA, et al. Elevated Leptin Concentrations in growth Hormone-Deficient Hypopituitary Adults. *Clinical Endocrinology (Oxford)*. 1997 Aug;47(2):153–9.

Bartke A, Brown-Borg H. Life Extension in the Dwarf Mouse. *Current Topics in Developmental Biology*. 2004;63:189–225.

Bartke A. Growth Hormone, Insulin and Aging: The Benefits of Endocrine Defects. *Experimental Gerontology*. 2011;Feb–Mar;46(2–3):108–11.

Bartke A. Pleiotropic effects of Growth Hormone Signaling in Aging. *Trends in Endocrinology and Metabolism*. 2011 Nov;22(11):437-42..

Beshyah SA, et al. Abnormal Body Composition and Reduced Bone Mass in growth Hormone Deficient Hypopituitary Adults. *Clinical Endocrinology (Oxford)*. 1995 Feb;42(2):179–89.

Child CJ, et al. Prevalence and Incidence of Diabetes Mellitus in GH-Treated Children and Adolescents: Analysis from the GeNeSIS Observational Research Program. *Journal of Clinical Endocrinology and Metabolism*. 2011;Jun;96(6):E1025–34.

Cornford AS. Rapid Suppression of Growth Hormone Concentration by Overeating: Potential Mediation by Hyperinsulinemia. *Journal of Clinical Endocrinology and Metabolism*, March 2011, 96(3):824–830.

Cuatrecasas G. High Prevalence of Growth Hormone Deficiency in Severe Fibromyalgia Syndromes. *Journal of Clinical Endocrinology and Metabolism*, September 2010, 95(9):4331–4337.

Green J, et al. Height and Cancer Incidence in the Million Women Study: Prospective Cohort, and Meta-Analysis of prospective studies of Height and Total Cancer Risk. *Lancet Oncology*. 2011;Aug;12(8):785–794.

Lee HW, et al. Long-term Growth Hormone Administration Increased Hepatic Insulin Resistance, but Not Muscle Insulin Resistance, in Healthy Older Men And Women. *Endo Pharmaceuticals* 2011;Abstract OR27-4.

Makimura H, et al. Reduced Growth Hormone Secretion in Obesity Is Associated with Smaller LDL and HDL Particle Size. *Clinical Endocrinology (Oxford)*. 2011;Aug 5. doi: 10.1111/j.1365-2265.2011.04195.x.

Mukherjee A, et al. Impact of Growth Hormone Status on Body Composition and the Skeleton. *Hormone Research*. 2004;62 Suppl 3:35–41.

Murray RD, et al. Adults with Partial Growth Hormone Deficiency Have an adverse Body Composition. *Journal of Clinical Endocrinology and Metabolism*. 2004 Apr;89(4):1586–91.

Ozbey N, et al. Serum Lipid and leptin concentrations in Hypopituitary Patients with Growth Hormone Deficiency. *International Journal of Obesity and Related Metabolic Disorders*. 2000 May;24(5):619–26.

Salman S, et al. Serum Adipokines and Low Density Lipoprotein Subfraction Profile in Hypopituitary Patients with Growth Hormone deficiency. *Pituitary*. 2011;Jul 21.

Van Bunderen, CC, et al. Does Growth Hormone Replacement Therapy Reduce Mortality in Adults with Growth Hormone Deficiency? *Endo Pharmaceuticals* 2011;Abstract OR27-2.

Vance ML, Mauras N. Growth Hormone Therapy in Adults and Children. *New England Journal of Medicine*. 1999 Oct 14;341(16):1206–16.

Woodhouse LJ, et al. The Influence of Growth Hormone Status on Physical Impairments, Functional Limitations, and Health-Related Quality of Life in Adults. *Endocrine Reviews.* 2006 May;27(3):287–317.

Practical Weight Loss Tips and Tools References

Alberga AS, Sigal RJ, Kenny GP. A Review of Resistance Exercise Training in Obese Adolescents. *Physician and Sportsmedicine.* 2011;May;39(2):50–63.

Aldabal L, Bahammam AS. Metabolic, Endocrine, and Immune Consequences of Sleep Deprivation. *Open Respiratory Medicine Journal.* 2011;5:31–43.

Alvarez GG, Ayas NT. The Impact of Daily Sleep Duration on Health: A Review of the Literature. *Progress in Cardiovascular Nursing.* 2004;Spring;19(2):56–9.

Anton SD, et al. Effects of a Weight Loss Plus Exercise Program on Physical Function in Overweight, Older Women: A Randomized Controlled Trial. *Journal of Clinical Interventions in Aging.* 2011;6:141–149.

Antunes–Correa LM, et al. Exercise Training Improves Neurovascular Control and Functional Capacity in Heart Failure Patients Regardless of Age. *European Journal of Cardiovascular Prevention & Rehabilitation.* 2011 Jun 22. [Epub ahead of print]

Arble DM, et al. Circadian Timing of Food Intake Contributes to Weight Gain. *Obesity.* 2009;17(11):2100–2102.

Arsenescu V, et al. Polychlorinated Biphenyl-77 Induces Adipocyte Differentiation and Proinflammatory Adipokines and Promotes Obesity and Atherosclerosis. *Environmental Health Perspectives.* 2008;Jun;116(6):761–768.

Axelsson J, et al. Beauty Sleep: Experimental Study on the Perceived Health and Attractiveness of Sleep Deprived People. *British Medical Journal.* 2010;Dec 14;341:c6614. doi: 10.1136/bmj.c6614.

Ayala GX, et al. Away-from-Home Food Intake and Risk for Obesity: Examining the Influence of Context. *Obesity (Silver Spring).* 2008;May;16(5):1002–1008.

Babu AR, et al. Type 2 Diabetes, Glycemic Control and Continuous Positive Airway Pressure in Obstructive Sleep Apnea. *Archives of Internal Medicine.* 2005;165:447–452.

Balducci, S. Effect of an Intensive Exercise Intervention Strategy on Modifiable Cardiovascular Risk Factors in Subjects with Type 2 Diabetes Mellitus. *Archives of Internal Medicine.* 2010;Nov 8;170(20).

Baron KG, Reid KJ, Kern AS, Zee PC. Role of Sleep Timing in Caloric Intake and BMI. *Obesity (Silver Spring).* 2011;Jul;19(7):1374–1381. doi: 10.1038/oby.2011.100.

Beccuti G, Pannain S. Sleep and Obesity. *Current Opinion in Clinical Nutrition & Metabolic Care.* 2011;Jul;14(4):402–412.

Benedict C, et al. Acute Sleep Deprivation Reduces Energy Expenditure in Healthy Men. *American Journal of Clinical Nutrition.* 2011;Jun;93(6):1229–1236.

Blundell JE, Stubbs RJ, Hughes DA, Whybrow S, King NA. Cross Talk between Physical Activity and Appetite Control: Does Physical Activity Stimulate Appetite? Proceedings of the *Nutrition Society.* 2003;Aug;62(3):651–661.

Brainard GC, et al. Sensitivity of the Human Circadian System to Short-Wavelength (420-nm) Light. *Journal of Biological Rhythms.* 2008;Oct;23(5):379–386.

Brondel L, et al. Acute Partial Sleep Deprivation Increases Food Intake in Healthy Men. *American Journal of Clinical Nutrition*. 2010;Jun;91(6):1550–1559.

Broom DR, Batterham RL, King JA, Stensel DJ. Influence of Resistance and Aerobic Exercise on Hunger, Circulating Levels of Acylated Ghrelin, and Peptide YY in Healthy Males. *American Journal of Physiology - Regulatory, Integrative, and Comparative Physiology*. 2009;Jan;296(1):R29–R35.

Buison A, et al. Augmenting Leptin Circadian Rhythm Following a Weight Reduction in Diet-Induced Obese Rats: Short- and Long-Term Effects, *Metabolism*. 2004;Jun;53(6):782–789.

Canapari CA, et al. Relationship between Sleep Apnea, Fat Distribution, and Insulin Resistance in Obese Children. *Journal of Clinical Sleep Medicine*. 2011;Jun 15;7(3):268–273.

Carey DG. Quantifying Differences in the Fat Burning Zone and the Aerobic Zone: Implications for Training. *Journal of Strength & Conditioning Research*. 2009;Oct;23(7):2090–2095.

Carhuatanta KA, et al. Voluntary Exercise Improves High-Fat Diet-Induced Leptin Resistance Independent of Adiposity. *Endocrinology*. 2011;Jul;152(7):2655–2664. Epub 2011;May 17.

CDC Exercise Guidelines. http://www.cdc.gov/physicalactivity/everyone/guidelines/index.html.

Chaput JP, Després JP, Bouchard C, Tremblay A. Longer Sleep Duration Associates with Lower Adiposity Gain in Adult Short Sleepers. *International Journal of Obesity (London)*. 2011;Jun 7. doi: 10.1038/ijo.2011.110.

Chaput JP, Klingenberg L, Sjödin A. Do All Sedentary Activities Lead to Weight Gain: Sleep Does Not. *Current Opinion in Clinical Nutrition & Metabolic Care*. 2010;Nov;13(6):601–607.

Charlier C, Desaive C, Plomteux G. Human Exposure to Endocrine Disrupters: Consequences of Gastroplasty on Plasma Concentration of Toxic Pollutants. *International Journal of Obesity and Related Metabolic Disorders*. 2002;Nov;26(11):1465–1468.

Christakis NA, Fowler JH. The Spread of Obesity in a Large Social Network over 32 Years. *New England Journal of Medicine*. 2007;July;357(4): 370–379.

Church TS, et al. Trends over 5 Decades in U.S. Occupation-Related Physical Activity and Their Associations with Obesity. *PLoS One*. 2011;6(5):e19657.

Church TS., et al. Effects of Aerobic and Resistance Training on Hemoglobin A1c Levels in Patients with Type 2 Diabetes: A Randomized Controlled Trial. *Journal of the American Medical Association*. 2010;304:2253–2262.

Dattilo M, et al. Sleep and Muscle Recovery: Endocrinological and Molecular Basis for a New and Promising Hypothesis. *Medical Hypotheses*. 2011 Aug;77(2):220-2

De Souza RW, et al. High-Intensity Resistance Training with Insufficient Recovery Time Between Bouts Induce Atrophy and Alterations in Myosin Heavy Chain Content in Rat Skeletal Muscle. *Anatomical Record (Hoboken)*. 2011;Jun 28. doi: 10.1002/ar.21428.

Desvergne B, Feige JN, Casals-Casas C. PPAR-Mediated Activity of Phthalates: A Link to the Obesity Epidemic? *Molecular and Cellular Endocrinology*. 2009;May 25;304(1–2):43–48. Epub 2009;Mar 9.

Diamanti-Kandarakis E, et al. Endocrine-Disrupting Chemicals: An Endocrine Society Scientific Statement. *Endocrine Reviews*. 2009;Jun;30(4):293–342.

Ding Q, Ying Z, Gómez-Pinilla F. Exercise Influences Hippocampal Plasticity by Modulating Brain-Derived Neurotrophic Factor Processing. *Neuroscience*. 2011;Jun 29.

Dirinck E, et al. Obesity and Persistent Organic Pollutants: Possible Obesogenic Effect of Organochlorine Pesticides and Polychlorinated Biphenyls. *Obesity (Silver Spring)*. 2011;Apr;19(4):709–714.

Drake CL, et al. Shift Work, Shift Work Disorder, and Jet Lag. In: Kryger MH, Roth T, Dement WC, eds. *Principles and Practice of Sleep Medicine*. 5th ed. Philadelphia: Saunders, 2010:784–798.

Drake CL, et al. Sift Work Sleep Disorder: Prevalence and Consequences Beyond That of Symptomatic Day Workers. *Sleep*. 2004;27(8):1453–1462.

Duhigg, C. Debating How Much Weed Killer Is Safe in Your Water Glass. *New York Times*. August 22, 2009. http://www.nytimes.com/2009/08/23/us/23water.html?

Eastman CI, et al. Dark Goggles and Bright Light Improve Circadian Rhythm Adaptation to Night-Shift Work. *Sleep*. 1994;17(6):535–543.

Elder CR. Impact of Sleep, Screen Time, Depression and Stress on Weight Change in the Intensive Weight Loss Phase of the LIFE Study. *International Journal of Obesity*. Advance online publication, 2011;Mar 29;doi: 10.1038/ijo.2011.60.

King JA, et al. Differential Acylated Ghrelin, Peptide Yy3-36, Appetite, and food Intake Responses to Equivalent Energy Deficits Created by Exercise and Food Restriction. *Journal of Clinical Endocrinology and Metabolism*. 2011;Apr;96(4):1114–1421.

Environmental Working Group. http://www.ewg.org/foodnews/.

Erdmann J, et al. Plasma Ghrelin Levels during Exercise: Effects of Intensity and duration, *Regulatory Peptides*. 2007;Oct 4;143(1–3):127–135.

Escobar C, et al. Scheduled Meals and Scheduled Palatable Snacks Synchronize Circadian Rhythms: Consequences for Ingestive Behavior. *Physiology & Behavior*. 2011;Sep 26;104(4):555–561.

Feigenbaum MS, Pollock ML. Prescription of Resistance Training for Health and Disease. *Medicine & Science in Sports & Exercise*. 1999;Jan;31(1):38–45.

Field T, Tai Chi Research Review. *Complementary Therapies in Clinical Practice*. 2011;Aug;17(3):141–146.

Folland JP, Williams AG. The Adaptations to Strength Training : Morphological and Neurological Contributions to Increased Strength. *Sports Medicine*. 2007;37(2):145–168.

Gabriel DA, Kamen G, Frost G. Neural Adaptations to Resistive Exercise: Mechanisms and Recommendations for Training Practices. *Sports Medicine*. 2006;36(2):133–149.

Garaulet M. et al. Ghrelin, Sleep Reduction and Evening Preference: Relationships to CLOCK 3111 T/C SNP and Weight Loss. *PLoS One*. 2011;Feb 28;6(2):e17435.

Gooley JJ. Exposure to Room Light before Bedtime Suppresses Melatonin Onset and Shortens Melatonin Duration in Humans. *Journal of Clinical Endocrinology and Metabolism*, 2011;doi:10.1210/jc.2010–2098.

Grün F, Obesogens. *Current Opinions in Endocrinology, Diabetes and Obesity*. 2010;Oct;17(5):453–459.

Grün F, Blumberg B. Endocrine Disrupters as Obesogens. *Molecular and Cellular Endocrinology*. 2009;May 25;304(1–2):19–29.

Grün F, Blumberg B. Environmental Obesogens: Organotins and Endocrine Disruption via Nuclear Receptor Signaling. *Endocrinology*. 2006 Jun;147(6 Suppl):S50–S55.

Guerra B, et al. Is Sprint Exercise a Leptin Signaling Mimetic in Human Skeletal Muscle? *Journal of Applied Physiology*. 2011;Jun 9.

Gupta S. Dear (food) diary. A new study shows that dieters can double their weight loss by Jotting Down What Foods They Eat. *Time*. 2008;Aug 4;172(5):70.

Harrison CL, Stepto NK, Hutchison SK, Teede HJ. The Impact of Intensified Exercise Training on Insulin Resistance and Fitness in Overweight and Obese Women with and without Polycystic Ovary Syndrome. *Clinical Endocrinology (Oxford)*. 2011;Jun 28. doi: 10.1111/j.1365–2265.2011.04160.x.

Hart CL, et al. Zolpidem-Related Effects on Performance and Mood during Simulated Night-Shift Work. *Experimental and Clinical Psychopharmacology*. 2003;11(4):259–268.

Hayes AL, Xu F, Babineau D, Patel SR. Sleep Duration and Circulating Adipokine Levels. *Sleep*. 2011;Feb 1;34(2):147–152.

He K. et al. Consumption of Monosodium Glutamate in Relation to Incidence of Overweight in Chinese Adults: China Health and Nutrition Survey (CHNS). *American Journal of Clinical Nutrition*. 2011;Jun;93(6):1328–1336.

Hollis JF, et al. Weight Loss during the Intensive Intervention Phase of the Weight-Loss Maintenance Trial. *American Journal of Preventive Medicine*. 2008;Aug;35(2):118–126.

Hopps E, Caimi G. Exercise in Obesity Management. *Journal of Sports Medicine and Physical Fitness*. 2011;Jun;51(2):275–282.

Horne JA, et al. Sleep Related Vehicle Accidents. *British Medical Journal*. 1995;310:565–567.

Hotchkiss AK, et al. Fifteen Years after "Wingspread": Environmental Endocrine Disrupters and Human and Wildlife Health: Where We Are Today and Where We Need to Go. *Toxicological Sciences*. 2008;Oct;105(2):235–259.

Howe CM, Berrill M, Pauli BD, Helbing CC, Werry K, Veldhoen N. Toxicity of Glyphosate-Based Pesticides to Four North American Frog Species. *Environmental Toxicology and Chemistry*. 2004 Aug;23(8):1928–1938.

Hsu YW, et al. Aging Effects on Exercise-Induced Alternations in Plasma Acylated Ghrelin and Leptin in Male Rats. *European Journal of Applied Physiology*. 2011;May;111(5):809–817.

Huang W, Ramsey KM, Marcheva B, Bass J. Circadian Rhythms, Sleep, and Metabolism. *Journal of Clinical Investigation*. 2011;Jun 1;121(6):2133–2141. doi: 10.1172/JCI46043.

Ide BN, et. al. Time Course of Strength and Power Recovery After Resistance Training with Different Movement Velocities. *Journal of Strength & Conditioning Research*. 2011;Jul;25(7):2025–2033.

Ivanova EA, et al. Altered Metabolism in the Melatonin-Related Receptor (GPR50) Knockout Mouse. *American Journal of Physiology—Endocrinology and Metabolism*. 2008;Jan;294(1):E176–E182.

Janesick A, Blumberg B. Endocrine Disrupting Chemicals and the Developmental Programming of adipogenesis and obesity. *Birth Defects Research Part C: Embryo Today*. 2011;Mar;93(1):34–50. doi: 10.1002/bdrc.20197.

Janesick A, Blumberg B. Minireview: PPAR? as the target of obesogens. *Journal of Steroid Biochemistry and Molecular Biology*. 2011 Oct;127(1-2):4-8 Epub 2011 Jan 18.

Jobst KA. You Are What You Eat: Stress, Survival Anxiety, the Environment, and Chemical Obesogens. *Journal of Alternative and Complementary Medicine*. 2002 Apr;8(2):101–102.

Johns MW. A New Method for Measuring Daytime Sleepiness: The Epworth Sleepiness Scale. *Sleep*. 1991 Dec;14(6):540–545.

Ka He, Shufa Du, Pengcheng Xun, Sangita Sharma, Huijun Wang, Fengying Zhai, and Barry Popkin, Consumption of Monosodium Glutamate in Relation to Incidence of Overweight in Chinese Adults: China Health and Nutrition Survey (CHNS). *American Journal of Clinical Nutrition* June 2011;93 no. 6 1328–1336.

Karatsoreos IN, et al. Disruption of Circadian Clocks Has Ramifications for Metabolism, Brain, and BehavioR. *Proceedings of the National Academy of Science of the United States of America*. 2011;Jan 25;108(4):1657–1662.

Karmaus W, et al. Maternal Levels of Dichlorodiphenyl-Dichloroethylene (DDE) May Increase Weight and Body Mass Index in Adult Female Offspring. *Occupational and Environmental Medicine*. 2009;Mar;66(3):143–149.

King JA, et al. Differential Acylated Ghrelin, Peptide YY3-36, Appetite, and Food Intake Responses to Equivalent Energy Deficits Created by Exercise and Food Restriction. *Journal of Clinical Endocrinology and Metabolism* 2011 Apr;96(4):1114-21.

King NA, Burley VJ, Blundell JE. Exercise-Induced Suppression of Appetite: Effects on Food Intake and Implications for Energy Balance. *European Journal of Clinical Nutrition*. 1994 Oct;48(10):715–724.

Kirchner S, et al. Prenatal Exposure to the Environmental Obesogen Tributyltin Predisposes Multipotent Stem Cells to Become Adipocytes. *Molecular Endocrinology*. 2010;Mar;24(3):526–539.

Klem ML, Wing RR, McGuire MT, Seagle HM. Hill JO. A Descriptive Study of Individuals Successful at Long-Term Maintenance of Substantial Weight Loss. *American Journal of Clinical Nutrition*. 1997;66;239–246.

Knutson KL, Van Cauter E. Associations between Sleep Loss and Increased Risk Of Obesity and Diabetes. *Annals of the New York Academy of Sciences*. 2008;1129:287–304.

Knutson KL. Sleep Duration and Cardiometabolic Risk: A Review of the Epidemiologic Evidence. *Best Practice & Research: Clinical Endocrinology & Metabolism*. 2010;Oct;24(5):731–743.

Konturek PC, Brzozowski T, Konturek SJ. Gut Clock: Implication of Circadian Rhythms in the Gastrointestinal Tract. *Journal of Physiology and Pharmacology*. 2011;Apr;62(2):139–150.

Korkmaz A, Topal T, Tan DX, Reiter RJ. Role of Melatonin in Metabolic Regulation. *Reviews in Endocrine and Metabolic Disorders*. 2009;Dec;10(4):261–270.

Lee DH, et al. Polychlorinated Biphenyls and Organochlorine Pesticides in Plasma Predict Development of Type 2 Diabetes in the Elderly: The Prospective Investigation of the Vasculature in Uppsala Seniors (PIVUS) Study. *Diabetes Care.* 2011;Jun 23. 2011 Aug;34(8):1778-84.

Leproult R, Van Cauter E. Effect of 1 Week of Sleep Restriction on Testosterone Levels in young healthy men. *Journal of the American Medical Association.* 2011;Jun 1;305(21):2173–214.

Leproult R, Van Cauter E. Role of Sleep and Sleep Loss in Hormonal Release and Metabolism. *Endocrine Development.* 2010;17:11–21.

Li X, Ycaza J, Blumberg B. The Environmental Obesogen Tributyltin Chloride Acts via Peroxisome Proliferator Activated Receptor Gamma to Induce Adipogenesis in Murine 3T3-L1 Preadipocytes. *Journal of Steroid Biochemistry and Molecular Biology.* 2011;Mar 21.

Ligibel JA, et al. Impact of a Mixed Strength and Endurance Exercise Intervention on Levels of Adiponectin, High Molecular Weight Adiponectin and Leptin in Breast Cancer Survivors, *Cancer Causes & Control.* 2009;Oct;20(8):1523–1528.

Lira FS, et al. Exercise Training Improves Sleep Pattern and Metabolic Profile in Elderly People in a Time-Dependent Manner. *Lipids in Health and Disease.* 2011;Jul 6;10(1):113.

Lo MS, Lin LL, Yao WJ, Ma MC. Training and Detraining Effects of the Resistance vs. Endurance Program on Body Composition, Body Size, and Physical Performance in Young Men. *Journal of Strength and Conditioning Research.* 2011;Aug;25(8):2246-54

Martin, A. Chemical Suspected in Cancer Is in Baby Products. *New York Times.* May 17, 2011. http://www.nytimes.com/2011/05/18/business/18chemical.html

Martins C, Morgan LM, Bloom SR, Robertson MD. Effects of Exercise on Gut Peptides, Energy Intake and Appetite. *Journal of Endocrinology.* 2007 May;193(2):251–258.

Martins PJ, Marques MS, Tufik S, D'Almeida V. Orexin Activation Precedes Increased NPY Expression, Hyperphagia, and Metabolic Changes in Response to Sleep Deprivation. *American Journal of Physiology—Endocrinology and Metabolism.* 2010;Mar;298(3):E726–E734.

McConnell, R, et al, Association of BMI with Combustion Products from Secondhand Smoke Exposure and Vehicular Exhaust. *Obesity.* 2011;Abstract 449-P.

Meador JP, et al. Tributyltin and the Obesogen Metabolic Syndrome in a Salmonid. *Environmental Research.* 2011;Jan;111(1):50–56.

Melnick, Meredith. Study: Can Exercise Keep Us from Aging? *Time.* March 3, 2011. http://healthland.time.com/2011/03/03/study-can-exercise-keep-us-from-aging/

Melov S, Tarnopolsky MA, Beckman K, Felkey K, Hubbard A. Resistance Exercise Reverses Aging in Human Skeletal Muscle. *PLoS ONE,* 2007;2(5): e465. doi:10.1371/journal.pone.0000465.

Melzer D, Galloway T. Bisphenol A and Adult Disease: Making Sense of Fragmentary Data and Competing Inferences. *Annals of Internal Medicine.* 2011;Sep 20;155(6):392–394.

Mitchell PJ, et al. Conflicting Bright Light Exposure during Night Shifts Impedes Circadian Adaptation. *Journal of Biological Rhythms*. 1997;12(1):5–15.

Morgenthaler TI, et al. Practice Parameters for the Clinical Evaluation and Treatment of Circadian Rhythm Sleep Disorders. An American Academy of Sleep Report. *Sleep*. 2007;30(11):1445–1459.

Nedeltcheva AV, et al. Sleep Curtailment Is Accompanied by Increased Intake of Calories from Snacks. *American Journal of Clinical Nutrition*. 2009;Jan;89(1):126–133.

Newman AB, et al. Progression and Regression of Sleep-Disordered Breathing with Changes in Weight: The Sleep Heart Health Study. *Archives of Internal Medicine*. 2005;165:2408–2413.

Ning G, et al. Relationship of Urinary Bisphenol A Concentration to Risk for Prevalent Type 2 Diabetes in Chinese Adults: A Cross-sectional Analysis. *Annals of Internal Medicine*. 2011;Sep 20;155(6):368–374.

Owen, N. Sedentary Behavior: Emerging Evidence for a New Health Risk. *Mayo Clinic Proceedings*. 2010;Dec;85(12):1138–1141.

Plotnikoff RC, et al. Predictors of Physical Activity in Adults with Type 2 Diabetes. *American Journal of Health Behavior* 2011;May;35(3):359–370.

Poirier P, Després JP. Exercise in Weight Management of Obesity. *Cardiology Clinics*. 2001;Aug;19(3):459–470.

Porcu S, et al. Performance, Ability to Stay Awake, and Tendency to Fall Asleep during the Night After a Diurnal Sleep with Temazepam or Placebo. *Sleep*. 1997;20(7):535–541.

Rajkovic V, Matavulj M, Johansson O. Studies on the Synergistic Effects of Extremely Low-Frequency Magnetic Fields and the Endocrine-Disrupting Compound Atrazine on the Thyroid Gland. *International Journal of Radiation Oncology*. 2010;Dec;86(12):1050–1060.

Ratey JJ, Loehr JE. The Positive Impact of Physical Activity on Cognition during Adulthood: A Review of Underlying Mechanisms, Evidence and Recommendations. *Review of Neuroscience*. 2011;22(2):171–185.

Reynolds CF, et al. Depressive Psychopathology in Male Sleep Apneics. *Journal of Clinical Psychiatry*. 1984;45:287–290.

Richards CA, Rundle AG. Business Travel and Self-Rated Health, Obesity, and Cardiovascular Disease Risk Factors. *Journal of Occupational and Environmental Medicine*. 2011;Apr;53(4):358–363.

Riu A, et al, Peroxysome Proliferator-Activated Receptor-*y* Is a Target for Halogenated Analogues of Bisphenol-A. *Environmental Health Perspectives*. 2011;2011 Sep;119(9):1227–32.

Rudel RA, et al. Food Packaging and Bisphenol A and Bis(2-ethyhexyl) Phthalate Exposure: Findings from a Dietary Intervention. *Environmental Health Perspectives*. 2011;Jul;119(7):914–920.

Sack RL. Jet Lag. *New England Journal of Medicine*. 2010;362(5):440–446.

Schmid SM, et al. Short-Term Sleep Loss Decreases Physical Activity under Free-Living Conditions but Does Not Increase Food Intake Under Time-Deprived

Laboratory Conditions in Healthy Men. *American Journal of Clinical Nutrition*. 2009;Dec;90(6):1476–1482.

Shepstone TN,et al. Short-Term High- vs. Low-Velocity Isokinetic Lengthening Training Results in Greater Hypertrophy of the Elbow Flexors in Young Men. *Journal of Applied Physiology*. 2005 May;98(5):1768–1776.

Simpson NS, Banks S, Dinges DF. Sleep Restriction Is Associated with Increased Morning Plasma Leptin Concentrations, Especially in Women. *Biological Research for Nursing*. 2010;Jul;12(1):47–53.

Skene DJ, Optimization of Light and Melatonin to Phase-Shift Human Circadian Rhythms. *Journal of Neuroendocrinology*. 2003;Apr;15(4):438–441.

Steiger A, et al. Effects of Hormones on Sleep. *Hormone Research*. 1998;49(3–4):125–130.

Steiger A, et al. Ghrelin in Mental Health, Sleep, Memory. *Molecular and Cellular Endocrinology*. 2011;Jun 20;340(1):88–96.

Steiger A. Sleep and the Hypothalamo-Pituitary-Adrenocortical System. *Sleep Medicine Reviews*. 2002 Apr;6(2):125–138.

Stoewsand GS, Bioactive Organosulfur Phytochemicals in Brassica Oleracea Vegetables—A Review. *Food and Chemical Toxicology*. 1995 Jun;33(6):537–543.

St-Onge MP, et al. Short Sleep Duration Increases Energy Intakes but Does Not Change Energy Expenditure in Normal-Weight Individuals. *American Journal of Clinical Nutrition*. 2011;Jun 29.

Tabb MM, Blumberg B. New Modes of Action for Endocrine-Disrupting Chemicals. *Molecular Endocrinology* 2006 Mar;20(3):475–482.

Tanaka T., et al. Congener-Specific Polychlorinated Biphenyls and the Prevalence of Diabetes in the Saku Control Obesity Program. *Endocrine Journal*. 2011;May 7.

Tang-Péronard JL, et al. Endocrine-Disrupting Chemicals and Obesity Development in Humans: A Review. *Obesity Review*. 2011;Apr 4. doi: 10.1111/j.1467-789X.2011.00871.x.

Terman S, et al. Light Therapy for Seasonal and Non-seasonal Depression: Efficacy, Protocol, Safety, and Side Effects. *CNS Spectrum*. 2005;10(8):647–653.

The National Weight Control Registry Database. http://www.nwcr.ws/default.htm.

Van Cauter E, et al. Impact of Sleep and Sleep Loss on Neuroendocrine and Metabolic Function. *Hormone Research*. 2007;67 Suppl 1:2–9.

Van Cauter E, Knutson KL, Sleep and the Epidemic of Obesity in Children and Adults. *European Journal of Endocrinology*. 2008;Dec;159 Suppl 1:S59–S66.

von Schantz M. Phenotypic Effects of Genetic Variability in Human Clock Genes on Circadian and Sleep Parameters. *Journal of Genetics*. 2008;Dec;87(5):513–519.

Walsh JK, et al. Physiological Sleep Tendency on a Simulated Night Shift: Adaptation and Effects of Triazolam. *Sleep*. 1988;11(3)251–264.

Walsh, B. Flame Retardants in Everyday Products May Be a Health Hazard, Scientists Say, *Time*, October 28, 2010. http://healthland.time.com/2010/10/28/chemical-safety-scientists-come-out-against-chemical-flame-retardants-in-ordinary-products/

Watkins DJ, et. al. Exposure to PBDEs in the Office Environment: Evaluating the Relationship Between Dust, Handwipes, and Serum. *Environmental Health Perspectives.* 2011 Sep;119(9):1247-52.

West KE, et al. Blue Light from Light-Emitting Diodes Elicits a Dose-Dependent Suppression of Melatonin in Humans. *Journal of Applied Physiology.* 2011;Mar;110(3):619–626.

Wyatt HR, Phelan S, Wing RR, Hill JO. Lessons from patients who have successfully maintained weight loss. *Obesity Management.* 2005;1:56–61.

Yamada M, et al. Effect of resistance training on Physical Performance and Fear of Falling in Elderly with Different Levels of Physical Well-Being. *Age and Ageing.* 2011 Sep;40(5):637–41.

Yang J, et al. Functional Evolution of Leptin of Ochotona curzoniae in Adaptive Thermogenesis Driven by Cold Environmental Stress. *PLoS One.* 2011;6(6):e19833.

Young T, et al. Risk Factors for Obstructive Sleep apnea in Adults. *Journal of the American Medical Association.* 2004;291:2013–2016.

Young T, The Occurrence of Sleep-Disordered Breathing among Middle-Aged Adults. *New England Journal of Medicine.* 1993;328:1230–1235.

Zee PC, Goldstein CA. Treatment of Shift Work Disorder and Jet Lag. *Current Treatment Options in Neurology.* 2010;Sep;12(5):396–411.

Zelasko CJ. Exercise for Weight Loss: What Are the Facts? *Journal of the American Dietetic Association.* 1995 Dec;95(12):1414–1417.

Zirlik S, et al. Leptin, Obestatin and Apelin Levels in Patients with Obstructive Sleep Apnoea Syndrome. *Medical Science Monitor.* 2011;Feb 25;17(3):CR159–64.

Index

V

vaginal dryness, 219, 238, 244, 249
Valium, 97
valproate, 146–147
valsartan, 141
vanadium, 131
Vaniqa, 227
varicocele, 271
vasculitis, 157
vasectomies, 272
Vasotec, 141
vegetables, 47, 53, 195, 382
vegetarian pasta sauce, 378–379
venlafaxine, 96, 142–143
ventromedial hypothalamus, 82
Veterans Affairs Diabetes Trial (VADT), 137
Viagra, 265
Victoza, 100, 135
Vimpat, 146
Viracept, 145
virilism, 210
visceral fat, 11, 238
vitamins,
    A, 197
    B complex, 206
    B12, 167, 186, 191
    biotin (B7), 129–130
    C, 207
    D, 109, 186, 252
    E, 133, 207
    folic acid (B9), 132
    niacin (B3), 132, 138–139, 140, 144
vitiligo, 157
voice, softening of, 267
Vytorin, 140

W

water, 68
waxing, hair, 2297
weakness, 290
Wegener's granulomatosis, 157
weight,
    adrenal gland and, 287–289, 290
    androgen and, 216, 267
    diet and, 333–337
    exercise and, 337–345
    genetics and, 13–14
    guidelines for losing, 327, 328–329, 330, 334–335
    and insulin resistance, 126
    sleep and, 346–352
    stress and, 287–289
    thyroid and, 152, 157, 162, 182–183
    women and, 203–205
WelChol, 139
Wellbutrin, 96, 143
Westhroid, 193–194
white fat, 19, 20
white mulberry leaf, 133
whole wheat bread, 44
wild rice and chicken salad with broccoli cole slaw, 374–375
Wilson, E. Denis, 176
Wolever, Thomas M. S., 45
Wolff-Chaikoff disease, 155
women *see* androgen excess; estrogen; menopause; pregnancy
Women's Health Initiative, 242, 244, 245, 246
World Health Organization, 7, 113, 154

X

Xanax, 97
Xenical, 63, 144

Y

Yasmin, 223, 224
yawning, 162–163
Yaz, 223, 224
yeast infections, 111, 296
yoga, 305

Z

Zestril, 141
Zetia, 139
zinc, 160, 196–197
Zocor, 136–138
Zoloft, 58, 95, 207
Zonegran, 143
zonisamide, 143
Zovia, 225
Zyprexa, 147

About the Author

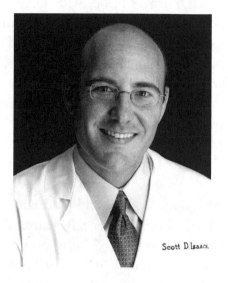

Scott Isaacs, M.D., F.A.C.P., F.A.C.E., is a board-certified endocrinologist in Atlanta, Georgia, and is widely considered to be one of the leading weight loss experts in the country. Dr. Isaacs is a faculty member at Emory University School of Medicine and the medical director for Atlanta Endocrine Associates and their award-winning weight loss program.

Dr. Isaacs has been honored with numerous awards, including listings in Castle Connolly Top Doctors for the past four years. His peers voted him Best Physician in *Lifestyles* magazine in 2011 and 2012. The online *Citysearch Guide* announced Dr. Isaacs's weight loss program as its 2009 "Best of Citysearch" winner.

Noted author Jillian Michaels called Dr. Isaacs the "guru of all things hormonal" and referenced his books in her *New York Times* best-selling book, *Master Your Metabolism*. Dr. Isaacs has been profiled on CNNHealth.com, livestrong.com, WebMD.com, and many other websites. The American Association of Clinical Endocrinologists lists Dr. Isaacs's books as a resource for practicing endocrinologists.

He has also been featured in national publications including *Ladies Home Journal, Better Homes and Gardens, Fitness, Shape, Parents, Red Book, Family Circle,*

Men's Health, Better Health and Living, Good Housekeeping, Glamour, the *Chicago Tribune,* the *Atlanta Journal Constitution, Atlanta, First Health, Lifetime, Prevention, Women's World,* and others. Dr. Isaacs has provided expert commentary on radio and television news programs including CNN Headline News, CNN Health, National Public Radio, and local NBC, ABC, CBS, and Fox news affiliates. He appeared as a weight loss expert on TBS Superstation's *Movie and Makeover.*

Dr. Isaacs is actively involved with the American Association of Clinical Endocrinologists at a national level, serving on several committees. He serves on the board of directors for the Atlanta chapter of the American Diabetes Association, as a medical advisor for Cushing's Help and Support Group, and is past president of the Georgia chapter of the American Association of Clinical Endocrinologists.

Dr. Isaacs attended Emory College and graduated magna cum laude and Phi Beta Kappa with a degree in psychology. Research from work in the Emory Honors Program resulted in his first publication on hormones and the brain in 1991. He went on to Emory University School of Medicine, continuing for his residency in internal medicine and fellowship in endocrinology, lipids, diabetes, and metabolism, where he received a research grant from the National Institutes of Health and won an award from the American College of Physicians for published research on diabetes and obesity.

He has published clinical and basic science research on diabetes, obesity, and bone metabolism. His publications in peer-reviewed medical journals include the *Journal of Endocrinology and Metabolism, Diabetes Care, Journal of Cellular Physiology,* and the *Journal of Critical Care.* His articles have been referenced and cited in many subsequent publications, including a listing as a primary reference in the 2012 *Endocrine Society Clinical Practice Guideline: Management of Hyperglycemia in Hospitalized Patients.*

A frequent speaker to national and international groups, Dr. Isaacs is a diplomate of the American College of Physicians and a fellow of the American College of Physicians and the American College of Endocrinology.

Dr. Isaacs lives with his wife and five-year-old daughter in Atlanta. He enjoys taking walks in Atlanta, hiking, swimming, fishing, cooking, and learning Spanish.

Visit www.IntelligentHealthCenter.com, Hungry Hormones.com, and www.YourEndocrinologist.com for more information about Dr. Isaacs.